THE PARKINSON'S DISEASE
TREATMENT BOOK

The Parkinson's Disease Treatment Book

◆ ◆ ◆

Partnering with Your Doctor
to Get the Most from Your Medications

J. ERIC AHLSKOG, PH.D., M.D.

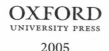

OXFORD
UNIVERSITY PRESS

2005

OXFORD

UNIVERSITY PRESS

Oxford University Press, Inc., publishes works that
further Oxford University's objective of excellence
in research, scholarship, and education.

Oxford   New York
Auckland   Cape Town   Dar es Salaam   Hong Kong   Karachi
Kuala Lumpur   Madrid   Melbourne   Mexico City   Nairobi
New Delhi   Shanghai   Taipei   Toronto

With offices in
Argentina   Austria   Brazil   Chile   Czech Republic   France   Greece
Guatemala   Hungary   Italy   Japan   Poland   Portugal   Singapore
South Korea   Switzerland   Thailand   Turkey   Ukraine   Vietnam

Copyright © 2005 by Mayo Foundation for Medical Education and Research
Illustrations Copyright © 2005 by The Mayo Clinic

Illustrations by David A. Factor, Medical Illustrator, Mayo Clinic

Published by Oxford University Press, Inc.
198 Madison Avenue, New York, NY 10016
www.oup.com

Oxford is a registered trademark of Oxford University Press

Library of Congress Cataloging-in-Publication Data
Ahlskog, J. Eric.
The Parkinson's disease treatment book : partnering with your doctor
to get the most from your medications / J. Eric Ahlskog.
p. cm.
ISBN-13: 978-0-19-517193-9
ISBN-10: 0-19-517193-4
1. Parkinson's disease—Treatment—Popular works. I. Title.
RC382.A365   2005
616.8'3306—dc22
2004061687

1 3 5 7 9 8 6 4 2
Printed in the United States of America
on acid-free paper

♦ ♦ ♦

Contents

Part Four
The Cause and Progression of Parkinson's Disease

Part Five
The Movement Problems of Parkinson's Disease: Medication Rationale and Choices

Part Six
Beginning Treatment of Parkinson's Disease: Medication Guidelines

Part Seven
The Early Years on Medications

Part Eight
Later Medication Inconsistency: Motor Fluctuations and Dyskinesias

Part Nine

Other Treatment Problems: Not Just a Movement Disorder

Part Ten

Nutrition, Exercise, Work, and Family

Part Eleven

Surgery and Procedures for Parkinson's Disease: Present and Future

Part Twelve

Parkinson's Disease Information Sources

◆ ◆ ◆

Acknowledgments

I must first acknowledge and thank my teachers. This especially includes my patients, many of whom have become dear friends over the years. A doctor learns as much from the people he cares for as from medical texts. My mentors and colleagues at the Mayo Clinic continue to provide me with countless pearls of wisdom, long after they first taught me as a green neurology resident physician in the late 1970s. I am humbled and honored to be working with many outstanding Mayo clinicians who practice medicine with true compassion.

Of my many mentors, two deserve special recognition and thanks. During my neurology residency and early years on the Mayo staff, Professor Manfred Muenter was an endless source of knowledge and insight about Parkinson's disease. His legendary early published studies of the levodopa response formed the basis for what he taught me. He could take complex therapeutic problems and make them simple. I still use the principles of treatment that he taught me in my daily practice. I am deeply indebted to Professor Bartley G. Hoebel, who was my mentor, thesis adviser, and friend when I was a young Ph.D. student at Princeton University. During the three years I spent in Professor Hoebel's laboratory, I matured in many ways and saw the doors open for my life's work. From him I learned that neuroscience is as exciting as a ninth inning, game-winning home run. I also saw and experienced firsthand how a wise mentor nurtures and guides a novice and naive student. Bart is one of the kindest, most thoughtful people I have ever met and has been a stellar role model as I pursued my career in medicine.

I have had the good fortune of outstanding collaborators in the publication of this book. All of the figures are original drawings by David Factor, Mayo medical illustrator. David became a good friend in this endeavor. Before putting pencil to paper, he read each chapter to understand what each illustration needed to communicate. He transformed my crude stick figure drawings into pictures worth at least a thousand words. What a pleasure to work with someone so talented! I am also indebted to my friend Dr. Stephen Reich, associate professor of neurology at the University of Maryland, who took the time to read and edit this book. Dr. Reich, an internationally recognized expert on the treatment of Parkinson's disease, offered invaluable insights and suggestions. I also had the good fortune to have Joan Bossert, vice president and associate publisher, Oxford University Press, edit this book. She honed my writing skills and helped keep my message clear and concise. She and others at Oxford, Norman Hirschy, Maura Roessner, Chrisona Schmidt, and Joellyn Ausanka, were models of efficiency who facilitated every step.

The love and help of my family, in my career in medicine and in writing this book, have been critical. Doctors don't get home on time and they are not always there when their family needs them. In our household, my chair at the dinner table is usually empty. Despite my long days and absences, my wife and my sons shower me with love and support. Without their unconditional love, the work I have done for those with Parkinson's disease, including this book, would never have been accomplished. To my beautiful wife, Faye, and to my sons, Mike, John, and Matt, I dedicate this book.

J. Eric Ahlskog, Ph.D., M.D.

THE PARKINSON'S DISEASE TREATMENT BOOK

1

◆ ◆ ◆

Background and Rationale

Parkinson's disease (PD) is a treatable condition. Medical treatment increases longevity and allows most people with PD to remain active and productive for many years. We don't have a cure (yet), but some of the responses to available drugs are striking and occasionally border on the miraculous. PD is one of the most treatable of all neurological conditions.

The medical treatment of PD, unfortunately, is not always simple. There are multiple medications and they can be used in a variety of ways. The choice of the drug, the dose, and the timing often are crucial; therapy must be individualized to meet each person's unique requirements. Also, the distinction between PD symptoms and medication side effects frequently causes confusion, with potential for ineffective or inappropriate treatment. Sometimes, treatable symptoms are not even recognized as part of PD. The difference between optimal versus ineffective therapy may be the difference between a nursing home and independent living. The goal of this book is to help each and every person with PD achieve the best treatment.

Numerous texts have been published on PD, targeting either the patient or the physician. Many texts written for patients and families provide excellent information but address treatment in only a general sense. They describe medications but do not explain how and when to use them, dosage, or which problems they are prescribed for. Specific treatment guidelines are confined to texts written for physicians. Even many books for physicians, however, are written in general terms because for any given problem a variety of treatment strategies may be appropriate. Hence a general, nonspecific overview avoids offending those with different treatment philosophies.

In this book I offer a new approach: this is a nuts-and-bolts treatment book directed to the person with PD and family; however, the audience also includes the physician. After all, physicians and patients (including family) are on the same team. If patients have a good understanding of not only their disease but also appropriate drugs, doses, and the rationale for using them, optimal treatment should be facilitated.

Writing a technical book addressing the nuances of medical therapy is challenging; the language of medicine must be translated into words the layperson understands. Yet watering down the content would defeat the purpose of the book. But does the patient really need to cross into the domain of the physician? Why not let the doctor handle everything? Indeed, passive reliance on the physician works well for people who have simple problems. PD, however, is not a simple problem. Complex problems require complex solutions, which opens the possibility for misunderstanding and miscommunication.

People with PD often misinterpret symptoms or describe them ambiguously. This is challenging to the treating physician, especially given a typically busy practice that forces him or her to maximize efficiency. This book is meant to provide knowledge about the complex symptoms of PD that people need to assist their physician in this process. Proactive patients and families who are good observers and recognize treatment principles can help maximize therapeutic outcomes. This book is not intended to make patients into their own doctors but to open avenues of informed communication, stimulate discussion, and streamline the decision-making process.

Are the guidelines and recommendations provided in this book the best strategies for treatment of PD? As you might expect, several therapeutic solutions often exist for the same problem. In this text I have included the ones that have worked best for my patients and have withstood the test of time. They have been distilled from over twenty years of experience treating people with PD at the Mayo Clinic. I gained this experience both as a full-time practicing neurologist and as a clinical investigator responsible for PD treatment protocols. Early in my career I recognized the importance of listening to the people I was treating. They have taught me invaluable lessons about PD that cannot be found in medical textbooks. Where there is more than one reasonable approach, I try to present the alternative strategies, with the arguments for each. For example, the choice of initial medication for PD therapy continues to be debated. The arguments can become extremely complex while lacking definitive answers. In this instance, I err on the side of being dogmatic. Although I do not disavow all other treatment strategies, I assume (correctly or not) that presenting too many options introduces ambiguity and uncertainty. I want to avoid paralysis by analysis.

This book has one more goal: to help the layperson wade through the morass of information about PD in the lay press and on the Internet. Seem-

PART ONE

◆ ◆ ◆

Basic Facts about the Brain and Parkinson's Disease

2

◆ ◆ ◆

A Primer on the Brain

A text on Parkinson's disease (PD), a disorder of the brain, should start with a discussion of the brain, an incredibly complex organ. Not only is brain structure complicated, but so is human thought and action. How amazing that the human brain can derive complex mathematical equations, compose great novels, and direct the swing of a baseball bat toward a curving baseball thrown at ninety miles per hour! Although we are not close to understanding how the brain mediates the genius of a mathematician or the artistry of a composer, we do understand many elementary things about brain function. What we have learned has led to breakthroughs in the medical treatment of many neurological conditions.

PD stands as a shining example of how an understanding of brain function provided a rational basis for effective treatment. Over decades, many scientists and clinicians contributed insights, piecing together the PD brain puzzle. From these aggregate efforts, effective symptomatic treatment of PD was predicted and later confirmed in clinical trials. We now are able to treat PD based on our knowledge of brain mechanisms. We continue to build on these scientific principles, and thus the treatment of PD remains a work in progress.

This chapter outlines elementary principles about the brain and how it is organized. You will be introduced to twenty-five terms in the medical language of PD, which are also included in the glossary at the end of this book.

Neurons:
The Primary Component of the Brain

The brain is in many ways like your computer, which has small electronic components that are interconnected and integrated in complex circuits. Computers perform complicated tasks through multiple series of electrical processing.

The primary unit of the brain is the brain cells, or neurons, which are analogous to computer microchips. The normal brain contains approximately 10 billion neurons. Each is capable of receiving and sending electrical signals in complex brain circuits. One neuron transmits signals to as many as 10,000 other neurons in these circuits.

To see what neurons look like, glance at figure 2.1. Neurons are brain cells and share many of the properties of all other cells in the body. You may recall from your biology classes that all cells have a nucleus. The blueprints for cell function (DNA) are stored and activated in the nucleus. All cells have metabolic machinery for producing the structural building blocks making up the cell. They also have metabolic machinery for producing energy necessary for cell function. As you can see from figure 2.1, at one end of the neuron is the cell body that contains the nucleus and most of the metabolic machinery. This is also the area where most of the signals from other neurons are received.

Electrical circuits need wires; the neuron has a wire-like extension called the axon (fig. 2.1). These axons may be quite long, allowing signals to be transmitted across broad expanses of brain and spinal cord. The signal that starts in the cell body of a neuron passes down the axon by electrical transmission.

On the end of the wire-like axon are small bulbs called terminals. They contain a specific brain chemical called a neurotransmitter. These neurotransmitters are released to signal the next neuron in the circuit. Each type of neuron releases one primary neurotransmitter. The neurons are sometimes named according to the neurotransmitter they secrete (adding the suffix "ergic"). For example, neurons that secrete dopamine as the neurotransmitter are called dopaminergic; those that release acetylcholine are called cholinergic; when glutamate is the neurotransmitter, the neurons are called glutamatergic.

A single neuron may receive these chemical messages from hundreds or even thousands of other neurons. Most of these incoming signals are received on the dendrites (shown in fig. 2.1) or the cell body. These dendrites often form a bushy reception network for these incoming signals.

To recap, when the cell body portion of the neuron is activated by another neuron, an electrical signal is initiated and transmitted to the other end, down the axon. When the electrical signal passes down the axon and reaches the terminals, it causes release of the neurotransmitter. This neurotransmitter activates the next cell in the circuit. Signals pass from one brain cell to the next electrically until the very end; the final step involves chemical transmission.

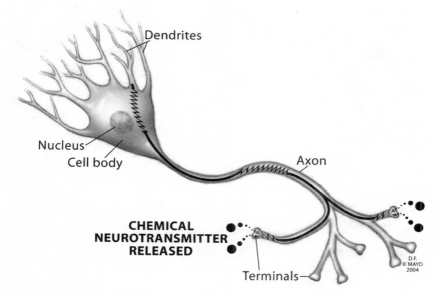

2.1 The neuron. Signals generated from this neuron are electrically propagated from the region of the cell body down the wire-like process called the axon. To signal the next neuron, a chemical is released from the terminals at the end of the axon. This chemical is called a neurotransmitter. Incoming signals from other neurons are primarily received at the level of the dendrites or the cell body.

Neurotransmitters and Receptors

The neurotransmitter released by one neuron binds to a specific site on the next brain cell; this is where the chemical signaling occurs to complete the transmission. The second brain cell is not activated by just any neurotransmitter. Only the specific neurotransmitter used in that circuit is effective. Why doesn't just any neurotransmitter work? Because there is a specific receptor for every neurotransmitter. That receptor is located in large numbers on the receiving end of neurons. Other chemicals in the area do not activate that receptor; it must be the specific neurotransmitter employed in the brain computer circuit (see fig. 2.2). Once that neurotransmitter activates the receptor, electrical signals are generated in the next neuron. If enough of these receptors are stimulated on that brain cell, the electrical signal passes down the axon to the terminal. The terminal then releases a certain amount of neurotransmitter and the sequence starts in the next neuron in the circuit. These neurotransmitters are contained in discrete packages called vesicles and are stored in the terminal until they are released.

The site where terminals release their neurotransmitter to activate the receptor is called the synapse. Thus a synapse includes the presynaptic terminal, the postsynaptic receptor, and the tiny space in between.

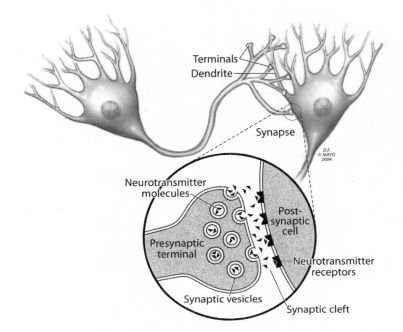

2.2 Site of neurotransmitter release, the synapse. The neurotransmitter is packaged into vesicles and released into the synaptic cleft, where it activates a specific receptor on the next neuron.

An External View of the Brain

Now that you have a sense of brain components at the microscopic and sub-microscopic level, we will take a step back and look at the bigger picture. Figure 2.3 illustrates two views of the brain, one from the side (revealing the connection with the spinal cord) and the other sliced through the middle.

- Note the cortex, which is the thick region of outermost brain circuitry shown in figure 2.3. The cortex is most highly developed in humans, less developed in monkeys, and even less developed in lower species. Complex human thought and language are presumed to originate largely within the cortex. Some neurological conditions (e.g., Alzheimer's disease) result in widespread damage to the cortex that may impair the ability to think, remember, and communicate (dementia).

- At the back of the brain, just above where the neck meets the skull, is the cerebellum. It is shaped like a tree in full leaf. This area integrates with other brain regions and is a coordination center. This is spared in Parkinson's disease (PD) but degenerates in some disorders that resemble PD. Incoordination due to cerebellar damage is called ataxia.

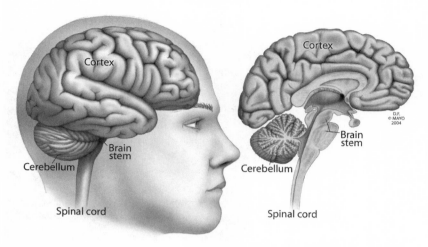

2.3   External view of the brain (left figure) showing cortex, cerebellum, brainstem, and connection to spinal cord; on the right is the midline view sliced through the middle.

- The brain stem is located under the cerebellum, as shown in figure 2.3. At the top of the brain stem is the substantia nigra, which we will examine in detail in subsequent chapters. The substantia nigra degenerates in Parkinson's disease and is primarily responsible for the tremor, slowness, and other movement symptoms. Other collections of brain cells are also located in the brain stem. Many mediate elementary functions such as breathing, eye movements, swallowing, jaw opening, and so on. Also, information passing from the spinal cord to the brain, and vice versa, goes through the brain stem. This is conducted along cable systems containing countless axons. These cable systems are called tracts.

- The spinal cord is a continuation of the brain stem (fig. 2.3). This is the final common pathway for translating thoughts and intentions into goal-directed movements of trunk and limbs. The decision to wave good-bye, throw a ball, or jump from a step originates in the cortex. The thought activates motor programs in the cortex and centers beneath the cortex (the subcortex). The brain computer code for the specific movement(s) is then conducted downstream via the tracts passing through the brain stem into the spinal cord. Neurons in the spinal cord are then activated in the proper sequences to move muscles appropriately. The spinal cord also sends information in the opposite direction. When we stub a toe, sensors in the skin and joint are stimulated. These sensors send signals up nerves in the leg to the spinal cord. Some processing of these signals occurs in the spinal cord. Passage of these signals, triggered by the stubbed toe, continue up to the brain. The pain signals activate groups of neurons at several levels of the brain including brain stem, subcortex, and cortex.

Brain Centers Directly Affected by Parkinson's Disease

Now that you have a sense of the general design of the brain, we can focus on the areas responsible for many of the symptoms of Parkinson's disease (more will be said about this in the next chapter). Neurons in the brain are organized into well-delimited regions called nuclei. Many nuclei are visible to the naked eye in a brain slice. Early anatomists sometimes named these nuclei based on their appearance. Hence certain nuclei have descriptive names, such as the "superior and inferior olives" (shaped like olives) or red nucleus, named because of its reddish tint.

The nucleus that degenerates in those with PD and is responsible for many of the symptoms is the substantia nigra. This is located at the top of the brain stem (midbrain region), as shown in figure 2.4. The substantia nigra neurons contain a black pigment and hence the name, which means "black substance."

The darkly pigmented cell bodies of the substantia nigra send axons to another area of the brain, the striatum, as shown in figure 2.5. The striatum is actually two nuclei—the putamen and caudate.

Three other brain nuclei are shown in figure 2.5: the thalamus, globus pallidus, and subthalamic nucleus. They are intimate components of movement control circuits. Although they are not directly damaged in Parkinson's disease, they are the three primary sites for PD brain surgery, which is addressed in chapter 33.

I already described how groups of neurons release a common neurotransmitter, which signals the next set of neurons. The neurotransmitter for the

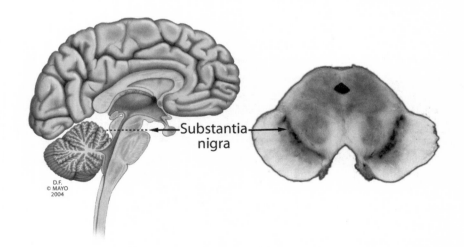

2.4 On the left is shown the site of the midbrain, including the substantia nigra. A slice through this region is shown on the right, displaying the darkly pigmented neurons of the substantia nigra.

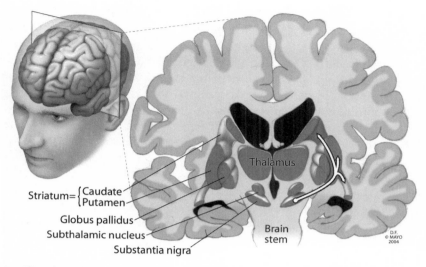

2.5 Slice through the brain to reveal the locations of the caudate, putamen, and other nuclei. These caudate and putamen make up the striatum. The substantia nigra is shown sending projections to the striatum. Other structures relevant to PD are also labeled: thalamus, globus pallidus, and subthalamic nucleus.

substantia nigra projections to the striatum is dopamine; hence they are called dopaminergic neurons. In PD, these substantia nigra cells degenerate; consequently, dopamine levels plummet in the striatum. These dopaminergic substantia nigra cells are key in PD, as I explain further in the next chapter.

Brain Circuits Relevant to Parkinson's Disease

In a basic sense, the connections of these brain nuclei may be conceptualized as an electrical wiring diagram. The brain movement control circuits are actually more complex than this, but the major connections (projections of axons) are often thought of as electrical circuits.

The programming of walking and other movements partially occurs in the striatum. Projections from the striatum are primarily to the globus pallidus. The globus pallidus is a crucial output nucleus of this system, which processes and relays the signals to other brain nuclei. The globus pallidus is also called the pallidum.

A major connection from the globus pallidus is to the thalamus. The thalamus is at the very center of the brain and contains numerous subdivisions. It is sometimes conceptualized as a relay station to and from the large expanse of cortex. The thalamus has widespread, large projections to all areas of the cortex.

To summarize, the striatum is a nodal point for brain movement programs. It sends output to the globus pallidus, which projects to the thalamus, and ultimately the thalamus projects to the cortex. Signals from the cortex are transmitted back to the striatum, forming a complete loop; this allows the cortex to modulate activity in the striatum. The dopaminergic substantia nigra exerts influence through its connections to the striatum.

The subthalamic nucleus is another relay station in these subcortical movement control circuits. It receives input from the striatum and projects to the globus pallidus. It is located just below the thalamus, but its function is distinct from that of the thalamus. This nucleus has an interesting history. For decades, it has been recognized that a stroke in the subthalamic nucleus causes an unusual syndrome characterized by wild, flailing, involuntary movements in the limbs on the opposite side of the body (known as hemiballismus). This nucleus has become a target for the neurosurgeon treating PD, as will be discussed in chapter 33.

General Terms Relating to PD Brain Circuits

Two other anatomic terms are frequently encountered in readings about PD: basal ganglia and extrapyramidal. The precise definitions of these terms vary slightly, depending on the author. They refer to the brain motor control systems discussed above. "Basal ganglia" is an encompassing term for both the striatum (caudate and putamen) and the globus pallidus. Both the substantia nigra and subthalamic nucleus have intimate connections with the striatum and globus pallidus, and they are typically thought of as part of the basal ganglia. Thus the core nuclei of the basal ganglia are striatum and globus pallidus, plus their interconnected nuclei, the substantia nigra and subthalamic nucleus.

"Extrapyramidal" is often used interchangeably with "basal ganglia." It primarily refers to the basal ganglia nuclei plus their connections (which also includes connections with the cortex). Clinicians often use this term when referring to symptoms and signs caused by damage to these circuits, for example, "The patient had an extrapyramidal gait." The major motor control systems originating in the cortex are sometimes called "pyramidal" pathways (on cross-section of the brain stem, shaped like a pyramid). Hence other motor control systems are called extrapyramidal.

3

♦ ♦ ♦

Parkinson's Disease:
Changes in the Brain and Beyond

Parkinson's disease (PD) is a disorder characterized by slowness, stiffness, and often tremor. It is a disorder of brain motor systems ("motor" implies movement and action). In this chapter we consider how PD fits in the larger context of all brain disorders. We will then review what is occurring inside the brain, both microscopically and biochemically, resulting in the symptoms of PD. An understanding of this is crucial, since treatment principles are based on this knowledge.

Neurodegenerative Disease

A variety of disorders may damage the brain and cause it to malfunction, for example, strokes, tumors, brain infections (encephalitis), and trauma. One category of brain disorders is neurodegenerative disease. These diseases affect specific groups of brain cells, which slowly die (degenerate). Neurodegenerative disease encompasses a variety of conditions, most of which occur for unknown reasons, such as Alzheimer's disease and Lou Gehrig's disease (amyotrophic lateral sclerosis, or ALS). Parkinson's disease is a neurodegenerative disease.

The loss of brain cells in these neurodegenerative disorders is a very slow process that takes years. The degeneration of these specific brain regions is typically incomplete and not every cell dies. Furthermore, the degeneration is confined to limited brain areas; much of the brain is spared. Which neurons degenerate and which are spared depends on the specific neurodegenerative disease. For example, in Alzheimer's disease, thinking, language, and memory neurons are selectively lost. In ALS, the neurons activating the muscles degenerate. In Parkinson's disease, most of the symptoms are due to degeneration of the substantia nigra, a brain nucleus crucial for movement.

What causes neurodegenerative diseases is largely unknown, although clues are now starting to surface. Undoubtedly there will be a different cause for each type of neurodegenerative disorder. However, we are beginning to recognize some common themes, and what we learn about one disorder may help us understand the others.

The Substantia Nigra, Dopamine, and PD

The substantia nigra, which degenerates in PD, is a pivotal part of movement control systems in the brain. It sends axons throughout the striatum, where it regulates the firing rate of neurons in movement circuits. We call this the nigrostriatal pathway, which is a contraction of two words, nigra and striatum. The two components of the striatum, the caudate and putamen, are not equally affected, with the putamen being more profoundly depleted of input from the substantia nigra.

Signaling from one neuron to the next is by release of a neurotransmitter, which in the nigrostriatal system is dopamine. Thus, when a substantia nigra neuron is normally activated, dopamine is released in the striatum and we categorize these neurons as dopaminergic.

The neurons in the striatum have specific receptors that recognize and respond to dopamine. These receptors are not activated by other neurotransmitters and, conversely, different neurotransmitters are inactive at these dopamine receptors.

When the substantia nigra cells are lost in PD, dopamine levels plummet within the striatum. When there is no dopamine, striatal cells don't activate properly and the symptoms of PD result. This can be demonstrated experimentally in animals. When a monkey or rat is given a drug that lowers brain dopamine levels, the animals walk and move just like people with PD. Conversely, drugs that restore these animals' brain dopamine levels reverse these symptoms.

Medical treatment of PD capitalizes on the recognition that loss of brain dopamine is primarily responsible for the movement problems of PD. The major drugs used to treat PD symptoms either elevate brain dopamine levels or substitute for the lost dopamine.

What Is a Lewy Body and Why Should I Care?

The first important insight into the underpinnings of PD occurred nearly a century ago. In 1913 Dr. Frederick Lewy described unique microscopic changes in the brains of people with PD. He noted that brain cells from those with PD contained small, round collections of some type of material. These have since been known as Lewy bodies. They are found in certain areas of the brain, most notably in the substantia nigra of people with PD. They are now recognized as the hallmark of PD. Pathologists look for them when asked to determine after death whether someone truly had PD. Lewy bodies cannot be seen with the naked eye.

In typical PD, Lewy bodies are found in certain specific brain areas and are associated with loss of neurons in these regions. The substantia nigra is obviously one critical area where these Lewy bodies are found. Presumably, the process causing PD generates Lewy bodies and ultimately results in brain cell death.

Although Lewy bodies occur in only limited brain areas in typical PD, they are widespread in another condition, Diffuse Lewy Body disease (or dementia with Lewy bodies). This is a disorder in which thinking and memory problems are among the early and primary symptoms, although there are also symptoms of PD. More is said about this in chapters 6 and 23.

A Brain Protein: Alpha-Synuclein

Because Lewy bodies mark the areas of degeneration, they are presumed to hold a key to the understanding of PD. What is contained in these Lewy bodies? A variety of component substances have been identified over the years, but until recently nothing surfaced that provided insight to the underlying disorder. This changed with the discovery of the gene that caused parkinsonism in several Italian–Greek families.

For many years, one large Italian family with parkinsonism was the focus of scientific investigation. In this family, parkinsonism was passed from one generation to the next. This was recognized as exceptional, since typical PD is not passed from generation to generation. Through laborious and detailed genetic investigations, the gene abnormality causing this condition was identified. The abnormal protein that was miscoded by this gene turned out to be a brain protein, alpha-synuclein.

Initially little was known about alpha-synuclein and almost nothing about its normal role in the brain. Early enthusiasm was dampened when it was found that no one with typical PD carried this genetic abnormality. This genetic mutation was restricted to a few families in Italy and Greece. So how could this be relevant to PD in general? The importance became apparent when a special stain was developed that marked where alpha-synuclein is found within the brain: alpha-synuclein is found in high concentrations in Lewy bodies! Although this is not the abnormal alpha-synuclein like that of the Italian–Greek families, the high concentrations in Lewy bodies suggest a role for alpha-synuclein in typical PD. Scientists now speculate that there may be something abnormal about the production and metabolism of alpha-synuclein that predisposes to PD. More is said about this in chapter 8.

Lewy Bodies in Normal People

Are Lewy bodies found only among those with PD or those with Diffuse Lewy Body disease? In fact, Lewy bodies are found on postmortem examination in about 10 percent of "normal" people. This is ten times the incidence of Parkinson's disease. Would these normal individuals have developed PD if they had lived longer? Is PD actually a common condition that only a fraction of those predisposed develop? This is food for thought.

Why Are the Symptoms of PD Asymmetric (More on One Side Than the Other)?

People with PD typically experience their initial symptoms predominantly or exclusively on one side of their body, perhaps in only one limb. Why is that? Shouldn't the degeneration of PD be uniform? In fact, the loss of the substantia nigra cells is somewhat haphazard. Even with progression, PD remains asymmetric, affecting one side of the body more severely than the other. Why some substantia nigra cells succumb and others survive is unknown.

PD Symptoms Outside the Motor System

Although the problems with movement and tremor have received most of the publicity in PD, nonmovement symptoms also occur frequently. Some of these nonmovement symptoms have their origins outside the nigrostriatal dopaminergic system. In other words, the nigrostriatal system is not the only brain circuit to degenerate. It is the most crucial in that it is primarily responsible for the movement problems. These nonmotor symptoms are detailed in later chapters; however, we will briefly consider a few to gain some anatomic perspective.

- Depression (feeling blue most of the time) is common in PD and often is not simply a psychological reaction to the life changes caused by PD. There is a neurochemical basis and the deficiency of dopamine may play a role. However, reduction of other brain neurotransmitters, especially serotonin, may be more important. Neurons releasing serotonin are located primarily in the midline of the brain stem. These serotonergic neurons degenerate in PD, although less severely than the substantia nigra. Depression in people without PD has also been linked to insufficient serotonin activity. The newer antidepressant medications capitalize on this and activate brain serotonin systems.

- A variety of sleep disorders affect those with PD. Dopamine deficiency underlies some but not all of these sleep problems. Since sleep centers are located primarily in the brain stem, degeneration in these areas is probably responsible.

- With advancing PD, thinking and memory problems can occur; up to a third of people in PD clinics have dementia. Although slowness of thinking relates to loss of the dopaminergic nigrostriatal system, more substantial problems (dementia) reflect degeneration that is more widespread, especially including the cortex.

- Problems with bowels, bladder, and low blood pressure are common in PD. These are due to degeneration in the autonomic nervous system, the circuits that unconsciously control bladder, bowels, sweating, heart rate, and blood pressure.

Although movement problems from nigrostriatal dopamine deficiency take center stage in PD, other brain circuits are also affected, resulting in additional symptoms.

Not All Movement Problems Are Due to Dopamine Deficiency

Most of the movement problems of PD respond to medications that replenish dopamine, but some respond incompletely or not at all. Late in the course, this may increase. Imbalance in advanced PD is a prime example; whereas other aspects of walking may be well controlled with dopamine replenishment, balance problems are often much less responsive. If degeneration of the dopaminergic substantia nigra were responsible for all the movement symptoms, none would be refractory. In fact, other brain movement control circuits degenerate to a limited extent.

Brain Circuits Connected to the Dopaminergic Systems

Treatment of the motor symptoms of PD has focused on the dopamine deficiency and dopamine replenishment is the foundation of treatment. However, the dopaminergic neurons are part of a complex brain motor-control circuit and medications have also been directed at other links in this circuit. Two of the many brain systems connected with the nigrostriatal pathway have been targeted for PD drug treatment—circuits containing neurotransmitters acetylcholine and glutamate.

The striatum contains many neurons that release acetylcholine as the neurotransmitter and hence are called cholinergic. These cholinergic neurons have short axons that are confined to the striatum; they don't extend outside its borders. They seem to have a function that is opposite to that of the dopaminergic nigrostriatal system. Consequently drugs that block acetylcholine improve certain aspects of parkinsonism. In fact, cholinergic-blocking drugs (anticholinergic) were the first medications used for the treatment of PD. Anticholinergic drugs have a very limited role in the current treatment of PD.

The other circuit targeted for therapy in PD is the cortical system releasing the neurotransmitter glutamate. These neurons in the cortex send their axons to the striatum, where they interact with the dopaminergic system. Like the cholinergic system, they have a function that is opposite to the nigrostriatal system. Hence drugs that block glutamate tend to improve parkinsonism. However, drugs that block glutamate usually induce major side effects and these drugs too have only a limited role in the treatment of PD.

Changes Outside the Brain: The Autonomic Nervous System

The symptoms of PD include problems with bladder, bowels, sexual functioning, and low blood pressure, reflecting involvement of the autonomic nervous system.

THE AUTONOMIC NERVOUS SYSTEM

A series of monitoring devices in our internal organs constantly take readings on basic body functions, such as blood pressure, heart rate, and so on. These sensors are part of complex reflexes that make adjustments in response to what is being detected. This is done without our awareness. This internal regulatory network is called the autonomic nervous system. It regulates bowels, bladder, sweat glands, sexual functioning, heart rate, and blood pressure. When it senses that we are too hot, we sweat. When it senses that the stomach is full, a valve opens and allows food to pass into the small intestine. When we stand, there is a tendency for the blood to be pulled into our legs by gravity; when this is internally sensed, blood is redistributed throughout the body, keeping the blood pressure constant. Thus the autonomic nervous system continuously monitors internal systems and makes adjustments to meet our body's needs.

The autonomic nervous system is a large network with centers in the brain and circuits distributed throughout the body. Brain centers are located in the hypothalamus (an area just below the thalamus) and the brain stem. Broad-ranging nerve circuits connect these areas with the heart, blood vessels, stomach, intestines, genitalia, and sweat glands. Sensors and effectors

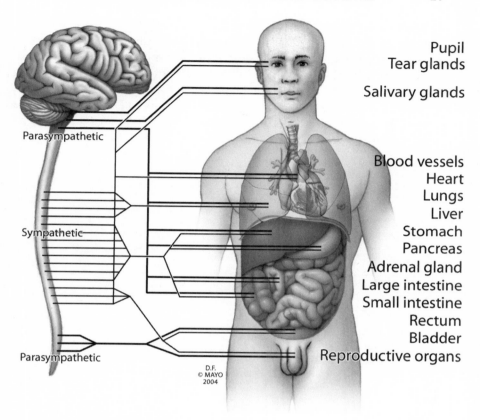

Pupil
Tear glands

Salivary glands

Parasympathetic

Blood vessels
Heart
Lungs
Liver
Stomach
Pancreas
Adrenal gland
Large intestine
Small intestine
Rectum
Bladder
Reproductive organs

Sympathetic

Parasympathetic

D.F.
© MAYO
2004

3.1   The autonomic nervous system regulates the function of the internal organs. This system is involved to variable degrees in PD.

of the autonomic nervous system are located throughout the body. A general schematic is shown in figure 3.1. As you can see, this is divided into two primary components—the sympathetic and parasympathetic autonomic nervous systems.

THE AUTONOMIC NERVOUS SYSTEM AND PD

Problems of the autonomic nervous system are common in those with PD. They are often mild or minimal early in the course. With time they become more prominent. Furthermore, medications used to treat PD or other conditions often aggravate these problems.

Damage to the autonomic nervous system is part of the neurodegenerative process of PD. As we have already learned, this neurodegeneration is not confined to the dopaminergic neurons of the substantia nigra. Lewy bodies like those found in the substantia nigra are also found in neurons of the autonomic nervous system. However, the chemistry of the autonomic nervous system is quite different from that of the substantia nigra. Hence, replenishing dopamine, which reverses the movement problems due to substantia nigra degeneration, does not improve autonomic symptoms.

Recent evidence suggests that PD may affect the autonomic nervous system very early in the course, even before the movement problems. Typically, however, these autonomic symptoms remain mild until PD is well established. Common symptoms referable to autonomic dysfunction in PD are summarized in table 3.1. These are described in more detail in subsequent chapters.

Table 3.1.   Autonomic Nervous System Involvement in PD

Organ	Problem	Symptoms
Blood pressure regulatory systems	Low blood pressure when standing (orthostatic hypotension)	Lightheadedness, faintness when standing; if severe, fainting or near fainting
Bowels	Slowed transit through the large intestine	Constipation
Stomach	Delayed passage of food from the stomach to the small intestine	Bloating, gas, heartburn
Bladder	1. Excessive bladder contraction	1. Urinary urgency and frequency (strong urges to void and void often); incontinence
	2. Poor bladder contraction	2. Hesitant and delayed voiding; susceptibility to urinary tract infections; incontinence
Sweating	Reduced or inappropriate sweating	Heat intolerance; excessive sweating
Male genitalia	Erectile dysfunction	Impotence

PART TWO

◆ ◆ ◆

Parkinson's Disease: Diagnosis and Prognosis

4

◆ ◆ ◆

How Do I Know If I Have
Parkinson's Disease?

The diagnosis of Parkinson's disease (PD) is not always simple. Even seasoned physicians may be troubled by certain cases. For the person with PD, recognizing that something is wrong may take months. The onset is insidious and symptoms may blend into the routine. Although tremor may provide a clear signal, many people do not experience this as one of their initial symptoms. Some of the manifestations of PD may be so subtle and nonspecific that they are not even appreciated as being abnormal. For example, they may be written off to age: "Of course I'm slowing down; I'm getting older." Or some other explanation may seem plausible: "I walk bent over because my back hurts." On the other hand, certain signs may be incorrectly attributed to PD. Not all tremor represents PD, and in fact the majority of people with tremor do not have PD.

Parkinson's disease is a clinical diagnosis made in the doctor's office. The story plus examination findings provide the evidence. There are no laboratory tests that identify PD. The tests are primarily for the purpose of excluding other disorders and are often not needed (see chapter 7 on testing). In this chapter, we focus on the clinical clues that point us to the diagnosis.

Parkinsonism Versus Parkinson's Disease

The symptoms and signs of PD include slowness, tremor, and stiffness. However, not everything that looks like PD is PD, and these outward signs may occur in other conditions. The term "parkinsonism" characterizes the appearance of PD (but not necessarily true PD). Thus there are various causes for parkinsonism, including PD.

The History and Examination

The diagnosis of PD is primarily made by the physician's interview and examination. There are three logical steps in correctly identifying someone with PD via this history and examination.

1. Parkinsonism must be present (the specific findings are discussed below).

2. There should be no unusual features that suggest another condition. Parkinsonism due to another cause typically can be identified by additional and unexpected findings. For example, severe imbalance with falls early in parkinsonism argues against typical PD. We will review red flags that point to other disorders.

3. The parkinsonism should markedly improve with medications that replenish brain dopamine (or substitute for brain dopamine). Why? Because the fundamental basis for most PD symptoms is loss of brain dopamine. If the parkinsonian symptoms markedly improve with dopamine replenishment, this usually confirms the diagnosis of PD. With other parkinsonian conditions, the brain degenerative changes are more widespread (not simply confined to dopaminergic systems) and usually are not very responsive to dopamine replenishment therapy.

Thus, if you have parkinsonism, the odds are that you have PD, but steps 2 and 3 above provide confirmatory evidence that it is PD.

Is it necessary to start treatment on everyone to prove the diagnosis of PD? No. The decision whether to start a medication and choice of medication should be based on whether the symptoms are interfering with your life. If the symptoms are mild and do not demand treatment or require only a mild treatment, patience is in order. This will sort itself out in time.

Symptoms of PD

People with PD experience a wide variety of symptoms. Some of these are unique and suggestive of the diagnosis, whereas others are less specific. A list of common symptoms is shown in table 4.1. If you recognize several symptoms from this list, the suspicion of parkinsonism and hence PD is raised.

The initial entries in table 4.1 relate to tremor. How do we define "tremor"? Tremor is a repetitive, rhythmic movement that precisely repeats itself. It is a

Table 4.1. Parkinson's Disease Symptoms*

Common Symptoms Very Suggestive of PD

Tremor	• Resting hand tremor (tremor when the hand is relaxed or at one's side when walking) • Resting thumb or finger tremor (observed when the hand is resting in the lap) • Chin or lip tremor (also a "resting" tremor, meaning that it is seen when sitting quietly but not talking or chewing) • Tremor of a leg when seated (also a resting tremor)
Feet and gait	• Toes curling or turning up • Feet get stuck ("freezing") • Shuffling gait
Loss of automatic movements	• Less animated (facial appearance not expressive, poker-faced, reduced blinking, loss of expressive movements of the hands) • Reduced arm swing
Slowness	• Slowed movements (takes longer to do things)
Speech and writing	• Softer voice and less distinct speech • Smaller handwriting

Other Common Symptoms That May Have Other Explanations

General	• Sense of overall weakness • Fatigue • Sense of restlessness, nervousness • Stiffness, neck or limbs
Gait, stance, and trunk	• Mild imbalance • Stooped posture • Difficulty rising from seated position • Difficulty turning over in bed
Hand function	• Difficulty buttoning buttons, using eating utensils • Difficulty brushing teeth
Cognition	• Slowed thinking
Saliva	• Drooling or sense of increased saliva

*Among those with early PD, the symptoms are often on only one side of the body or are asymmetric (more on one side than the other). This asymmetry persists throughout life.

back-and-forth movement that goes on and on and on. We have all seen tremor in hands. However, tremor may involve other areas of the body.

Neurologists categorize hand tremor on the basis of whether it is present when the hand is active versus "at rest." If your hand is tremulous in your lap or at your side when you are walking, this is classified as at rest. Tremor at rest is typical of PD. Tremor of your hand when using it, such as writing or bringing a fork to your mouth, is termed an action tremor; action tremors are not typical of PD. Sometimes a parkinsonian rest tremor affects only the thumb or the fingers; an old term for this is a pill-rolling tremor. This is because the rhythmic movements of the fingers give the appearance of a pill being rolled back and forth between the thumb and fingers. Note that table 4.1 also includes a rest tremor of the chin or lip as suspicious for PD. Similarly, a parkinsonian rest tremor in the legs may be apparent when seated; you may see your knee going up and down if your feet are resting on the floor. Or a foot may move back and forth if your feet are dangling off the floor.

Another foot symptom suspicious for PD is involuntary curling of the toes, as if in spasm. We all experience cramps at times and, rarely, our toes may cramp. However, if involuntary spasms and curling of the toes are recurrent, this is suspicious for parkinsonism. This is not to be confused with hammer toes, where the toes naturally assume a bent position. Hammer toes are not a sign of PD.

Certain walking abnormalities suggest parkinsonism. If your feet stick to the floor when attempting to take a step, this suggests gait freezing, a symptom of PD. However, the classic gait abnormality of parkinsonism is a "shuffling" gait. Normally when we walk, we take a step by cocking up our lead foot and planting the heel in front of us. We then push off with the ball and toes of that foot as we continue with the step. This alternates from one foot to the other to generate a typical human gait. In contrast, the "shuffling" gait is characterized by loss of the normal heel strike; rather, the foot tends to slide along the floor, one foot after the other. In addition, the length of the stride shortens with this classic shuffling gait.

Parkinsonism is also associated with loss of normal facial animation. Humans are very expressive in their facial appearance. We smile, frown, grimace, and convey a variety of subtle communications with our faces. This tends to be dampened or lost in PD. This is what is meant by facial masking. One component is a reduction in the normal blink rate, which produces the appearance of staring. Facial masking is rarely appreciated by the person with parkinsonism, but others notice it. People who are depressed also tend to have bland facial expressions. They don't smile and convey the sentiment that nothing is of interest. This shouldn't be confused with the facial masking of parkinsonism.

A corollary of facial masking is the loss or reduction of normal spontaneous and expressive movements of the hands, such as gesturing when talking or swinging one's arms while walking. This parallels the loss of facial expression.

Slowness of movement—bradykinesia in the language of physicians—is a highly characteristic feature of parkinsonism. Movements are made as if done in a swimming pool, slow and laborious. The slowness may predominantly or exclusively affect one limb; thus it may be hard to button with one hand. Similarly, one leg may lag behind the other when walking. Bradykinesia may affect the entire body, giving the appearance of moving in slow motion.

Particular changes in the voice and speech may also suggest the diagnosis. First, the voice tends to get softer. Second, speech may be less precise and may take on a subtle stammering quality. Third, the normal inflections of speech diminish and speaking may be in a monotone. Often the spouse complains of not being able to hear what his or her mate is saying.

Writing is often a clue to parkinsonism. Handwriting may start out normal but become progressively smaller by the end of a long word or a sentence. This is known as micrographia.

The bottom half of table 4.1 includes a variety of symptoms that are less specific for PD; that is, they also occur in other disorders or with normal aging. For example, fatigue is present in many conditions and physicians hear this complaint many times a day in their general practice. Mild imbalance or a stooped posture is common with normal aging. The arthritis of aging (osteoarthritis) may cause stiffness of limbs or difficulty buttoning, and so on. Hence these less specific symptoms listed in table 4.1 may be manifestations of parkinsonism but could have other explanations as well.

Signs That Point to PD

In the language of medicine, "signs" are what the physician finds by observing and examining and hence they constitute objective evidence. They are to be distinguished from symptoms, which patients experience and subjectively report to their physician. I just described the symptoms of PD; now I will address what the physician sees.

Although physicians perform a formal examination, the observation of the patient starts as soon as the doctor enters the room. Physicians are trained to be good observers, and parkinsonism may be suggested early in the visit by subtle clues. We will break down our strategy for analyzing the signs of PD from the perspective of a physician meeting and evaluating the patient. No special tools are required. Imagine that you are the doctor and you enter the room where your patient, Mr. Jones, has been waiting.

- Does he have trouble rising from his chair to greet you? Difficulty rising from the seated position is common in PD. The legs are strong but the problem is with programming the movements in the brain.

- Do you get a sense of overall slowness? Those with PD may move as if they are in a bowl of molasses.

- Is he poker-faced with little facial animation? Loss of facial expression is a hallmark of PD.

- Is there a tremor of the hand that is in his lap? Note that this could be subtle, for example, only a thumb moving back and forth. A tremor of the hand when it is relaxed, or even just the thumb or fingers, is a tell-tale sign of parkinsonism. The same is true for a chin or lip tremor.

- Is one arm and hand stiffly held in the lap? Asymmetric immobility of a limb is a clue to parkinsonism.

- Is his voice soft? Is his speech less articulate than normal? Does he speak in a monotone? A decline in voice volume is common in parkinsonism, as is loss of the normal inflections and precision of speech.

- Does he lack animation, such as not gesturing when talking? Those with parkinsonism lose their automatic movements. This includes gesturing when speaking, arm swinging when walking, and facial animation.

These initial observations are summarized in table 4.2 and matched with the formal medical term for the corresponding sign of parkinsonism.

Once you have visited with Mr. Jones (and made your observations), you can proceed to the more formal parkinsonism examination, analyzing whether someone does indeed have parkinsonism. It requires no tools, just open eyes. You are now the doctor. Here is what to ask Mr. Jones to do, what to look for, and how to interpret what you are seeing.

Table 4.2. Signs of Parkinsonism Apparent from Simple Observation
(What your doctor observes when first greeting you and talking to you)

Sign	Medical Term
Trouble standing up from the seated position	
Moves slowly	Bradykinesia
Poker-faced	Facial masking or hypomimia
Tremor when hand is in lap (also tremor of chin, leg, or foot when in relaxed posture)	Rest tremor
Arm and hand held stiffly in lap or at the side	Rigidity (stiffness) and bradykinesia (slowness and reduced spontaneous mobility)
Voice is softer and speech is less articulate, often devoid of inflections (monotone)	Hypokinetic dysarthria or hypophonic voice (parkinsonian speech)
Lack of gesturing when talking	Loss of automatic movements

(1) Have him stand up. Is he slow? Does he require several tries to get up? Does he need help?

(2) Have him walk through the office door, down the hall, turn and come back. Analyze the different components of gait.

- Did he hesitate with the first step or when walking through the doorway? Do his feet seem stuck to the floor when he tries to take a step? *Comment:* Those with parkinsonism may have trouble taking the initial step, as if their feet were glued to the floor. This is called freezing. Typically it abates once they get going but may recur when they approach doorways or make a turn.

- Observe the posture when walking. Is he stooped? *Comment:* As we age we may get a little stooped. However, with parkinsonism, it may be more than expected for age.

- Is he slow as he walks down the hall? *Comment:* Bradykinesia (slowness) is a cardinal sign of parkinsonism. Obviously not everyone moves as fast as the next person. However, those with parkinsonism typically move more slowly than expected for age.

- Observe the details of his foot placement as he walks. Is the stride length shortened? Are the feet moving parallel to the floor instead of planting with the heel and pushing off with the ball of the foot? Is this occurring to the extent that the gait appears shuffling? Does one foot lag behind? *Comment:* In those with parkinsonism, the amplitude of foot movements dampens. As described above, the normal heel strike may be lost and the stride length is often shortened. When severe, the foot never leaves the floor; this constitutes shuffling.

- Watch the hands when walking. Is arm swing normal? Is a subtle tremor (rest tremor) present in a hand, thumb, or fingers? *Comment:* Reduced arm swing is typical of parkinsonism. PD tends to be an asymmetric disorder and often there is a substantial difference in arm swing between the two sides. Observation during walking is also one of the best times to observe the hand rest tremor. Since PD is an asymmetric condition, that tremor may be present in only one hand.

- Watch Mr. Jones turn. Instead of pivoting, does he take several steps to turn? Is there gait freezing? *Comment:* Instead of making a smooth pivot, those with parkinsonism often will need to stop and replant their feet several times to complete the turn. This may also unmask the tendency for freezing, with the feet briefly getting stuck in place.

- Is there unsteadiness? *Comment:* Early in PD balance is usually preserved or only mildly impaired. It may be more of a problem later. Severe imbalance early in parkinsonism suggests a parkinsonism look-alike condition.

(3) Test balance by the "pull test" once Mr. Jones has completed his walk. To do this, stand behind Mr. Jones and tell him to resist being pulled backward. You then pull back on his shoulders. The pull should be forceful enough to pull the shoulders back slightly, but not so vigorous that it would cause a normal person to fall back.

- Does he fall backward into your arms? (Be prepared to catch him.) *Comment*: People with parkinsonism often have mild imbalance and this is often primarily manifest as a tendency to fall backward, termed retropulsion.

The remainder of the examination is conducted with Mr. Jones seated on the examining table (or a chair).

(4) Assess for rigidity, which is stiffness of the limbs, as well as trunk and neck. To properly interpret this, you must do this on normal people to get a sense of normal limb tone. Rigidity can be assessed wherever there is a joint. To test for rigidity, move the joint back and forth, asking Mr. Jones to relax that limb. Start with the wrist, then elbow, shoulder, and then repeat on the other side. Next, rigidity can be similarly assessed at the knee joints. After the limbs have been examined, gently move the neck, again asking Mr. Jones to relax as best he can.

- Is there resistance to movement of these joints? Do they feel stiff? *Comment:* Increased limb tone is one of the hallmark features of parkinsonism. A normal joint should move like a well-lubricated hinge. Rigidity feels like a rusty hinge; there is resistance to moving it. Sometimes the rigidity of PD has a tremulous quality, which is termed cogwheel rigidity. Obviously Mr. Jones must do his best to relax to allow this to be properly assessed. Minor degrees of rigidity may be difficult to determine. If there are major joint problems (arthritis), then this cannot be analyzed easily.

(5) "Alternate motion rate" testing is the last set of tasks (also called rapid alternating movements). Ask Mr. Jones to rapidly perform repetitive tapping maneuvers with his fingers, hands, and then feet. Focus on the speed of movements as well as the amplitude (amplitude implies the width of the excursions of movement).

Analyzing one hand at a time, have Mr. Jones repetitively tap the tips of his thumb and index finger together, back and forth. Ask him to do this rapidly and with wide excursions. Have him continue to do this for about ten seconds.

- Is he slow? Does the amplitude of the movement (the excursion) diminish with continued tapping? Is there a substantial difference, comparing one hand to the other? *Comment:* Those with parkinsonism will often slow down when doing this, and the amplitude of the movement will diminish with repetition. For example, Mr. Jones may perform the first few excursions normally, but as he continues, he may not separate his thumb and finger as widely as initially. It may dampen to the extent that they barely separate or even freeze in place. Also, because PD is an asymmetric condition, one hand often performs better than the other.

(6) Now have Mr. Jones pat his knee with his hand, alternating between the palm and the back of the hand (so-called pronation-supination). Do this one hand at a time.

- Is he slow? Is he able to do this continuously, or does the movement break down? Is there a substantial difference, comparing one hand to the other? *Comment:* Those with parkinsonism may do this slowly and with breakdown of the movements (stopping-starting).

(7) Finally, have Mr. Jones tap his foot repetitively and rapidly (as if listening to music). Do this one foot at a time.

- Is he slow? Is he able to do this continuously, or does the movement break down? Is there a substantial difference, comparing one foot to the other? *Comment:* Like hand movements, this may be slowed and the amplitude of the movements may be limited. Note that if Mr. Jones has a leg tremor, the repetitive foot tapping may be driven by the tremor. In that case, have him tap his heel instead.

Our formal parkinsonism examination is summarized in table 4.3. To that may be added a handwriting sample to look for micrographia.

Once we have completed this assessment of parkinsonism, we consider the totality of our results. This includes our initial observations, plus what we witnessed on the formal examination. Those with PD will not necessarily display all the signs described above. We are looking for enough of these signs to put Mr. Jones into the parkinsonism category. Only one or two of these signs, especially some of the less specific ones, will usually not support a diagnosis of parkinsonism. For example, a mildly stooped posture may be due to age and reduced arm swing could reflect a shoulder problem. Thus one needs to look at the big picture. Parkinsonism may be diagnosed only if there are enough of these signs that, especially, cannot be written off to other causes.

Some findings carry more weight than others. For example, a resting tremor of the hand is extremely suspicious; it typically cannot be attributed to other factors. However, mild slowness in tapping the foot, especially if not accompanied by many other signs, may not be very informative. In sum, the physician must be convinced by the number of symptoms and signs, while at the same time factoring in whether there is another explanation, such as age or joint problems.

Table 4.3.   The Formal Parkinsonism Examination

Task	Things to Look For That Suggest Parkinsonism
Standing up from sitting	• Hesitant, slow; requires help; may have to push off with hands (nonspecific sign since lower limb pain or weakness might also impair standing)
Walking	• Hesitant (gait freezing; feet get stuck to the floor) • Stooped posture • Slowness (bradykinesia) • Does not plant heel, then push off the ball of the foot with each step; feet move parallel to floor (when pronounced, gait is shuffling; feet don't leave the floor) • Stride length shortened • Reduced arm swing • Hand, thumb, or finger tremor (rest tremor) • Turns with several steps rather than smooth pivot (cannot turn on a dime) • Imbalance (should not be severe early in PD)
Pull test	• Falls backward with moderately forceful tug on shoulders
Assess rigidity	• Movement of the joints encounters resistance (the person being tested must relax); if superimposed tremor, this gives it a ratchety feel, termed cogwheel rigidity
Alternate motion rate testing (tapping of finger-thumb, hands, feet)	• Slow • Amplitude of the excursions is reduced (sometimes apparent only after 5-10 seconds of repetitions); hesitation or lack of rhythmicity

There are four cardinal signs of parkinsonism:

• Resting tremor

• Rigidity

• Bradykinesia (includes general body slowness and slowness in just one limb, as evidenced in alternate motion rate tasks)

• Imbalance

Two of the four are sufficient to constitute parkinsonism. Bear in mind, however, that prominent imbalance with falls is not an early sign of PD; it suggests another parkinsonian disorder (discussed in chapter 6).

Occasionally the signs are mild and the physician is unable to say for certain whether parkinsonism is truly present. Time sorts this out. With evolution of the condition over the ensuing six to twelve months, the exam will probably be a little worse and the diagnosis more obvious.

Specialists employ a scoring system for PD—the Unified Parkinson's Disease Rating Scale (UPDRS). In this scheme, each of the observations and tasks we just considered are given a rating on a 4-point scale. You can add the score and come up with a number that correlates with the severity of parkinsonism. This is primarily a research tool for investigators. They use this as a reference point in studies of medical or surgical treatments, repeating the examination after a new drug has been added or surgery performed.

Additional Signs Evaluated by the Physician

The evaluation described above will tell us if parkinsonism is present. The next step is to determine whether there are any other symptoms or signs to suggest another type of parkinsonian disorder besides PD (see also chapter 6). Hence, additional neurologic examination is necessary, which I will briefly summarize. Since some of this requires special tools and clinical experience, a detailed discussion is beyond the scope of this book.

Once the physician recognizes the findings of parkinsonism, the examination is expanded to determine whether other brain systems are involved. These other systems can be broken down into distinct categories:

- Corticospinal tract: Are there signs of spasticity with abnormal reflexes?

- Cerebellar: Are there signs of incoordination (ataxia)?

- Praxis: Are complex movements of the hands (or feet) impaired?

- Eye movements: Is movement of the eyes impaired (especially looking down)?

- Cognition: Are thinking and memory impaired?

If you have PD, there should not be any substantial abnormalities in these areas. Basic assessment of these categories is summarized in table 4.4.

The physician may also learn facts during the initial interview which suggest that the parkinsonism may not be PD. Just like the signs listed above, the patient may describe features that point to another disorder. Some of the more common elements that physicians look for in this setting are summarized in table 4.5.

Certainly the physician will review the medication list. A variety of drugs may cause parkinsonism, which resolves when the drug is stopped. This is discussed in detail in chapter 6.

Table 4.4. The Extended Neurological Examination*

Brain System	Evidence Found by the Neurologist
Corticospinal tract	• Increased tendon reflexes (assessed with a reflex hammer) • Babinski sign (response of the great toe when the bottom of the foot is scratched: reflexively goes up instead of down) • Characteristic changes in gait and certain unique changes in limb tone
Cerebellar	• Imprecision when asked to point back and forth from nose to examiner's finger (incoordination) • Garbled speech (ataxic dysarthria) • Unsteady gait with legs spread apart (so-called wide-base gait)
Praxis	• Inability to perform patterned movements correctly, such as the throwing motion, waving good-bye, and so on
Eye movements	• Inability to move the eyes, especially downward
Cognition	• Prominent and early thinking and memory problems

*Assessment of other brain systems that should be spared in Parkinson's disease but may be involved in other parkinsonian disorders. If you have prominent signs in one or more of these categories, your parkinsonism may not be due to PD.

Table 4.5. Features That Raise Suspicion That Parkinsonism Is Not PD

Category	Symptoms	Alternate possibilities
Age at onset	• First symptoms before age 40	Although this still could be PD, very young onset indicates need for more thorough investigation.
Time course	• Sudden changes	Sudden onset of symptoms raises question of stroke.
	• Rapid deterioration	Some other disorder or some second factor, such as super-imposed pneumonia.
	• Symptoms began after starting a medication	Medication could be responsible.
Gait	• Many falls, early in the course	Progressive supranuclear palsy, multiple system atrophy or other cause.*
Autonomic nervous system	• Low blood pressure leading to faints or near-faints (plus prominent other autonomic symptoms)	Multiple system atrophy, if medications are not the cause for the low blood pressure.*

*See chapter 6 for more details.

Testing

Are there tests we can use to confirm our diagnosis? Actually, tests will not tell us if someone has PD, but they may be used to determine if the parkinsonism is due to some other cause. Since degeneration of the substantia nigra does not change the normal contours of the brain, brain scans are typically normal in PD; however, they may be abnormal in other conditions. Similarly, blood studies may exclude other causes for certain symptoms, such as the fatigue due to a low thyroid state. Testing may not be necessary when the symptoms and signs are typical of PD. We consider testing in more detail in chapter 7.

Diagnostic Confirmation: The Response to Medications

The symptoms and signs of PD primarily reflect a deficiency of dopamine in the brain. Hence, if we administer a medication that restores dopamine (or the dopamine effect), the symptoms should reverse. Thus the treatment turns out to also be a useful diagnostic test.

The two classes of drugs used to restore dopamine or the dopamine effect are levodopa and dopamine agonists. These will be examined in detail in later chapters. Levodopa is a natural substance that brain cells can convert directly to dopamine. It is combined with carbidopa, which prevents nausea and allows more of the levodopa to enter the brain. The generic form of this medication is carbidopa/levodopa and the brand name is Sinemet. Dopamine agonist drugs act like synthetic forms of dopamine, although they are not as potent. There are four dopamine agonists available in the United States: bromocriptine (Parlodel), pergolide (Permax), pramipexole (Mirapex), and ropinirole (Requip).

An excellent response to one of these drugs tells us that a brain dopamine deficiency state is present but other brain circuits are intact. If non-dopaminergic brain circuits are additionally impaired, therapy directed at dopamine would likely be insufficient. Many disorders that look like PD (such as progressive supranuclear palsy described in chapter 6) reflect degeneration in other brain circuits besides those containing dopamine. Hence levodopa and dopamine agonist therapies are typically not highly effective in those settings.

Which drug should you take to test the response, levodopa or a dopamine agonist? Levodopa is more potent and thus is a better test. However, an excellent response to a dopamine agonist drug also confirms the diagnosis of PD. One caveat is in order. Occasionally people with PD fail to respond to one of these drugs because the dose was too low or the drug was incorrectly taken. This is especially common with the dopamine agonist drugs. They must be started at very low doses to avoid side effects. The usual dosage escalation scheme requires about six to eight weeks of increments. Sometimes people get stuck on the initial low doses and never escalate the dosage into the therapeutic range. Levodopa (carbidopa/levodopa) may also be incorrectly administered, resulting in a failed response. There are two ways this may occur. First, as with the dopamine agonists, the dose must be raised sufficiently high to capture a good effect. Second (in contrast to the dopamine agonists), carbidopa/levodopa must be taken on an empty stomach to assure passage into the brain. Details about the dosage of all of these drugs are found in later chapters.

Does an initial response to these drugs guarantee that PD is the diagnosis? Usually this is the case, but there are exceptions. Some of the conditions that resemble PD respond partially and briefly (see chapter 6). In PD, the beneficial response is substantial and sustained.

Review of the Steps to Diagnose PD

There is a logical order of analysis necessary to arrive at the diagnosis of PD. This is the sequence of thinking used by the physician.

1. Is parkinsonism present on the basis of the office interview and examination? Remember, parkinsonism is not necessarily PD.

2. If yes, are there other symptoms or signs to suggest the parkinsonism is not truly PD (tables 4.4 and 4.5)? Is a prescription medication causing the parkinsonism (see chapter 6)? If there are no unusual or unexpected features, then testing may be unnecessary (discussed in chapter 7).

3. Is there an excellent response to medical treatment? This can only be assessed if adequate doses of appropriate drugs are utilized. Where there is uncertainty, levodopa therapy is the most reliable means for assessing this (dosing described in later chapters).

But I Don't Have Tremor

In the minds of many, tremor is synonymous with PD. However, many with PD do not have tremor, and hence absence of tremor is not an argument against the diagnosis. Conversely, tremor occurs in other disorders. The most frequent cause of tremor is not PD but essential tremor. Although essential tremor is present with action and not at rest, there are rare exceptions. This is discussed further in chapters 6 and 14.

One-Sided PD

PD is occasionally confused with other neurologic conditions because of the asymmetry of symptoms and signs. PD often starts in one limb and is restricted to that limb for a period of time. Often this will be one arm. With progression, the remaining limb on that same side of the body (arm or leg) becomes symptomatic. At this point, half the body will be normal and the other half affected. If the typical resting tremor is present, the diagnosis is usually apparent. However, without the tremor to give away the diagnosis, stiffness and slowness in one limb or one side of the body may raise concerns about a variety of other disorders. This may get more difficult to diagnose if there is pain or aching in that limb, as often occurs with PD. If symptoms are in just one limb, the initial thought may be a pinched nerve or some arthritic condition. If one side of the body is slow moving and stiff, this might erroneously be thought to represent spasticity, suggesting a stroke or multiple sclerosis.

The asymmetry of PD is curious and unexpected in a neurodegenerative disorder. Seemingly such a degenerative process should be more uniform and affect both sides of the body and all four limbs at the same time. The reason for the asymmetry is unexplained.

As PD progresses, the other side eventually will become involved. However, PD typically remains an asymmetric condition; the first side to be affected remains a little worse than the other side. Sometimes this is minimal, but often not.

Is PD more likely to start on the right side of the body? The left side? Or in the right arm in right-handed people? The answer to all these questions is no. It seems to be a random process. It may start on either side, regardless of whether one is right- or left-handed.

What About My Other Symptoms?

PD encompasses more than just problems with movement and tremor. There are a wide variety of additional symptoms that may be experienced as direct manifestations of PD; the most common of these symptoms are listed in table 4.6. You need to know that these may be PD-related so that treatment is appropriately tailored to the problem.

AUTONOMIC SYMPTOMS

As explained in chapter 3, the autonomic nervous system organizes and programs the workings of many internal organs. Autonomic problems are common in PD but typically are not severe early in the course and sometimes never.

GASTROINTESTINAL PROBLEMS: CONSTIPATION, BLOATING

The digestive system processes food in successive stages. Food is propelled from the mouth down to the stomach, where the digestive process starts.

Table 4.6. Nonmovement Symptoms of PD

Category	Symptom
Autonomic nervous system	
Gastrointestinal	• Constipation • Bloating • Heartburn (reflux)
Swallowing	• Impaired swallowing • Drooling
Bladder	• Hesitant urination • Sudden uncontrollable urges to void (urgency) • Incontinence • Need to urinate frequently, including at night (nocturia) • Frequent urinary tract infections
Genitalia	• Male impotence
Blood pressure	• Orthostatic hypotension (low blood pressure when standing; faintness, fatigue or faints when standing, walking)
Psychiatric	• Depression • Anxiety • Inner restlessness (akathisia) • Panic attacks
Cognitive	• Slowed thinking (bradyphrenia) • Dementia • Hallucinations, delusions
Sleep	• Insomnia • Daytime sleepiness • Acting out dreams (REM sleep behavior disorder) • Restless legs syndrome
Sensory symptoms	• Sciatica or other limb pain • Pain or discomfort in neck, trunk, or abdomen • Numbness, tingling • Cramps (painful) • Sensation of heat or cold
Other symptoms	• Fatigue • Shortness of breath

From there, it is passed to the small intestine, where nutrients enter the blood-stream. Waste from the food passes to the colon (large intestine) to form feces. Contractions of the stomach and intestines keep things moving. These contractions are programmed by the autonomic nervous system. When this system malfunctions, things back up. A sensation of abdominal bloating oc-curs if food cannot get out of the stomach or move downstream through the intestines. Heartburn may develop if the stomach contents back up into the esophagus (the tube through which food passes from mouth to stomach). On the other end, constipation occurs when the colon does not contract nor-mally to produce bowel movements. Constipation is extremely common in PD, whereas the other gastrointestinal symptoms occur to variable degrees.

DIFFICULT SWALLOWING AND DROOLING

The first step in the process of propelling food through the digestive system is swallowing, and difficulty in swallowing may be a symptom of PD. Typically, however, this is not severe and often improves with medicines for PD (levodopa or dopamine agonist therapy). Major swallowing problems early in the course of PD raise a question of a parkinsonism look-alike condition, such as pro-gressive supranuclear palsy or multiple system atrophy (see chapter 6).

Drooling is common in untreated PD. This is not due to excessive saliva, but because of a reduction in the reflexive swallowing rate. Saliva is swal-lowed unconsciously. However, this automatic swallowing often diminishes in PD. This is similar to the reduction of other automatic movements in PD, such as blinking, arm swing when walking, or gesturing when talking. Drool-ing, like arm swing and facial masking, typically improves with medications for PD (levodopa, dopamine agonist drugs).

BLADDER: HESITANT URINE FLOW
OR LOSS OF CONTROL

The bladder is the reservoir where urine is stored after it has been produced by the kidneys. Neurological reflexes are triggered when the bladder is full, priming it to contract and expel the contents (hopefully into the toilet). Sig-nals also reach our brain indicating that we need to get to the bathroom. Normally we are able to suppress these urges until we are ready. When the autonomic control of the bladder malfunctions in PD, one of several symp-toms may occur, including:

- Difficulty passing the urine (hesitant urination)

- Sudden compulsions to void (urgency)

- Incontinence (inability to prevent expulsion of urine, with involuntary wetting)

- The need to urinate frequently, even when the bladder is only slightly full; this may require trips to the bathroom at night (nocturia)

- Frequent urinary tract infections (due to poor urine outflow, with the stagnant urine being a source of infection)

Sometimes it is not certain whether the urinary symptoms are due to PD.

It is common for men over sixty to experience prostate problems and a slowed urinary stream. Women who have given birth often experience so-called stress incontinence, meaning that physical stress or straining (for example, coughing, sneezing, or other straining) may inadvertently cause urine to leak. Urologic testing can help determine whether bladder problems are due to PD and guide appropriate treatment, as discussed in chapter 27.

IMPOTENCE

Male erectile dysfunction is common in PD and may be caused by problems of the autonomic nervous system, medications, or both. Also, difficulty maintaining an erection is common with normal aging and a variety of medical conditions. Sometimes the psychological stress of a failed erection adds to the problem in future sexual encounters. There are a variety of measures that can be tried for treatment of male impotence, as outlined in chapter 28.

Female sexual dysfunction may also occur in PD, although this has been poorly studied. It also is addressed in chapter 28.

LOW BLOOD PRESSURE WHEN STANDING

PD may predispose to a low blood pressure when standing. Furthermore, the medications used to treat PD may exacerbate this tendency. Occasionally it may be so severe that fainting or near fainting results. The medical term for this is "orthostatic hypotension" ("orthostatic" means standing erect; "hypotension" means low blood pressure). Besides faints or near-faints, orthostatic hypotension may result in fatigue, lightheadedness, or tiredness when up and about.

Orthostatic hypotension may go undetected. Symptoms are sometimes subtle and may not be recognized for what they represent. Furthermore, blood pressure is conventionally measured only in the sitting position. Among those with orthostatic hypotension, the sitting blood pressure may be normal, whereas the standing pressure may be extremely low. If you think that you may be experiencing symptoms of orthostatic hypotension, read chapter 21.

Psychiatric Conditions and PD

DEPRESSION

Depression is common among those with PD. In the mildest form, this may simply be feeling blue most of the time. In more severe forms, people may be disabled by hopelessness and despair. They may completely lose interest in things that previously brought them pleasure.

A variety of symptoms are spin-offs of depression, including loss of appetite, weight loss (sometimes weight gain), insomnia (or excessive sleep), fatigue, loss of initiative with poor energy, inability to concentrate, irascibility, loss of self-esteem, and even impotence. Among those with PD, however, these symptoms may have other origins, complicating the diagnosis. For example, poor appetite, weight loss, or impotence may be due to medications or problems in the autonomic nervous system. Weight loss may also be caused by the increased energy expenditure from involuntary movements (tremor, dyskinesias). Insomnia and fatigue are often the direct consequence of PD. Also, physicians recognize that people with PD tend to lose their facial expression ("masking"), which makes them appear depressed even if they don't actually feel that way.

Depression may have more than one cause among people with PD. They may be discouraged by their illness, with reduced abilities and capacities. Hobbies may no longer be possible or enjoyable; golf scores may increase or competitive tennis may no longer be feasible. Depression, however, is frequently due to chemical changes in the brain caused by PD. We previously noted that brain dopamine is reduced, as well as the neurotransmitter serotonin. Both of these brain chemicals are important for experiencing happiness and pleasure. Serotonin may be crucial, and most of the newer drugs developed for treating depression are tailored to increase brain serotonin activity.

Most important, depression is treatable, but it must first be recognized. Strategies for treating depression are found in chapter 22.

ANXIETY AND PANIC ATTACKS

Anxiety is a common symptom of PD, although it is often attributed to other causes. Perhaps it receives little recognition since it cannot be seen (unlike tremor or shuffling gait) and cannot easily be measured. In its mildest form it may be experienced as simple nervousness or a sense of foreboding that seems out of proportion for the circumstances. At the other extreme are frank anxiety states and sometimes even panic attacks, which may be primary symptoms of PD.

People with PD also experience a sense of inner restlessness, termed akathisia. They describe feeling tense and uncomfortable when sitting still or lying in bed. Sometimes this is difficult to distinguish from anxiety, since the lay term for each of these is often "nervousness."

Not everyone with anxiety can blame this on PD. Obviously, anxiety is a common disorder in general. However, when the anxiety state begins simultaneously with parkinsonian symptoms (or after), PD may be the cause.

Because anxiety is often unrecognized as caused by PD, the most effective treatments may not be employed. Anxiety due to PD often responds to the same medications that we use to treat the other symptoms of PD, as will be discussed in chapter 19.

Cognitive Functions and PD

SLOWED THINKING

Like slowness of movements experienced by those with PD, thinking may be similarly slowed. The medical term for this is bradyphrenia. Those with bradyphrenia will typically come up with correct answers to questions, but it takes longer. Bradyphrenia improves with the usual medications for PD (such as levodopa therapy). Bradyphrenia is not an early sign of dementia and does not indicate that major cognitive problems are imminent.

DEMENTIA

Major thinking and memory problems (dementia) may develop among those with PD. However, this spares many with PD and, if it occurs, typically appears much later in the course. It is more likely among seniors, and probably aging contributes to this tendency, as it does in the general population. When dementia develops, the typical onset is many years after the development of PD.

Dementia needs to be distinguished from the mild memory problems that are a part of normal aging as well as from bradyphrenia. Other causes of brain dysfunction must also be excluded, as will be discussed in chapter 23.

HALLUCINATIONS AND DELUSIONS

Hallucinations—seeing things that aren't there—may be caused by PD. However, in most cases, this is primarily due to the medications we use to treat parkinsonism. The mildest form may include seeing bugs or some nondescript, shadowy image in the periphery of vision. However, hallucinations of people, children, or animals may also intrude on consciousness. Hallucinations are uncommon in early and even intermediate stages of PD; they tend to be late manifestations. When they do occur, there are a variety of strategies that can be employed to treat them, as will be addressed in chapter 24.

Delusions are beliefs that have no validity and often are nonsensical. Like hallucinations, delusional thinking tends to occur late in PD, if it occurs at all. This is not common but may be troublesome when it develops. Some delusions are benign, such as being convinced that company is coming for supper. Others may be disruptive, such as believing that one's spouse is unfaithful, or bizarre, such as thinking that this same spouse is a secret agent. Delusions, like hallucinations, tend to be caused or exacerbated by the medications used to treat PD. They respond to the same drugs that are used to treat hallucinations (see chapter 24).

Sleep

INSOMNIA

Insomnia is common in the general population but is much more common among those with PD. People with PD frequently experience problems both getting to sleep and staying asleep. Most often this is secondary to a variety of symptoms that are linked to PD, which include the following:

- Anxiety
- Akathisia
- Restless legs syndrome (see below)
- Sense of stiffness (rigidity)
- Tremor (present at rest)
- Difficulty turning in bed to get into comfortable position
- Night cramps (see below)

Since these are primary manifestations of PD, they respond to levodopa and related medications, as discussed in chapter 20.

DAYTIME SLEEPINESS

People with PD may experience daytime drowsiness. This is usually caused by some other primary factor, including:

- Insomnia with poor nighttime sleep (leaving them drowsy during the day)
- Medications
- Inability to achieve deep sleep; this may be due to disordered breathing (sleep apnea) or other reasons

Daytime sleepiness is discussed in detail in chapter 20.

ACTING-OUT DREAMS (REM SLEEP BEHAVIOR DISORDER)

Normally when we dream, our body remains in a relaxed state; we don't move. Although we may be experiencing a very vivid dream, we lie still in bed. This is because once the dream starts, the connection between the brain's dreaming center and the rest of the brain is switched off. In those with PD, this connection tends to remain open; the dreaming brain remains partially connected to brain movement centers. Thus people with PD tend to act out their dreams. The medical term for this is REM sleep behavior disorder. REM stands for rapid eye movement. REM sleep is a deep stage of sleep where much dreaming occurs. The body is normally limp and unmoving during this sleep stage, except for our eyes. Thus the normal person acts out dreams with the eyes only. However, among those with PD, a vivid dream may provoke a variety of vigorous nighttime behaviors known only to the sleep partner. Not only is REM sleep behavior common in PD, it may precede the usual PD symptoms by many years. See chapter 20 for more details.

RESTLESS LEGS SYNDROME

Sleep may be prevented by a creepy-crawly, tingly sensation in the legs. It typically occurs in a relaxed state or at bedtime. It provokes the urge to get up and walk, and walking tends to relieve it. Restless legs syndrome is common in the general population but is more common among those with PD. Chapter 20 covers this in more detail, including treatment.

Sensory Symptoms

NUMBNESS AND TINGLING

People with PD often experience a variety of uncomfortable or unusual sensations, especially in the limbs. Descriptions include numbness, tingling, pins and needles, or a nondescript sense that something is not right in that area of the body. A feeling of heat or cold may also be experienced. These sometimes respond to the medications used to treat parkinsonism.

PAIN AND CRAMPS

Pain is common among those with PD but does not get much publicity. A common type of parkinsonian pain is a cramp-like sensation. This typically represents a parkinsonian state that responds to levodopa or related medications. Limb pain characteristic of sciatica may be a symptom of PD, as may pain experienced in the neck, trunk, or abdomen.

Obviously pain is common and we should not jump to the conclusion that any and all pain is due to PD. Our body uses pain to tell us that something isn't right and other causes need to be investigated. However, if the pain completely resolves with levodopa treatment, it is likely due to PD.

Other Symptoms

FATIGUE AND WEAKNESS

Poor energy and loss of the usual stamina are typical of PD. People with PD find that they are less able to burn the candle at both ends. They may be able to function at moderate activity levels but cannot switch into high gear or work long hours as they could previously. Similarly, people with PD may complain of feeling weak, but without any true muscle weakness apparent on examination. The medications for PD are at least partially helpful in treating these symptoms.

SHORTNESS OF BREATH

Shortness of breath is common later in life and usually suggests heart or lung problems. However, shortness of breath may also be due to PD (see chapter 19). One shouldn't jump to the conclusion that PD is responsible, however; your physician must first consider other more common causes. Shortness of breath due to parkinsonism typically responds to PD medications.

SUMMARY OF NONMOVEMENT SYMPTOMS IN PD

A variety of nonmovement symptoms occur in PD. Some of the more common symptoms have been discussed above, but this is not an all-inclusive list. As a general rule of thumb, if a particular symptom goes away following treatment with levodopa and related medications, it may well represent a symptom of PD. This is especially likely if there is no other medical explanation.

5
◆ ◆ ◆
Prognosis

Initially being told that you have Parkinson's disease (PD) can be devastating. Often the first thing that comes to mind is an image of a relative or an acquaintance with terrible, end-stage problems. We tend to remember worst-case scenarios. Hearing Parkinson's disease may evoke a mental image of Uncle Frank with PD, who was in a wheelchair and died in a nursing home. However, someone in the workplace, still leading a full life after ten years of PD, may be forgotten. Furthermore, Uncle Frank may not have had PD but a disorder that only looks like PD, or possibly his course was complicated by a stroke. Also, Uncle Frank may have developed PD before effective medications became available.

Stories in the lay press may also raise worries about your future. Newspaper articles on PD frequently begin with statements such as, "The medicines for Parkinson's disease only work for a few years," leading you to worry that you will have no effective treatment within a few years. In fact, the press sometimes takes major liberties with the facts, at least when it comes to writing about PD. This may be necessary to make the story interesting. However, this can be disconcerting if you have PD.

What, then, are the facts? How will you do over the long term with PD? Although precise predictions are not possible, the collective experience with PD over the past several decades provides a framework for looking into your future.

Life Expectancy

Will I die from PD? Will it shorten my life? These are questions people often ask their doctor at diagnosis. Some neurodegenerative disorders cut life short. For example, people with Lou Gehrig's disease (ALS, amyotrophic lateral sclerosis) typically succumb to their disorder within a few years. Although PD is also a neurodegenerative disorder, it does not fall into this category.

You may have read that people with PD have a shorter life span. Whereas that is true, the average reduction in life span associated with PD is relatively small. Bear in mind that how long you are expected to live depends on your age. A normal person of fifty may be expected to live about thirty years; a person of thirty should live about fifty years. Consequently, any figures cited for PD must be relative to the age of the person.

We examined longevity among residents of Olmsted County, Minnesota, where the Mayo Clinic is located. Over a twenty-year span, from the mid-1970s to the mid-1990s, approximately two hundred Olmsted County residents were diagnosed with PD. These people lived an average of ten years after diagnosis. If you saw this figure in isolation, it might be a bit disconcerting if you are currently sixty years old. However, consider that the average age of this group was seventy-one years. In comparison, a group of Olmsted County residents without PD but of similar age lived only slightly longer on average, thirteen years. This difference was not dramatic, especially considering that both groups lived into their eighties, on average.

Levodopa and Longevity

In the mid-1960s, before we had effective medications for PD, the mortality rate for those with PD was not very good, although not as bad as for ALS. All studies from that era suggested that people with PD did not live nearly as long as the rest of us. The introduction of levodopa therapy around 1969–1970 changed all that. It revolutionized treatment, pulled people out of wheelchairs, and increased longevity. Over a half dozen independent studies examined mortality rates in the first several years after levodopa was introduced, compared to the years just prior. All found that mortality rates were substantially improved with the introduction of levodopa therapy. This is not surprising, given the often dramatic effect in reversing parkinsonian symptoms.

Progression of PD: The Levodopa Response

Unfortunately PD is not a static condition. We know that there is a slow progression within the brain that is reflected in the clinical course. When the initial symptoms of PD become apparent, the loss of dopaminergic neurons in the substantia nigra is reduced by 50–80 percent. In other words, 20–50 percent of these neurons remain alive and well. However, over the years, more die, and eventually fewer than 10 percent remain.

The continued loss of dopaminergic neurons in the substantia nigra ultimately tends to result in an unstable response to levodopa. This makes sense if you think about it (and if you recall what you read in chapter 3). It is the remaining substantia nigra neurons that mediate the levodopa benefit in those with PD. They take up administered levodopa and transform it into dopamine; then the nerve terminals release it to activate the dopamine receptors within the striatum. In PD, these remaining dopaminergic neurons work doubly hard to make up for the lost cells. This goes well for a number of years; however, at some point, the few of these substantia nigra neurons are unable to compensate for all of the losses. At that point, other neighboring brain cells come into the picture. Other neurons in the striatum have the capability of taking up levodopa and manufacturing it into dopamine. These other cells then take on most of the task. However, they are not ideally designed or positioned for this purpose. First, they are not located precisely at dopaminergic synapses, and released dopamine may need to diffuse over relatively long distances to reach the receptor. Second, they do not have the capability of modulating dopamine release; neither are they capable of removing excess dopamine. The result is inconsistent and erratic dopamine receptor stimulation. The receptor may see both dopamine insufficiencies and excesses.

What does all this mean for the person with PD? During the early years, the compensation from the surviving substantia nigra neurons allows a stable response to levodopa. These remaining neurons take up the administered levodopa, synthesize dopamine, release it at the site of the receptor, and control the concentrations there. The levels are neither too high nor too low. Because there are no sudden shifts in the dopamine concentrations at the receptor, there are no ups or downs in parkinsonism control. At this stage of PD, the timing of the levodopa doses is not critical. They can be taken earlier or later in the day without any noticeable difference. This is largely because there is adequate substantia nigra dopamine storage capacity and a well-regulated release rate at the receptor.

Over years, the situation changes. With few surviving dopaminergic nerve terminals to modulate dopamine levels, the clinical responses become erratic. Rather than precisely timed and programmed dopamine release and regulation, huge dopamine fluxes occur at the synapse. This is when the parkinsonism control starts to become unstable in two respects. First, because the amount of dopamine at the receptor can no longer be tightly regulated, it may be intermittently excessive. At times, too much dopamine stimulates the receptor. Then the slow movements of parkinsonism transform into excessive, involuntary movements called dyskinesias. In other words, the person with PD, who otherwise moves too slowly, now moves too much.

Second, dopamine is no longer being continuously released at the receptor site. These backup brain cells, which normally have nothing to do with dopamine, make and release it only when levodopa is administered. They are incapable of a slow regulated release or any long-term storage. For the person with PD, the benefits become tightly time-locked to each dose of levodopa. There no longer are continuous, long-lasting responses. With each dose of levodopa the benefit develops, persists for a few hours, and then wears off. This is the "short-duration" levodopa response. These ups and downs in parkinsonism control are called motor fluctuations. It also appears that these marked fluxes of dopamine inside the synapse lead to instability of downstream neurons, which develop labile firing patterns.

The extent to which these problems occur varies from person to person. Some with PD never experience very troublesome complications of this type. There are others where it is extremely difficult to maintain a consistently beneficial response.

What is the likelihood of developing these levodopa complications? This is extremely variable. In general, about four people in ten (40 percent) will experience levodopa-related dyskinesias after five years of treatment. Motor fluctuations will occur in a similar percentage (40 percent) by the time they have been treated for five years. Some have suggested that the stable responses can be saved for later by deferring levodopa treatment. However, there is no evidence that this strategy works. More is said about this in later chapters.

These levodopa complications (dyskinesias and fluctuating responses) are the basis for such statements in magazines as, "The medications for Parkinson's disease only work for a few years." In fact, the medications continue to work; however, it is the consistency of the response that is the problem. These consistency problems are the driving force for the development of many of the newer medications for PD. Bear in mind that these are by no means hopeless problems. Often they can be handled reasonably well with levodopa dosage adjustments and supplementary medications.

A reduced response to levodopa does tend to occur later in the course. Whereas the initial response may result in an almost normal appearance, this may be less complete after a number of years. This is not to say that the response is lost; in PD, that is rarely the case. However, after some years, parkinsonian symptoms and signs start to creep into the picture that do not respond adequately to medications. Imbalance may be one such problem. Some people require a cane or other gait aids ten years into their course. This is not universal, however; some maintain athletic activities for many years with PD.

Other Modes of Progression

PD may progress in other ways, although this can be quite variable. We discussed in the last chapter a number of nonmovement symptoms that may develop in PD. Most tend to occur later in the course. Again, it must be emphasized that any such progression is slow and takes years.

Dementia may slowly develop after a number of years, with a prevalence in the PD medical literature ranging from 10 percent to 40 percent. Some will also experience disordered perceptions and hallucinations. We have medications to treat hallucinations, but none that are very effective for major memory and thinking problems.

We also reviewed problems of the autonomic nervous system that can occur in PD (bowels, bladder, low blood pressure). Usually these are minimal during the early years but become more apparent over the subsequent course of PD. These are usually treatable to at least some extent and later chapters address therapy.

Early- Versus Later-Onset PD: Effect on Progression

Those who develop PD earlier in life tend to progress differently, on the average, than those with later-onset PD. When the symptoms begin very early, such as before age 40, levodopa complications tend to develop earlier. Dyskinesias and short-duration, fluctuating levodopa responses often become treatment problems in the first few years. However, when the levodopa effect is present, there may be almost complete resolution of parkinsonism. It is common among people with young-onset PD to remain in the mainstream of life for many years. They continue to cut the grass and play golf. However, they tend to be at the mercy of their medications, often requiring complex medication regimens.

At the other extreme, those that develop PD after age 75 usually do not experience substantial problems with dyskinesias or motor fluctuations. However, their response to levodopa may be incomplete; in other words, despite maximal levodopa therapy, they may still experience some parkinsonian symptoms, especially imbalance. This group is also more likely to experience cognitive problems.

Most people with PD fall somewhere in between these two extremes of age. However, given that PD is such a variable disease, there are many exceptional cases.

How Best to Prognosticate

We have learned about the progression of PD and discussed some general principles. What about you, however, the person with PD? How will you do over the next ten years or the next twenty years?

Medical prognostication is partially guesswork. Predictions based on the averages of others with PD are a starting point. However, we have already emphasized that PD is an extremely variable disorder. What is fairly consistent, however, is the course in any single person; your rate of progression tends to remain fairly consistent. Hence, one can predict how he or she will do, based on how parkinsonism has progressed up to that point in time. For example, if someone has had PD for five years and continues to do well, still playing tennis and working full-time, a good prognosis for the next five years is likely. On the other hand, if each year has brought substantial decline, there is less reason for optimism. Thus it may take a few years to sense the longer-term picture.

Much Is Spared in PD

We have addressed the problems that occur in PD. But is that all? What about other brain regions or other organs such as heart, liver, and kidneys? Are they affected by PD?

In most cases, the regions of the brain that degenerate in PD are quite restricted. This includes the substantia nigra and several other relatively small areas, but much of the remainder of the brain is spared. The exception is among those who develop dementia, as thinking and memory regions in the cortex are affected. In prevalence surveys of PD, however, people with dementia are in the minority.

People with PD also need to know that the internal organs, such as liver, heart, lungs, and kidneys, are not affected. Although shortness of breath can occur in PD, this does not reflect a primary lung or heart problem. If urinary difficulties develop, this is not a kidney problem but indicates reduced autonomic system control of the bladder. People with PD are not substantially more likely to experience heart attacks or strokes. Cancer rates have been debated among those with PD, with some studies suggesting a lower rate and others a higher rate; in the aggregate, however, no major trends in cancer incidence are suggested.

Medications and Long-Term Toxicities

For the most part, the medications we use to treat PD have no long-term toxicities. Levodopa has been the subject of debate, but the cumulative evidence over three decades has failed to reveal any long-term toxicity (see chapter 9). The drugs commonly used to treat PD do not carry substantial potential for liver or kidney damage or compromise blood counts, with a few exceptions; tolcapone has potential liver toxicity and requires monitoring of blood tests; pergolide and bromocriptine may cause inflammatory reactions of the lungs or heart. Otherwise, the medications we routinely use for PD appear to have no long-term adverse consequences.

Will I Develop All the Problems I Am Reading About?

Finally, do not assume that you are destined to experience all these symptoms. Many of them develop in only a minority of people with PD. You need to be aware of these diverse potential problems so that if they do occur, they can be recognized and appropriately treated. However, you may be spared many or most of them.

Will I Pass PD to My Children?

Could I have inherited Parkinson's disease? Will my children come down with PD? These concerns are voiced by many with PD. Fortunately, inherited parkinsonism, with many affected family members and a documented genetic basis, is extremely rare. This is not to say that genetic factors do not play a role in PD; as we will see in chapter 8, they may play a fundamental role. However, there does not appear to be a single gene responsible for typical PD. Rather, there may be multiple genes and perhaps environmental factors that interact. There is probably a complex interplay of factors and not any one gene that is passed to the next generation. Your having PD does not jeopardize your children. Having a parent with PD only modestly increases the risk; the lifetime probability of PD when a parent is affected is considerably less than 10 percent.

PART THREE

◆ ◆ ◆

Distinguishing Parkinson's Disease from Other Disorders

6

◆ ◆ ◆

Conditions Mistaken for Parkinson's Disease

Not every form of parkinsonism is PD. In this chapter we review disorders that are commonly confused with PD, including

- Prescription drugs that induce parkinsonism
- Essential tremor and other tremor syndromes
- Parkinsonism-plus syndromes that resemble PD but have additional features
- Parkinsonian gait disorders (lower-body parkinsonism)
- Dementias with parkinsonism
- Copper or manganese toxicity with parkinsonism, including Wilson's disease

Most of these conditions can be easily distinguished from PD, provided the clues are recognized.

Check Your Medications: Drugs That Cause Parkinsonism

A variety of medications (see table 6.1) may induce a reversible syndrome of parkinsonism that is identical to typical PD. Note that these all require a prescription; no over-the-counter medications cause parkinsonism.

Table 6.1.   Common Prescription Medications That May Induce Parkinsonism

Conditions	Drug	Brain Mechanism Causing Parkinsonism
Major psychiatric disorders, psychosis, schizophrenia; also used for Tourette's	Aripiprazole (Abilify) Chlorpromazine (Thorazine) Fluphenazine (Prolixin) Haloperidol (Haldol) Loxapine (Loxitane) Mesoridazine (Serentil) Molindone (Moban) Olanzapine (Zyprexa) in higher doses Perphenazine (Trilafon) Perphenazine with amitriptyline (Triavil) Risperidone (Risperdal) Thioridazine (Mellaril) Thiothixene (Navane) Trifluoperazine (Stelazine) Ziprasidone (Geodon)	Block dopamine receptors
Depression	Amoxapine (Asendin)	Block dopamine receptors
Nausea and related gastrointestinal problems; also used for migraine	Metoclopramide (Reglan) Prochlorperazine (Compazine) Thiethylperazine (Torecan) Promethazine (Phenergan) Chlorpromazine (Thorazine)	Block dopamine receptors
Seizures, migraine, psychiatric disorders	Valproic acid (Depakote)	Unknown
Heart rhythm disturbances	Amiodarone (Cordarone)	Unknown

DRUGS THAT BLOCK DOPAMINE

Most of the prescription drugs that cause parkinsonism block the action of dopamine in the brain by attaching to the dopamine receptor. If dopamine cannot bind to this blocked receptor, the effect is the same as having no dopamine. These blocking drugs are called dopamine antagonists; that is, they antagonize the dopamine signal. Contrast this to the dopamine agonist drugs we previously discussed, which activate the dopamine receptors after binding to them (much like dopamine). The antagonist drugs simply block the receptor without activation. For a review of this subject, see chapter 2.

Drugs that block dopamine receptors are commonly prescribed for several conditions:

- Major psychiatric disorders, such as psychosis or schizophrenia
- Tourette's syndrome (a disorder of twitches and tics)
- Nausea or problems with bowel motility
- Migraine with nausea

The specific dopamine blocking medications are listed in table 6.1. Note that most drugs used to treat depression do not block dopamine receptors except for amoxapine (Asendin) and the combination drug perphenazine/amitriptyline (Triavil).

When one of these dopamine-blocking drugs is discontinued, the parkinsonism usually does not resolve immediately. It may take several weeks. In rare cases it has taken up to six months to resolve.

Occasionally the parkinsonism never goes away after stopping the dopamine antagonist medication. In this case, the drug was probably not the primary cause of parkinsonism but rather unmasked PD that was destined to develop. There is no compelling evidence to indicate that permanent parkinsonism is caused by medications that block dopamine receptors.

It may not be appropriate to discontinue the offending medication in certain cases, especially if treating schizophrenia and other severe psychiatric problems. However, two other medications for psychosis and schizophrenia do not induce parkinsonism—quetiapine (Seroquel) and clozapine (Clozaril). In addition, olanzapine (Zyprexa) and aripiprazole (Abilify) have an intermediate risk of causing parkinsonism, less than the other drugs listed in table 6.1.

WHAT TO DO?

If you are taking one of these dopamine antagonist drugs and parkinsonism develops, how can you tell if the drug is at fault? Should you stop it? If you do, how long should you wait before expecting resolution? As we address these issues, let's consider a prototypical case:

> Mrs. Jones had been taking metoclopramide (Reglan) for several years to treat chronic nausea (a dopamine antagonist drug). Within the past year, she has developed parkinsonism. Coincidentally her nausea has improved with other medical treatment and she thinks that she could tolerate discontinuing the metoclopramide.

A few rules of thumb apply to this situation:

- Stop a drug only if it seems safe to do this. In Mrs. Jones's case, stopping the medication for nausea carried no substantial risk (only a possible recurrence of nausea). On the other hand, if she were taking a medication for a major psychiatric disorder, she would need to consult with her psychiatrist. Some drugs need to be tapered off rather than stopped abruptly; your physician should advise how to do this.

- Allow sufficient time to determine if the parkinsonism will resolve, which is usually about one month after the offending drug is discontinued.

- Do not start treatment of parkinsonism immediately after discontinuing the offending drug, since it may not be effective. These drugs block dopamine receptors; levodopa and dopamine agonist drugs must have unblocked receptors to work. If the parkinsonism is severe, it is acceptable to start the PD medication immediately; there is no danger in doing this. However, it may not be effective until the dopamine blocking drug has left your body.

In Mrs. Jones's case, it would be appropriate to observe for about a month after stopping the metoclopramide. If she still has signs of parkinsonism, a medication for PD could then be started.

DRUGS THAT REDUCE BRAIN DOPAMINE

We have considered drugs that block dopamine receptors. What about drugs that lower brain dopamine? There are only two prescription drugs that do this, reserpine and alpha-methyldopa. Years ago, these were commonly prescribed for high blood pressure, but today are rarely used for that purpose. Even when these two drugs were in common use, parkinsonism from them was rare.

OTHER DRUGS THAT CAUSE REVERSIBLE PARKINSONISM

Valproic acid (Depakote) is a medication for seizure disorders (epilepsy); it is also used in the treatment of migraine and certain psychiatric conditions. Valproic acid is notorious for causing or worsening tremor. Less commonly, it may also induce mild parkinsonism. The mechanisms by which this occurs are not known. If you have parkinsonism and are taking valproic acid, it is reasonable to consider substituting another medication. However, this needs to be discussed with your physician, since there may not be good medication alternatives or it may run the risk of upsetting control of your epilepsy. In that case, the valproic acid should be maintained and concurrent treatment of the parkinsonism can be initiated.

Amiodarone (Cordarone) is used in the treatment of serious heart rhythm disorders. It may produce a variety of neurological symptoms, including parkinsonism. This drug is used for life-threatening heart irregularities, and sometimes there are no other medications that can be safely substituted. Amiodarone has a long duration of action; if it is stopped because of neurological side effects, they may take many months to resolve.

The medical literature suggests that selective serotonin reuptake inhibitor medications (SSRI) may rarely cause parkinsonism. This class of drugs includes Prozac (fluoxetine), Zoloft (sertraline), Paxil (paroxetine), and others. This is an extremely uncommon complication from these drugs, probably occurring in less than one person out of a hundred. They serve an important role for those with PD who are depressed. The brain neurotransmitter serotonin is deficient in PD, parallel to the brain deficiency of dopamine. Reduced brain serotonin may cause psychological depression, which these drugs effectively treat by improving brain serotonin function. I do not hesitate to prescribe these medications for depression in someone with PD; my experience has been very favorable. For the rare person who experiences increasing parkinsonism time-locked to starting an SSRI drug, another medication may be considered.

Essential Tremor and Other Tremor Syndromes

The lay public often carries the mistaken impression that tremor is synonymous with PD. However, tremor has a variety of origins, and PD is not even the leading cause. The most common tremor disorder is essential tremor, which is often confused with PD.

Tremor is "essentially" the only symptom of essential tremor (ET). ET is not associated with slowness, stiffness, incoordination, walking problems, or any other neurological symptoms. Hence, it differs from PD, in which tremor is one of many symptoms. ET is common and occurs three to five times more frequently than PD. It may start in childhood, but more commonly begins in adulthood, and at any age. The majority of people with ET have another family member with tremor and a genetic cause is suspected.

The tremor of ET is different from PD. When ET affects the hands, it typically is absent with the hand at rest in the lap or at the side when walking. In other words, there is no resting tremor, which is the typical tremor of PD. In contrast, the typical hand tremor of ET appears when the hand is active, such as holding a cup to drink, writing, or eating with a utensil. Although not present when the hand is relaxed, it becomes apparent when the arms are outstretched in front of the body or when the hand is moving, such as reaching or pointing. In contrast, the hand tremor of PD markedly attenuates when the hand is moving; those with PD usually do not have a prominent tremor when holding a cup or bringing a fork to their mouth. PD hand tremor usually affects only one upper extremity in the beginning, which contrasts to ET, which typically involves both hands at the outset.

ET may also manifest as a head or voice tremor. Head and voice tremors are not a component of PD. Although a chin (or lower lip) tremor is common in PD, the entire head does not shake. These distinctions are summarized in table 6.2.

Occasionally people with PD also have the typical tremor of ET. In some cases, this may be a coincidence. Both ET and PD are common disorders and by chance may occur in the same person. In rare individuals, Parkinson's disease begins as ET and in a few years evolves into more typical PD. However, the vast majority of people with ET do not develop Parkinson's disease, and ET is not considered an early sign of this disorder.

**Table 6.2.   Essential Tremor Compared to
Parkinson's Disease with Tremor***

Tremor	Essential Tremor	Parkinson's Disease
Head	Yes	No
Voice	Yes	No
Hand tremor at rest	Rare	Yes
Hand tremor with movement	Yes	No or minimal
Jaw tremor or lower lip tremor	Rare	Common (minority)

*Some with Parkinson's disease have no tremor. On the other hand, both conditions are
common and occasionally occur together with signs of both in the same person.

A small minority of people with ET have a rest tremor, but it typically is
minor or occurs after decades. The exception is a rare disorder that includes
both a prominent resting hand tremor and the usual tremor of ET (prominent with movement). This has been called the resting-postural tremor syndrome and is a variant of ET. It includes no parkinsonian features (other than
the resting tremor). Like PD, however, there is often a prominent jaw tremor.
This resting tremor does not respond to the medications used to treat PD.

ET responds to different drugs than Parkinson's disease. The primary medications for essential tremor of the hands include mysoline (Primidone) and
drugs that block one type of adrenalin response (beta-blockers). Head and
voice tremor usually do not benefit from these drugs; however, they often
respond to injections of botulinum toxin into involved muscles (Botox or
Myobloc). More is said about treatment of tremor in chapter 14.

OTHER TREMOR SYNDROMES

Strokes, tumors, traumatic injuries, inflammation, or other insults to certain
specific brain regions may also cause tremor. Rarely are these confused with
PD, since the symptoms develop abruptly and often with features pointing to
another disorder. The brain scan is usually confirmatory, revealing the condition in brain areas known to cause tremor. Contrast this to PD, where the
brain scan is normal for age.

Tremor may also be caused by a variety of metabolic or toxic problems, such
as thyroid hormone excess or major systemic illnesses. Such medical causes
induce a tremor that resembles ET, rather than Parkinson's disease. Some drugs
also provoke this type of tremor, including medications that enhance adrenalin
responses (for example, certain asthma medications or high doses of caffeine).

Parkinson's-Plus Syndromes

Parkinson's-plus refers to a group of neurodegenerative disorders with prominent parkinsonism, plus other features not seen in PD. They also differ in

terms of the pattern of brain involvement, plus a usually poor response to medications and less favorable prognosis. Brain regions beyond the substantia nigra degenerate in these disorders, which gives them their unique clinical features. These PD imitators include:

- Multiple system atrophy
- Progressive supranuclear palsy
- Corticobasal degeneration

How can you distinguish these disorders from PD? Testing may help, but usually the physician's history and examination are key to making the correct diagnosis. These conditions are much less common than PD, and most people with parkinsonism do indeed have PD.

MULTIPLE SYSTEM ATROPHY (MSA)

Multiple system atrophy (MSA) is sometimes called the Shy–Drager syndrome, named after the physicians who initially described this disorder. It results in more widespread and varied damage to brain motor control systems than PD. Besides parkinsonism, people with MSA often display:

- Incoordination (ataxia) from cerebellar degeneration
- Signs of spasticity and increased tendon reflexes from damage to the corticospinal tract
- Prominent and early involvement of the autonomic nervous system, resulting in orthostatic hypotension (with fainting or near-fainting), bladder dysfunction, loss of erections, and other problems
- Stridor (abnormal breathing sounds) during sleep

Furthermore, the parkinsonism of MSA may not respond to levodopa therapy, or with a response that is unsustained or partial. These findings suggest that the diagnosis is not PD but may be MSA. We will now consider these in more detail.

Cerebellar Ataxia

Some with MSA have signs of cerebellar degeneration, resulting in ataxia (refer back to figure 2.3 in chapter 2 for a picture of the cerebellum). Ataxia is not seen in PD and, if identified, argues against the diagnosis of PD.

Ataxia means incoordination. This results in clumsy hand movements and a wide-based, unsteady gait resembling someone who is drunk. Speech may also resemble someone who is inebriated, due to difficulties coordinating lips, tongue, and palate. Physicians evaluate hand coordination by observing "finger-to-nose" movements, in which patients alternately touch their nose and then the examiner's outstretched finger; ataxia is apparent when these targets are missed. People with PD may be slow in doing this, but not imprecise. Similarly, people with PD may walk slowly or shuffle their feet, but distinct from the wide-based, clumsy gait of ataxia. In MSA, imbalance may be severe, resulting in falls, which is not expected during the early years of PD.

Corticospinal Tract Signs

The corticospinal tract is another motor control circuit frequently affected in MSA but spared in PD. If there are prominent corticospinal tract signs on examination, parkinsonism may not be PD. One clue is abnormally brisk (jumpy) reflexes when the physician uses the reflex hammer. For example, striking the knee with this rubber hammer normally elicits a slight kick of the leg; those with corticospinal tract problems kick high into the air. Also, scratching the bottom of the foot normally elicits reflexive curling of the toes downward; those with corticospinal tract problems extend their toe upward in response (Babinski sign).

Autonomic Dysfunction in MSA

The autonomic nervous system is often severely affected by MSA and early in the course. The earliest sign in men may be loss of erectile function, sometimes predating other symptoms by months. Bladder problems are also typically affected early, resulting in urinary urgency, hesitancy, or incontinence. The most obvious clue is often orthostatic hypotension, resulting in blood pressures so low (when standing) that fainting or near-fainting occurs. Of course, the physician must check the medication list to exclude drugs that cause low blood pressure (see chapter 21). These same problems do develop in PD, but are mild early in the course and only become troublesome much later. However, some people with PD defy this dictum and experience prominent autonomic dysfunction at the outset.

Stridor

MSA may result in stridor—a type of abnormal vocal cord movement. This occurs primarily or exclusively at night during sleep. This is not present in PD. Stridor is heard as a screeching, high-pitched sound while inspiring (breathing in). It is due to the vocal cords pulling together while inhaling (normally they should be separated to allow air to pass). Confirmation is necessary from breathing studies done during sleep (polysomnography; see chapter 7).

Two Types of MSA

MSA is subdivided into two categories, based on the primary manifestations, cerebellar ataxia (incoordination), or parkinsonism. The cerebellar form is usually not mistaken for PD, since the incoordination (ataxia) should provide telltale evidence. This cerebellar type of MSA is termed MSA-c (for cerebellum). When MSA presents with prominent parkinsonism, it is termed MSA-p (parkinsonism). This latter form is often misdiagnosed for PD, especially early in the course.

PARKINSONISM VARIANT OF MSA: STRIATONIGRAL DEGENERATION

The older term for MSA-p is striatonigral degeneration. In the initial stages, it may be identical to PD, except for the response to levodopa therapy. Because the neurodegeneration extends beyond the substantia nigra and includes the striatum, levodopa and related drugs may provide no benefit, or only a partial or short-lasting response. This is often the first clue that the diagnosis is MSA and not PD; however, the trial of levodopa must be adequate, as will be outlined in chapter 12. Also, if the parkinsonism is accompanied by unequivocal corticospinal tract signs, cerebellar ataxia, prominent autonomic problems or stridor during sleep, MSA-p should be strongly considered.

TESTING FOR MSA

MRI brain scans are often abnormal in MSA and may provide clues to the diagnosis. Some medical centers offer special tests of autonomic function that may be useful in distinguishing the more severe autonomic involvement of MSA. Sleep centers may document nighttime stridor, which may confirm MSA.

TREATMENT OF MSA

MSA is treatable but the therapies are limited, especially if levodopa provides no benefit. We have no good medications for cerebellar ataxia and the drugs for spasticity (corticospinal tract problems) help little or not at all. However, the autonomic symptoms are treatable (see chapters 21, 26–28). Stridor may result in serious breathing difficulties at night, but may be treated by sleep specialists.

PROGRESSIVE SUPRANUCLEAR PALSY (PSP)

Progressive supranuclear palsy (PSP) often strongly resembles PD in the early stages. Slowness (bradykinesia), stiffness (rigidity), and loss of normal animation (arm swing, facial animation) are typical of both disorders. PSP is commonly diagnosed as Parkinson's disease by experienced clinicians during the first few years.

PSP has also been called the Steele, Richardson, Olszewski syndrome, named after the three physicians who initially described it. The term "progressive supranuclear palsy" refers to eye movement abnormalities—palsies of eye movements. Specifically, people with PSP cannot easily move their eyes. "Supranuclear" is essentially a contraction of two terms, "supra" (above) and

Table 6.3.   Distinguishing Progressive Supranuclear Palsy from PD
(Parkinsonism Present in Both)

Symptom	Progressive Supranuclear Palsy	Parkinson's Disease
Eye movements	Often severely impaired; inability to look down is a hallmark feature	Able to move eyes in all directions, except occasionally looking up affected
Falls	Frequent early in the course	Rare until many years elapse
Resting tremor	Usually absent; if present, not very prominent	Occurs in majority
Eye blinking	Severely reduced; often prominent wide-eyed staring expression	Reduced, but not as much as PSP
Neck and trunk movement	Often marked neck rigidity, plus slow and impaired trunk movements; plop into chairs; severe difficulty rising from sitting	Mild to moderate rigidity and slowness of movement except for advanced disease
Response to levodopa therapy	No, or partial response that does not persist	Consistently very responsive

"nucleus," referring to the group of brain stem neurons that control the muscles of the eyes. The lowest level of eye movement control in the brain stem is intact, whereas higher-level ("supra") control of eye movements is lost.

PSP is distinguished from PD by appearances; the neurologic history and examination determine the diagnosis. There are a variety of clinical clues, several of which are summarized in table 6.3.

The limited eye movements of PSP may give away the diagnosis. Inability to look down is a hallmark of PSP, which compromises reading and eating; however, eye movements in all directions are affected. People with PSP may mistakenly think they need new glasses and often see the eye doctor first. Some with PSP do not develop prominent eye palsies until later in the course, making early diagnosis more difficult. In contrast, people with PD may have only mildly slowed or hesitant eye movements and not impaired down gaze.

A second important clue is falling. People with PSP usually have severe imbalance and fall frequently early in the course. They may repeatedly topple over while walking, tending to cross their legs and lose their balance. Contrast this with the first years of Parkinson's disease, when falls are rare or do not occur, even when imbalance is an early symptom. Late in PD, frequent falls may occur, but not during the first decade (except in the most elderly).

Only a minority of people with PSP have a rest tremor, in contrast to PD. When it is present, it typically is mild.

Facial appearance may help distinguish PSP from PD. People with PD have reduced facial animation (masking) and eye-blink rate. In PSP, however, facial animation tends to be severely reduced. Some with PSP have a striking wide-eyed, staring expression, giving the appearance of never blinking.

People with PSP also tend to have stiff-appearing trunk movements. When they sit, they plop into the chair. Conversely, they rise from the seated position with great difficulty. When engaged in conversation and looking from one person to another, they do this very stiffly and slowly. As they turn to speak, their whole upper body turns like a statue, instead of just the eyes or neck. Rigidity of the neck is often pronounced in PSP, exceeding that in PD.

The response to levodopa therapy is also an important clue. It is effective in perhaps 20 percent of people with PSP; even when it does work, the benefit wanes after a year or two. Again, this assumes that the carbidopa/levodopa trial was adequate, as will be discussed in chapter 12.

CORTICOBASAL DEGENERATION (CORTICOBASAL GANGLIONIC DEGENERATION)

Corticobasal degeneration is named for the brain areas that degenerate, which include the cortex and basal ganglia. Recall that the cortex is the outer portion of the brain, where thought, language, perception, and complex actions are organized at their highest level (see chapter 2). Not all the cortex is involved; the degeneration is primarily in limited areas of the front half, especially those involved in programming complex movements. This cortical damage results in apraxia, which implies inability to perform patterned movements, such as grasping a fork, saluting, or waving good-bye. This problem

Table 6.4. Corticobasal Degeneration Versus Parkinson's disease

Clue	Corticobasal Degeneration	Parkinson's Disease
Asymmetry	Pronounced; starts in one limb, which persistently is most affected	PD is asymmetric, but not to the degree seen in corticobasal degeneration
Rigidity (stiffness)	Marked limb muscle tension. With advancement, may result in a rigid, unmoving limb	Rigidity is less than the severe rigidity of corticobasal degeneration
Apraxia*	The hallmark of this disorder	Not seen in PD
Levodopa response	No substantial response	Prominent levodopa benefit

*This is most apparent in the hands and is characterized by an inability to easily perform simple tasks, such as waving or saluting, despite good strength.

lies in brain programming of muscle activity to generate such complex movements. Simple hand gestures, such as the thumbs-up sign, may take many seconds to perform, clumsily. People report that they cannot make their hand do what they want. To this problem is added parkinsonism, due to degeneration of certain portions of the basal ganglia; thus limb movements are stiff (rigid) and slow (bradykinetic).

For unknown reasons, corticobasal degeneration disproportionately affects one limb and often an arm. In the beginning, only one limb is typically compromised. With progression, the whole body is involved, but even then, the problems are most severe on one side and primarily in the initially affected limb. This marked asymmetry is more pronounced than in PD. The final clue is the lack of response to levodopa therapy; no medications significantly help this disorder. The features distinguishing corticobasal degeneration from PD are summarized in table 6.4.

Parkinsonian Gait Disorders (Lower-Body Parkinsonism)

Physicians occasionally encounter people with a shuffling gait, as in PD, but without other parkinsonian signs. They have no arm stiffness or slowness, their faces are not masked, and their voice is not soft. In other words, they have no symptoms above the waist. This has been called lower-half parkinsonism, although other names have been applied, such as frontal lobe gait or gait apraxia.

Among those with this lower-half parkinsonian syndrome, additional signs distinguish this from typical PD. First, the gait is often wide-based with the feet spread apart; this contrasts to PD, where the base is normal (narrow). Second, arm swing when walking is usually preserved, in contrast to the reduced arm swing of PD.

Although PD may rarely present as lower-half parkinsonism, it typically represents one of three other conditions:

1. Normal pressure hydrocephalus

2. Small strokes affecting basal ganglia brain circuits and their connections with the frontal lobes of the brain (hence the term "frontal gait")

3. A nonspecific neurodegenerative condition that affects the basal ganglia–frontal lobe brain circuits, which cannot be further characterized

Let's consider each.

NORMAL PRESSURE HYDROCEPHALUS (NPH)

Normal pressure hydrocephalus (NPH) is a condition that potentially has a neurosurgical cure. Hence, it is important to recognize this syndrome. The

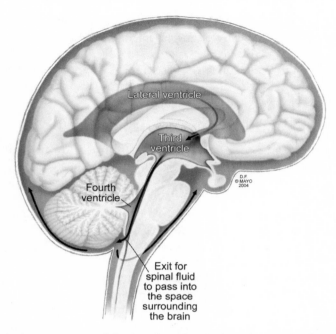

6.1 Ventricular system: Spinal fluid made within the lateral ventricles flows into the third, then fourth ventricles, exiting near the lower end of the brain stem. Ultimately, it passes back into the blood circulation. Thus, the brain floats in a large sack of spinal fluid.

problem is impeded flow of spinal fluid within the head. Normally most spinal fluid is produced inside cavities in the brain called ventricles, as shown in figure 6.1. There is a normal flow of spinal fluid passing from the large ventricles in the central part of the brain (lateral ventricles) down through the third and fourth ventricles. At the end of the fourth ventricle the spinal fluid exits into the space that surrounds the brain and spinal cord. Thus the brain floats in spinal fluid. Finally spinal fluid flows over the top of the brain and enters the bloodstream through special channels that function like one-way valves. This completes the dynamic circulation of spinal fluid.

In people with NPH, the flow of spinal fluid is partially obstructed, but not enough to raise the pressure inside the skull; hence the term "normal pressure." The term "hydrocephalus" translates into "water on the brain." Where is the obstruction to the flow of spinal fluid in NPH? Presumably this is external to the ventricular system, at the interface between the spinal fluid and blood stream, over the top of the brain.

Basically, NPH is a plumbing problem. However, there is no practical way to directly repair the obstruction to the flow. Thus treatment focuses on providing an alternative route to vent the spinal fluid. Neurosurgeons do this by inserting a tube into one of the ventricles, placing the other end elsewhere in the body where the excess spinal fluid can drain. This tube is called a shunt and contains a valve that allows appropriate amounts of fluid to exit, driven by the pressure that builds up.

The suspicion that someone might have NPH comes from the neurological history and examination. There are three primary features that suggest this diagnosis:

- A lower-half parkinsonian gait (typically wide-based)

- Urinary incontinence (unable to control urination with substantial leakage)

- Intellectual impairment (typically not severe)

This clinical picture will usually prompt the physician to order a brain scan, with attention to the brain ventricles. Since there is obstruction to flow of the spinal fluid, it will back up and the ventricles will enlarge. Thus the hallmark feature of NPH is large brain ventricles.

This diagnostic strategy sounds simple; however, the picture is often confused by the fact that normal aging results in enlarged brain ventricles. As we age, we slowly lose brain cells; over many decades, the brain shrinks and all the spaces in and around the brain get bigger. Thus ventricles enlarge with normal aging. The physician must decide whether the enlarged ventricles are disproportionately expanded or are enlarged in proportion to age-related brain shrinkage.

Shunting sounds simple but is not risk-free. Even with the most experienced neurosurgeons, bleeding inside the brain can occur, resulting in stroke-like symptoms. Fortunately this is uncommon, but problems can develop with the shunt, which can plug, become infected, or malfunction.

There are a variety of schemes for determining who truly has NPH and will respond to shunting. This includes lumbar puncture, where a large volume of spinal fluid is removed on a trial basis. Unfortunately, even with the best tests available, physicians cannot always predict who will respond to shunting. Sometimes the shunt fails to improve symptoms despite fulfilling all the diagnostic and predictive criteria.

TINY STROKES CAUSING LOWER-HALF PARKINSONISM

Multiple small strokes that go unrecognized may result in a parkinsonian gait (lower-half parkinsonism). Often this is associated with intellectual impairment and other neurological signs. The clues are on the MRI scan of the brain. Small discrete white areas representing tiny strokes are seen in the front half of the brain on certain MRI images (in a radiologist's terms, T2 images). These multiple tiny strokes are located in the basal ganglia and its connections with the frontal cortex.

Often this syndrome occurs in people with inadequately controlled high blood pressure. High blood pressure persisting over many years damages blood vessels, especially smaller blood vessels, causing atherosclerosis (hardening of the arteries). It is these small arteries in the front half of the brain that plug, ultimately resulting in the lower-half parkinsonism and/or intellectual impairment. Diabetes mellitus may also predispose to this problem. Some who fit this clinical picture, however, have not been hypertensive or diabetic.

When this clinical syndrome is identified, focus should be on control of atherosclerotic risk factors such as blood pressure, diabetes, and cholesterol. Although this is not PD, one might try levodopa therapy, using the guidelines in chapter 12. There is no downside to trying this and it can be discontinued if there is no benefit.

OTHER NEURODEGENERATIVE DISORDERS RESULTING IN LOWER-HALF PARKINSONISM

Occasionally people with lower-half parkinsonism do not have the other features of NPH, and the MRI brain scan does not reveal small strokes. There are three possible conditions this might represent:

1. Atypical PD
2. Another neurodegenerative disorder that might become apparent with passage of time
3. A nonspecific syndrome of brain aging occurring in people over age 75

Each of these conditions warrants a trial of levodopa therapy, as outlined in chapter 12; there is nothing to lose.

Dementias with Parkinsonism

Dementia is defined as a loss of intellectual abilities sufficient to interfere with activities of daily living, typically irreversible. This includes problems with memory, judgment, and abstract reasoning. Dementia is the central feature of certain neurodegenerative disorders, most noticeably Alzheimer's disease. With these neurodegenerative dementias, including Alzheimer's disease, signs of parkinsonism may additionally be present. What distinguishes these neurodegenerative dementias is that major thinking and memory problems are among the earliest symptoms. This differs from PD, since if dementia occurs, it is much later in the course (many years later). The later developing dementia of PD is discussed in chapter 23; here we will focus on disorders in which cognition is first affected.

ALZHEIMER'S DISEASE

Alzheimer's disease is the most common cause of dementia. Like PD, it tends to develop later in life. Also like PD, the onset is insidious and the progression is slow. Memory loss is often the most prominent early deficit. The diagnosis is based on the clinical features (history and examination), and testing is done to exclude other causes of confusion.

Signs of parkinsonism may occur in those with Alzheimer's disease. They are usually not prominent, although there are exceptions. Slowness (bradykinesia), stooped posture, and rigidity may insidiously develop, but usually these signs are not striking. Because dementia is the earliest and most prominent neurologic problem, it is rare that Alzheimer's disease is misdiagnosed as PD.

LEWY BODY DEMENTIA, DIFFUSE LEWY BODY DISEASE

Lewy body dementia is the second most common cause of dementia, second only to Alzheimer's disease. This disorder is sometimes confused with PD, and there is substantial overlap. The hallmark features of Lewy body dementia (also referred to as diffuse Lewy body disease) are the following:

- Dementia as an initial feature (often fluctuating in severity)

- Parkinsonism (often responsive to levodopa therapy)

- Hallucinations

Problems with the autonomic nervous system may also be present, such as bowel, bladder, or low blood pressure symptoms.

In this disorder, like PD, Lewy bodies are seen under the microscope. In PD, however, the Lewy bodies and associated degeneration are restricted to a few areas, such as the substantia nigra. In Lewy body dementia, Lewy bodies are diffusely present throughout much of the brain; hence the term diffuse Lewy body disease. This begs the question whether Lewy body dementia and PD have common origins. Are they a single disease with different manifestations? This is debated, but without any clear answers.

Treatment of Lewy body dementia parallels the treatment of Parkinson's disease. The same treatment strategies discussed in this book for PD are also appropriate for many aspects of Lewy body dementia. The major exception relates to treatment of the parkinsonism; in Lewy body dementia, carbidopa/ levodopa alone is advisable (guidelines in chapter 12). Avoid the dopamine agonist drugs, since they are more likely to induce hallucinations, which is a hallmark of Lewy body dementia. Other supplementary drugs for parkinsonism are best avoided for the same reason.

Copper or Manganese Toxicity with Parkinsonism

WILSON'S DISEASE

Wilson's disease is a disorder of copper metabolism. It is extremely rare but important to diagnose because it can cause irreversible brain damage and liver failure if unrecognized and untreated. In this condition, copper from the diet is not adequately excreted via the liver-biliary system (gall bladder). Normally the body excretes excess copper via the bile through gall bladder channels. In Wilson's disease, this malfunctions and more copper enters the body than leaves. Eventually the buildup of copper reaches toxic levels, primarily in the brain and liver.

The neurological syndrome typically includes tremor or parkinsonism. Most with Wilson's disease develop the neurological symptoms by early adulthood and certainly by age 55. Hence this is not a consideration in seniors. However, anyone with marked tremor or atypical parkinsonism, under age 55, should have this assessed. The workup includes a blood test (serum ceruloplasmin), urine test (24-hour urine collection for copper), and often an examination by an ophthalmologist. The ophthalmologist will use a magnifying device called a slit lamp to look at the surface of the eye. Copper accumulates in a ring pattern around the colored portion of the eye (iris). If there is any question about the diagnosis, a liver biopsy may be necessary to analyze the copper content.

MANGANESE TOXICITY

It has been known for decades that massive exposure to the metal manganese can induce parkinsonism. Usually the parkinsonism is different from typical PD and tends not to respond to levodopa and related drugs. This is an extremely rare cause of parkinsonism in the United States, where Occupational Safety and Health Administration (OSHA) standards minimize the likelihood of substantial manganese exposure in the workplace.

How can you tell that someone has manganese-related parkinsonism? One important clue is the MRI brain scan, with abnormalities in a very distinct pattern. Specifically, the globus pallidus becomes bright with certain MRI techniques (so-called T1 imaging); only rarely is this pattern seen in other disorders and never in PD. When this MRI finding is seen in someone with massive manganese exposure in conjunction with high blood manganese levels, then manganese is the probable cause of the parkinsonism.

Welding generates manganese fumes and there has been speculation that welders may be at increased risk for PD. However, scientists have not been able to document this with any degree of certainty. If welding was a frequent cause of PD, this should be obvious from MRI brain scans; however, the typical MRI signs of manganese toxicity are not seen in routine PD patients who have been welders. There are rare exceptions, however. I have encountered a few welders with parkinsonism who worked for years in unventilated environments and had evidence of manganese toxicity on brain imaging and blood work.

MANGANESE TOXICITY DUE TO LIVER FAILURE

Manganese toxicity is actually common in one clinical setting: liver failure. Manganese in trace amounts is present in almost everything we eat and drink.

Our body requires tiny amounts of manganese, and the excess is excreted through the liver's bile system. However, the bile system may not work properly among those with liver failure and manganese may accumulate in the body; it especially accumulates in the basal ganglia.

If you have liver failure and parkinsonism (or any similar neurological syndrome), an MRI brain scan is indicated to look for the pattern of manganese toxicity. If found, and if your blood manganese is elevated, this might be the cause of your parkinsonism.

How do you treat the manganese-related parkinsonism of liver failure? First, consult a dietitian for a special diet that limits foods and liquids high in manganese. Purging the manganese from your body by chelation therapy has been tried but appears ineffective. This should reverse with liver transplantation. Finally, the usual medications for parkinsonism may be tried, such as levodopa therapy.

7

◆ ◆ ◆

Testing: Blood Tests, X rays, and Scans

The diagnosis of Parkinson's disease (PD) is based on the symptoms and the neurological examination. Laboratory tests and scans have only a limited role in routine cases. However, when there are unusual or unexpected findings, these studies may be helpful. Also, testing is often appropriate in the evaluation and treatment of conditions linked to PD, such as urinary problems or memory impairment. We will divide our discussion along these lines, first addressing tests to establish the diagnosis and, second, laboratory evaluation of conditions related to PD.

Tests to Determine Parkinson's Disease Versus Another Disorder

The appearance of parkinsonism does not necessarily assure us that someone has PD. However, this is usually the case if there are no atypical or unusual features. Hence, in typical cases, limited or no testing may be appropriate. What constitutes a typical case of PD? If your condition meets the following criteria, the workup could be kept simple:

- Parkinsonism onset over age 55

- Symptoms and examination findings are only those of parkinsonism; that is, no ataxia, corticospinal tract signs, or apraxia, as discussed in chapter 4

- Balance adequate to avoid falling (except very late in the course)
- No major thinking or memory problems
- No sudden changes in symptoms (as occurs with strokes)
- No major problems with low blood pressure/orthostatic hypotension (unless explained by medications)
- No other active major medical problems

If you met these criteria, no neurological testing is usually necessary. However, I like to be assured that there are no general medical issues that might be contributing to the symptoms. Thus I also recommend a general physical examination by your internist or family physician, including routine blood studies, unless this has been done in the past year. Routine blood studies include a complete blood count, thyroid, and a chemistry panel. Also, the medication list should have been reviewed to make certain that there are no offending medications, as listed in chapter 6.

ONSET BEFORE AGE 55

PD frequently starts before age 55, but in this age group, additional tests are appropriate. For otherwise typical cases, these tests include a brain scan plus studies to exclude the copper toxicity of Wilson's disease, which I explained in the last chapter. Screening tests for Wilson's disease include serum ceruloplasmin (blood test), twenty-four-hour urine copper collection, and an eye examination by an ophthalmologist to look for copper deposits on the surface of the eyes. If Wilson's disease seems unlikely, often only a serum ceruloplasmin level is checked. If it is not low and if the routine blood work is within normal limits, this is typically sufficient.

What type of brain scan should be done? There are two scan types, CT (computed tomography) and MRI (magnetic resonance imaging). Either is appropriate in this setting, but the MRI scan is considerably more sensitive.

FURTHER TESTING BASED ON ATYPICAL FEATURES

Further testing is based on specific medical and neurological findings keeping company with parkinsonism. Some of the more common features that lead to additional testing are listed in table 7.1. This is not an exhaustive list and other clues may push the testing in different directions. As you review the table, consider the following comments about the listed conditions.

Sudden onset of major neurological symptoms, including parkinsonism, suggests a stroke; however, this is a rare cause of parkinsonism. The appropriate test in this setting is an MRI scan, which readily demonstrates any stroke-like events. Strokes causing parkinsonism typically damage other brain regions, resulting in additional symptoms and signs.

can be used to look beyond the throat into the esophagus, which is the passage-way between the throat and stomach (videofluoroscopic swallowing study).

DAYTIME SLEEPINESS

Drowsiness during the waking day is common in PD. Frequently this is due to poor sleep at night and may respond to levodopa and related treatment (see chapter 20). Alternatively, certain prescription drugs may also induce daytime drowsiness. However, daytime drowsiness may have other causes, unknown to the sleeper:

- Sleep apnea (intermittently not breathing during sleep)

- Frequent leg movements during sleep that intermittently partially arouse the sleeper (but not to the degree that he or she fully awakens)

In both of these conditions, the person perceives being asleep all night but awakens in the morning feeling unrested.

The specific test to evaluate this is called polysomnography. The person being assessed sleeps overnight in a sleep laboratory attached to a variety of breathing, brain wave, and muscle-sensing devices. Usually a video camera captures any movements. Disrupted breathing or frequent sleep-related move-ments can be correlated with brain waves.

SHORTNESS OF BREATH

Shortness of breath can be a consequence of PD, as explained in chapter 19. This does not reflect a primary problem with the lungs or heart. Rather, the normal involuntary breathing movements and breathing reflexes are impaired. This is not a dangerous problem for those with PD. When such symptoms are experienced, one should not simply jump to the conclusion that PD is the cause. Rather, the physician will want to make certain that there are no pri-mary heart or lung problems. A variety of breathing and heart tests can be employed and which are chosen depends on the person's symptoms and the physician's level of suspicion.

OSTEOPOROSIS

Weakening of the bones is not a problem directly linked to PD. However, this is common among seniors, who are typically the ones afflicted with PD. Also, those with PD may not produce enough of the active form of vitamin D (see chapter 30). Because PD may affect balance, one certainly wants to have strong bones in case of falls. How to evaluate bone strength? This is done with a special nuclear medicine bone density scan. A minimally radioactive substance that binds to bones is injected into a vein. The radioactivity is so slight that it is not dangerous. When this substance enters your bones, a scanner can measure how much is bound. This tells us whether the bone is dense or porous. This test is important for guiding therapy. Testing also includes limited blood and urine measurements of calcium and related substances.

Who among those with PD should have a bone density study? It might be considered in anyone over sixty years (especially if not a milk drinker), or if there is substantial risk of falling.

genetic causes are often the case (see below). Typical PD is rare among those in their forties, a little more common among people in their fifties, with the incidence rising steeply thereafter. Hence the aging process or perhaps some cumulative lifetime exposure or buildup of a noxious substance may be critical.

Men are more likely to develop PD. These gender differences are not dramatic, only a few percent. However, this has been a consistent finding in many studies. There has been speculation about the reason for this but no explanation to date. Are men more likely to be exposed to something in the workplace? Do female hormones (estrogens) reduce the risk of developing PD?

Those with an immediate family member who has PD are more likely to come down with it. In general, the risk for PD doubles when one first-degree relative (parent, brother, or sister) has PD. To put this into perspective, the lifetime risk for PD in general is around 2 percent (data, Olmsted County, Minn.); this doubles to 4 percent if one immediate relative is affected. Whether this represents a genetic factor or some common exposure is being debated.

Is PD More Likely in Certain Towns or Localities?

Epidemiologists look for clusters of people with a given disorder to provide them with clues. For example, if a disproportionately large number of people living near a toxic waste dump came down with PD, the clues would be obvious. However, despite an intensive search for such clusters, none have surfaced.

Practices and Habits Associated with PD

Large studies have examined lifestyles and exposures among people with PD, in comparison to those without PD of the same age and gender. What has been found is the following.

People who have smoked seem to be at a reduced risk to develop PD. This is by no means absolute; smokers also develop PD, but statistically at a lower rate than nonsmokers. At first glance, this suggests that there may be something in cigarette smoke that protects against PD. This is a very complex issue, however. Some have argued that smoking tends to shorten life and smokers are less likely to reach the age when PD is likely to develop. Others have suggested that the same inherent brain chemistry that confers a low risk of PD also makes smoking pleasurable. In other words, those destined to develop PD may have early life aversion to smoking or less enjoyment from smoking. There is no evidence, however, that smoking slows the rate of progression once PD has developed. Smoking, in general, is bad for the human body and no researcher advocates smoking as a treatment for PD.

Coffee drinking is also associated with a lower likelihood of PD. Some have argued that this may be analogous to smoking; there may be underlying brain chemistry conferring a lower risk of PD and also making coffee consumption pleasurable. Like nicotine, caffeine has effects in the basal ganglia. The internal chemistry of the brain that makes coffee drinking (or smoking) enjoyable may also make that person less susceptible to PD. There is no evidence that coffee or caffeine is a useful treatment for PD or slows the progression of PD once it starts.

Statistically, factors associated with rural living and farming appear to confer a higher risk of PD. Again, however, the associated risk from these factors is not substantial. Herbicide and pesticide exposure and perhaps drinking well water have been associated with a greater likelihood of PD. Pesticides and herbicides would seem to be good candidates for causing PD. If they kill bugs and plants, why not expect them to also kill vulnerable brain cells? However, if these are important factors, why has the incidence of PD been fairly stable over the past fifty years, a period when use of pesticides and herbicides has varied considerably? Although the recorded incidence of PD has risen slightly in recent years, it appears this is because physicians are better at diagnosing it; years ago, what was written off to aging is now correctly being diagnosed as PD. Allowing for that, it does not seem that PD incidence rose substantially coinciding with the introduction of farm chemicals.

Twin Studies

Epidemiologists have studied individuals with PD who have a twin. Twins come in two types—those who are genetically identical and those who are not. Identical twins carry the same genes. Nonidentical twins share only some genes, similar to any other set of brothers or sisters. Thus if a condition is purely the result of one abnormal gene, and if expressed in one identical twin, the other twin should also have that condition.

Several twin studies of PD have been published. The largest and most recent involved all the male twins who had served in World War II and were part of a large epidemiology registry. The investigators identified approximately seventy people in this registry with PD who had an identical twin and ninety with PD and a nonidentical twin. If PD is a genetic condition, then the identical twins should both have PD. However, PD was found in only 16 percent of both identical twins, which was not statistically different from the 11 percent concordance in the nonidentical twins. The conclusion was that genetic factors do not play a major role in causing PD. Earlier twin studies also found little evidence for a major genetic component.

Although these twin studies argue against inheritance being important in PD, this matter is still open to debate. Interpretation of twin studies is complicated by at least a couple of factors.

Someone carrying an abnormal gene may never develop the expected condition due to other overriding factors. This is called "incomplete penetrance" and occurs in many known genetic disorders. Incomplete penetrance implies that an abnormal gene results in the medical condition in some, but not all, who carry the gene. Presumably, something in one's environment or makeup compensates for the genetic abnormality.

Genetic disorders that tend to start late in life, such as PD, may be prevented from occurring by premature death. In other words, perhaps not all those predisposed to PD live long enough for this to develop. We can never precisely predict the age of onset of any genetic condition; for any given abnormal gene, there is a range of years, rather than a specific age, when it is likely to begin. As already noted, the likelihood of developing PD progressively increases with age. If there is a gene predisposing to PD, perhaps the range of years when it might start is extremely broad, extending beyond ninety years of age.

Thus the genetic potential to develop PD may be present and yet not obvious. This concept receives support from PET (positron emission tomography) studies. With special techniques, PET scans can measure dopamine stores in the brain. In fully developed PD, brain dopamine stores are low. PET scan evidence of mildly reduced brain dopamine (implying early PD) has been noted in several normal-appearing twins whose identical sibling has PD. Perhaps these individuals will eventually develop PD if they live long enough.

One caveat to consider: Does the fact that both twins (or others in the family) develop PD imply that their condition is inherited? Not necessarily, since if they lived in the same household, they were exposed to common environmental factors, which could conceivably be causative.

Although the twin studies seemingly argue against a major genetic contribution to PD, the role of inheritance is still unclear. Complex genetic factors, including multiple contributory genes, have not been excluded. Perhaps there are interactions between genetic makeup and environmental factors. The prospect of a genetic component takes on greater credibility when we consider what we are learning from studying rare families with genetically proven PD.

Families with Inherited Parkinsonism

Families in which parkinsonism is clearly inherited are extremely uncommon. Only a handful of such families have been recognized. These have been a focus of molecular biologic research, however, anticipating that what we learn about the cause in these cases may generalize to PD.

The biochemical problems responsible for several different types of inherited parkinsonism have been elucidated and are relevant to PD in general. The abnormal proteins coded by the respective genes in these families are alpha-synuclein (linked to two different types of inherited parkinsonism), parkin, and ubiquitin carboxy-terminal hydrolase. These are names for proteins contained in brain cells. There are common factors linking these inherited causes of parkinsonism and a theme is emerging: an inability of brain cells to dispose of certain substances that subsequently accumulate to toxic levels. Specific garbage may be accumulating inside brain cells that leads to their death or dysfunction. This type of buildup and insufficient disposal process seems to be involved in cases of inherited parkinsonism. Let's learn about each and then consider the bigger picture.

Alpha-Synuclein Mutations Causing Parkinsonism

Contursi is a beautiful village in southern Italy. Around the turn of the century a number of its sons and daughters emigrated to the East Coast of the United States. Some fifty to seventy-five years later, offspring started appearing in neurologic clinics with parkinsonism. Investigators from the Robert Wood Johnson Medical School in New Jersey astutely recognized the family ties. Through careful medical detective-work, they traced the condition back to two original Contursi families. The parkinsonism was nearly identical to typical PD, except that it started at an earlier age (mid-forties) and generally progressed more rapidly. Otherwise, it was similar, including responding to levodopa therapy plus the presence of Lewy bodies on microscopic examination of the brain. The passage from one generation to the next was typical of dominant inheritance. Hence, one abnormal gene was thought to be responsible.

The responsible gene was ultimately identified, which codes for the protein alpha-synuclein. Investigators subsequently looked for this abnormal alpha-synuclein gene in people with typical PD; however, it was not found in anyone with run-of-the-mill PD. Thus only a handful of families appeared to carry this gene and all had origins in Italy or Greece, with the exception of one family in Germany.

Little was known about alpha-synuclein at the time of this genetic discovery. What does this protein do in the normal person and how does it malfunction to cause parkinsonism? Answers started to come quickly. We now know that this protein is normally present in brain cells and especially in the synaptic terminal. As we learned in previous chapters, the synaptic terminal is at the end of the axon; the axon is the long, wire-like extension of the neuron, where the connection is made to the next brain cell in the sequence. Alpha-synuclein is widely present throughout the nervous system, but its function in normal brain cells remains unknown.

The general relevance became apparent when scientists started looking for alpha-synuclein in the brains of those with typical (noninherited) PD. They created a means of staining alpha-synuclein that allowed it to be identified in brain tissue at autopsy. What they found was a total surprise: alpha-synuclein was the major component of Lewy bodies! Recall that Lewy bodies are the microscopic markers of PD and are found in the brain substantia nigra when examined under the microscope. This was not the abnormal alpha-synuclein like that from the Contursi families; rather it was normal alpha-synuclein, but in large concentrations in these Lewy bodies. In other words, normal (not mutated) alpha-synuclein accumulates in the brain cells of those with PD forming Lewy bodies. Although a variety of other substances are also contained in Lewy bodies, it appears that alpha-synuclein is a major component.

Inherited Parkinsonism from Too Much Alpha-Synuclein

The relevance of alpha-synuclein to PD was highlighted by genetic investigations of a family in the Upper Midwest with inherited parkinsonism. This family also had a dominant inheritance pattern suggesting a single abnormal gene. Scientists discovered that the alpha-synuclein gene from this family was normal, but the gene itself was abnormally duplicated (actually triplicated). The extra copies of this gene resulted in overproduction of alpha-synuclein in brain cells. Presumably, more alpha-synuclein was being produced than could be disposed of by the brain cells.

What Are These Alpha-Synuclein-Linked Families Telling Us?

People with usual PD do not have it run in their families and have a normal alpha-synuclein gene pair. However, it appears that they do have excessive accumulation of alpha-synuclein and other proteins within diseased neurons in the form of Lewy bodies. Is this alpha-synuclein an innocent bystander along with other constituents of Lewy bodies, or is this a crucial factor? The fact that mutant or overexpressed alpha-synuclein causes parkinsonism in rare families suggests that we may be onto something. However, precisely what this is telling us is still uncertain.

We do know that normal alpha-synuclein is easily dissolved in cell fluids, like sugar in water. Under the right conditions, however, it becomes insoluble and tends to aggregate or clump. In fact, the mutant alpha-synuclein from those with Contursi family parkinsonism is more prone to develop these insoluble aggregates. Cells have difficulty disposing of this insoluble form; alpha-synuclein may then accumulate. Moreover, the accumulating alpha-synuclein may further impair the cell's capacity for disposing of it. In other words, it seems that when a lot of alpha-synuclein is in the cell, the mechanisms for disposing of it may not work right: the cell's metabolic machinery for degrading it tends to get gummed up. Once alpha-synuclein builds up, it may somehow disrupt cell function and ultimately lead to neuronal death.

In summary, alpha-synuclein may play a role in typical PD, even though it is not the abnormal type that is found in one of these rare families. How might it build up if the alpha-synuclein gene is normal in typical PD? One possibility relates to the cell's machinery for disposing of alpha-synuclein and other proteins. If this doesn't work properly, alpha-synuclein (or some similar protein) could accumulate to toxic levels. Is there any evidence that protein degradation is ever abnormal in PD? Read on.

Parkin Mutations Causing Parkinsonism

For years, Japanese investigators have been studying families in which parkinsonism developed at an early age. Unlike usual PD, affected people in these families often experienced the onset of symptoms before age twenty; hence, it was labeled "juvenile parkinsonism." Like typical PD, there was an excellent response to levodopa therapy.

The inheritance pattern in these families with juvenile parkinsonism was different from the Contursi and other families. It did not run from generation to generation but was often confined to one generation. This pattern suggested recessive inheritance. Recessive disorders require both genes, one from each parent, to be abnormal.

Japanese investigators recently identified the recessive genetic mutation causing inherited juvenile parkinsonism and named this gene "parkin." This genetic mutation turned out to explain many cases of early-onset parkinsonism around the world, even without a family history. It accounts for the about three-fourths of parkinsonism cases developing before age twenty, and for a distinct minority of cases with onset in the thirties. Although a pair of parkin mutations frequently is the cause of young-onset parkinsonism, it is uncommon for this to be found when parkinsonism starts after age forty-five years.

Interest is now focusing on those carrying a single parkin mutation (plus a normal parkin gene). The true inherited form of parkin-related juvenile parkinsonism requires both parkin genes to be abnormal. What happens if you have only one abnormal parkin gene? It appears that this may be one risk factor along with other factors in occasional later-onset PD. In other words, if you have one abnormal parkin gene you may never get PD, but it increases the likelihood.

Parkin Function

What is parkin? Everyone has parkin in all their brain cells, which normally plays a role in disposing of cell proteins that are no longer needed, are excessive, or are abnormal. Parkin is one component of a complex metabolic machine contained inside cells that is called the "ubiquitin-proteasome system"; this acts like a cellular recycling machine disposing of cell protein garbage. Proteins in cells that have outlived their usefulness or are abnormal are targeted for the ubiquitin scrap heap. The ubiquitin-proteasome system breaks down these targeted proteins into small fragments, which can then be easily eliminated by the cell. Thus inherited parkinsonism has been linked to both an abnormal (or excessive) protein, alpha-synuclein, and an abnormal protein degradation system, parkin. Is this just a coincidence?

Ubiquitin Carboxy-Terminal Hydrolase Mutation Causing Parkinsonism

In yet another type of inherited parkinsonism, the genetic abnormality was also identified in the ubiquitin-proteasome system. This genetic defect is in the part of the system where ubiquitin is recycled. This abnormal gene codes for ubiquitin carboxy-terminal hydrolase, which frees up the ubiquitin after the proteasome has done its work; chains of ubiquitin are unglued so that the ubiquitin can be used again. If this portion of the system is malfunctioning, there may be insufficient useable ubiquitin.

Abnormalities of the ubiquitin carboxy-terminal hydrolase gene have been identified in only one family. Although it is an extremely rare cause of parkinsonism, this finding lends further support to the notion that impaired breakdown of certain proteins in neurons may cause parkinsonism. Thus the ubiquitin-proteasome system and the proteins it degrades, especially alpha-synuclein, are moving toward center stage in our search for the cause of PD.

Relevance to PD

Evidence is now developing that ties these gene discoveries to the rest of the PD world. We already discussed the fact that carrying one abnormal parkin gene may be a risk factor for PD (recall that both parkin genes must be abnormal for the true inherited form to occur). Similarly, variations in these other genes may influence the risk of developing PD.

When the ubiquitin carboxy-terminal hydrolase gene was being studied, it was recognized that there are several forms of the normal gene. Scientists call different forms of a normal gene, polymorphisms. In fact, such polymorphisms are the rule in genetics; multiple types of a normal gene are typically found when screening large numbers of people. Thus it came as no surprise when several types of normal ubiquitin carboxy-terminal hydrolase were found. What was surprising, however, was that individuals having a specific type were found to be at a much lower risk for developing run-of-the-mill PD. Those carrying the polymorphic variant S18Y of the ubiquitin carboxy-terminal hydrolase gene were only about 50 percent as likely to have PD as those carrying other normal forms of this gene. Perhaps those with this S18Y variant have a more effective ubiquitin system. More importantly, it ties the ubiquitin-proteasome system to typical PD.

Polymorphisms of the normal alpha-synuclein gene have also been investigated among those with typical PD. One specific polymorphism of this gene (named Rep1) is found in normal people and those with PD. However, those with PD are significantly more likely to be carrying this gene. In other words, if you have this gene, you are at a greater risk of developing PD. This is similar to smoking and cancer; if you smoke, you may never get cancer, but your risk is significantly increased.

There now appears to be enough circumstantial evidence to suggest that lessons from inherited parkinsonism are indeed relevant to typical PD. What is unclear is the extent to which these inherited factors are playing a role in PD. Is inheritance a minor player that simply predisposes to PD when the right environmental factors are present? Alternatively, could there be a vast array of genetic contributions that, in the aggregate, are the primary cause of PD?

Parallels to Alzheimer's Disease

The cause of PD is far from being understood. However, the evidence cited above suggests that one or more insoluble proteins, such as alpha-synuclein, may be accumulating inside diseased neurons, which are unable to adequately dispose of them. This parallels the research in another neurodegenerative disorder, Alzheimer's disease. In that condition, we have even more convincing evidence that accumulation of a specific protein is the inciting factor. The particular protein that seems to be responsible for Alzheimer's disease, amyloid, was also initially identified through studying rare families. In these families the responsible genes coded for a certain form of insoluble amyloid. In garden-variety Alzheimer's disease, brain amyloid aggregates in discrete deposits (amyloid plaques), which are analogous to the Lewy bodies of PD. Alzheimer researchers are now studying ways to prevent the accumulation of amyloid. This gets at the source of the disease. Parkinson researchers may not be far behind.

Mitochondrial Abnormalities and Coenzyme Q_{10}

Scientists have consistently found abnormalities in the mitochondria of people with PD. Mitochondria are small structures contained inside all human cells. They are critical to the life of the cell and, in essence, are each cell's power plant. They burn fuel to generate energy. The fuel they burn is the product of our digestion (carbohydrates, fats, protein). Like a furnace where oxygen is necessary for the fire to burn, oxygen is critical to mitochondrial function. With this chemical interaction of digested fuels and oxygen, a critical high-energy molecule is produced, ATP (adenosine triphosphate).

The mitochondrial role in PD was recently given credibility by a preliminary report of relative improvement in parkinsonism with coenzyme Q_{10} treatment. Coenzyme Q is an important component of mitochondria.

The metabolic machinery of mitochondria is extremely complicated, with many components and subcomponents. There are four major metabolic engines in mitochondria, all linked, one to the next; they are named complexes I, II, III, and IV. Among those with PD, the problem primarily lies within mitochondrial complex I. Complex I does not operate efficiently and its biochemical output is less than normal. These mitochondrial abnormalities are present in muscles and blood cells as well as the brain. Speculation has focused on why such widespread mitochondrial dysfunction should be associated with the limited brain degeneration of PD. We still do not know how to integrate this into any general theory of the cause of PD. Perhaps this is simply a general susceptibility factor: it may not be the primary cause but limits the ability of neurons to survive when metabolically challenged. We now know that minor variability in the normal genetic codes for complex I can significantly influence your risk of developing PD—certain mitochondrial complex I polymorphisms confer a reduced risk of PD.

Not only is mitochondrial complex I function reduced in PD, but so are the concentrations of coenzyme Q. This suggested the obvious treatment strategy: administration of coenzyme Q to improve complex I function. A small clinical trial recently tested this hypothesis. Coenzyme Q_{10}, a specific form of coenzyme Q, was compared to placebo therapy (sugar pill) in people with PD. Remarkably, patients treated with the highest coenzyme Q_{10} dose, 1200 mg daily, had significantly better parkinsonian scores than those receiving placebo. This provides further confirmation that mitochondrial dysfunction plays a role in PD and opened the door to further trials of coenzyme Q_{10} therapy.

The Future

Research into the cause of PD has accelerated with recent breakthroughs and discoveries in molecular biology. It seems that we may be on the verge of a new era. If we can figure out the cause, more effective treatment, perhaps even a cure, should not be far behind.

9

♦ ♦ ♦

Are There Drugs and Strategies to Slow PD Progression?

PD slowly progresses over the years. Do we have drugs that target the underlying problem and change the course of PD? What about medications not just for treating symptoms but for protecting vulnerable neurons that might otherwise degenerate? The term "neuroprotection" has been used in this context.

Over the years, many drugs and strategies have been considered as means of slowing the progression of PD. Few, however, have actually been subjected to scientific investigation in people with PD. In this chapter, we will focus on drugs that have undergone at least some scientific scrutiny. To date, we have no medications with proven ability to slow PD progression. For some drugs, however, there is at least a modicum of circumstantial evidence, which we will consider.

The Problem: How to Assess Progression

With all the research focusing on PD, why can't medical science come up with drugs to stop the progression? Obviously, not knowing the cause of PD has been a primary limiting factor. Almost as important, however, is the difficulty in measuring the progression of PD. Why is this hard to measure?

- The progression of PD is very slow, over many years. Contrast this with testing drugs for cancer, where signs of progression often develop over months.

- Available medications (levodopa and dopamine agonists) effectively treat the symptoms and signs of PD, making it difficult to use these as indices of clinical progression. In other words, the progression is masked by symptomatic therapies.

- The progression rate is not the same from one person to the next; it may vary widely among people with PD. Moreover, the way PD progresses is also quite variable; for some, walking and balance deteriorate over time, whereas others may experience more decline in tremor control. Hence, progression must be assessed using large numbers of people to average out this variability.

- There are no blood tests or other simple biologic markers of disease progression. Contrast this with AIDS, where blood tests provide an index of progression, or kidney disease, where a blood test tells us how the kidneys are working.

Clinical Trials of Drugs to Slow PD Progression

Four drugs have been tested in large clinical trials, assessing their potential to slow PD progression. Selegiline and vitamin E were investigated over a decade ago. Parkinsonian symptoms and signs were measured to determine the rate of progression. More recently, two dopamine agonist drugs, pramipexole and ropinirole, were assessed using brain scanning techniques to monitor PD progression. Let's see what was learned from these clinical trials.

SELEGILINE (ELDEPRYL, DEPRENYL)

Nothing has been simple about this medication, including its name. For years, it was known as deprenyl; now the preferred generic name is selegiline (brand name, Eldepryl). This drug does many things in the body, but a primary function is to block an enzyme that breaks down dopamine, monoamine oxidase (MAO).

MAO is an enzyme that is present in the brain and elsewhere in the body. By breaking down dopamine and related substances, MAO prevents the levels from becoming excessive. In the normal brain, dopamine is constantly being made, degraded, and disposed. This is a balanced process that keeps the levels constant. MAO is present in two forms, MAO-A and MAO-B. Selegiline blocks the B form, and consequently results in a mild elevation of brain dopamine. Selegiline was initially used to enhance the levodopa effect, since MAO is one of the major ways the body breaks down dopamine.

The conjecture that selegiline might slow PD progression was based on two observations. First, selegiline reduces oxidative reactions in brain cells. As noted in a previous chapter, excessive oxidative reactions linked to dopamine metabolism have been hypothesized to cause PD, the so-called oxidative stress theory. Selegiline blocks monoamine oxidase, one route of oxidation; it also blocks at least one other dopamine oxidative reaction. (Of course, many oxidation reactions occur in all our cells; a variety of mechanisms are present to control these and prevent excessive oxidation.)

Second, selegiline blocks the toxicity of MPTP in animals and prevents them from developing parkinsonism. Recall from chapter 8 that people who had injected MPTP to get high developed parkinsonism, and this toxin is now used to make animal models of PD.

In the 1980s, a large clinical trial was conducted to assess a possible neuroprotective effect of selegiline in people with PD. Measurement of disease progression was by clinical measures, including questionnaires and examinations. Prior experience had suggested that selegiline administered alone (without levodopa) did not improve the symptoms of PD. Hence, it was thought reliable to use the symptoms and signs of parkinsonism as the index of the underlying disease process. The preliminary results generated excitement since it appeared to slow PD progression. However, further study and additional statistical analyses revealed that this could be explained by a direct effect on the symptoms and signs of parkinsonism. Thus the benefit appeared to be a symptomatic effect, like levodopa (or like taking aspirin for pain). Data gained from additional studies indicated that selegiline was probably treating the symptoms. There is ongoing debate about this subject. Some investigators continue to believe that there may be a favorable effect on the underlying disease process. However, this has been impossible to prove. What is clear is that even if present, any neuroprotective effect is modest at best.

ADMINISTRATION OF SELEGILINE

Some physicians continue to prescribe selegiline, based largely on faith. It is simple to use; one 5 mg tablet each morning is sufficient. The conventional dose is one tablet in the morning and one with lunch; however, the major pharmacologic effect, blocking the B form of MAO, is essentially complete with one tablet daily. More than two tablets daily should not be administered. When the dosage is increased substantially beyond that, all forms of MAO are blocked. This can be dangerous since certain chemicals in food are not properly metabolized, potentially resulting in severe hypertension.

The major downside of selegiline is the expense, around $2 per tablet. When it is taken without other drugs for PD, side effects are usually not a problem. It can cause insomnia, but this usually does not occur if it is taken in the morning. Rarely, it interacts with other medications, notably the narcotic meperidine (Demerol), as well as with most of the antidepressant medications (except for bupropion; brand name, Wellbutrin). The interactions with these other drugs can be serious, but they are extremely rare. Many people have been concurrently treated with selegiline and these antidepressants without experiencing problems.

When selegiline is used with carbidopa/levodopa, it enhances both the benefits and side effects. This includes increasing the potential for dyskinesias and hallucinations. In someone with hallucinations or delusions, selegiline should generally be discontinued.

Selegiline has a long duration of action in the brain. Blockade of MAO-B continues for weeks after it is stopped (reduced by an average of 50 percent forty days after discontinuation). Hence, if a decision is made to discontinue it, stopping abruptly is acceptable, since the effects will linger and slowly phase out. Because of this long duration of action, any side effects may take awhile to abate. Occasionally people stopping selegiline will experience a decline in control of their PD symptoms some weeks after stopping it, rather than right away.

Should you take selegiline as a neuroprotective agent? My view is that the data are insufficient to support this practice. Although it does have a mild symptomatic effect, this benefit is minor when compared to the more potent drugs we have for treating PD symptoms.

VITAMIN E AND OTHER ANTIOXIDANTS

The oxidant stress theory of PD predicts that antioxidant medications might slow disease progression. Antioxidant medications include vitamins E and C, beta-carotene, and others. These drugs are easier to assess in clinical trials since they do not affect the symptoms of PD, in contrast to selegiline. Only one antioxidant has been evaluated in such a clinical trial, vitamin E, also known as alpha-tocopherol.

Vitamin E was evaluated in the same clinical trial that assessed selegiline. Approximately 400 people with PD received 2000 units of vitamin E daily and another 400 received a placebo. Note that this is a relatively high dose of vitamin E; compare this to the standard 400-unit tablet found on pharmacy shelves. After one to two years of treatment, the progression of parkinsonism was similar, regardless of whether people received the real vitamin E or placebo. This result dampened the enthusiasm for antioxidant vitamin therapy in PD.

Vitamin C is another antioxidant vitamin that is commonly used. No clinical trials have evaluated this in PD. Even if beneficial, the appropriate dose is anyone's guess. In the laboratory, using very high doses, the antioxidant effect may actually reverse and facilitate oxidation. The bottom line is that we do not know if the oxidative stress theory of PD has any merit and there is no compelling evidence that antioxidants benefit PD.

There was a long hiatus after the selegiline and vitamin E experience when no drugs were tested in clinical trials of PD progression. The difficulty in measuring progression by assessing the symptoms and signs of PD was clearly illustrated in these prior investigations.

Assessing PD Progression with Brain Scans

More recently, nuclear medicine brain scanning has been proposed to measure PD progression. Special scanning techniques can image dopaminergic neurons in the brain. A special radioactive agent is injected by vein and passes into the brain, where it attaches to the dopaminergic cells. The scanning device measures the radioactive signal. With the progression of PD, fewer and fewer dopaminergic neurons survive, and this can be demonstrated with scanning repeated over months to years.

Two types of scanning devices are used—positron emission tomography (PET) and single photon emission computed tomography (SPECT). The injected agent employed with PET scanning is fluorodopa, a form of radioactive levodopa. With SPECT scanning, different radioactive agents are employed, which bind to a brain protein called the dopamine transporter; this dopamine transporter protein is unique to dopaminergic cells. One commonly used radioactive agent that binds to this dopamine transporter goes by the name of beta-CIT.

With these techniques, the radioactive signal from the striatum can be numerically measured; numbers are generated that allow comparisons to be made. This signal is also displayed in picture form. Normal people have very bright striatal images on these brain scans, in contrast to those with PD.

Using these scans to measure the effects of drugs on PD progression is a huge undertaking, quite expensive, and only limited studies of this type have been done. Many people with PD must be studied and the assessments must be done over years to measure the progression.

The reason that many study subjects are required relates to the variability of the scan results. There is variability of the measured brain signal from one person to the next, and from one scan to the next. To offset these inconsistencies, many PD patients are enrolled and statistics are employed to identify significant medication effects. Statistical measures can tell us whether any measured differences were simply due to chance.

The Dopamine Agonist Imaging Trials

Two recent large clinical trials used these techniques to monitor PD progression, generating enormous interest and controversy. These studies assessed the long-term effect of a dopamine agonist compared to levodopa treatment. Dopamine agonists not only act like synthetic forms of dopamine, but in test tubes appear to have favorable effects on brain cells. One of these trials assessed pramipexole (Mirapex) and the other, ropinirole (Requip). The results of each study revealed that patients chronically administered the dopamine agonist medication ultimately displayed more prominent brain dopaminergic imaging; this is consistent with better preservation of dopaminergic neurons.

Unfortunately, interpretation of these studies is seriously confounded. PET and SPECT scanning provide fairly reliable estimates of dopaminergic neurons in the brain only as long as drugs are not administered. The medications used in the treatment of PD, levodopa and the dopamine agonists, can directly influence the scanning values. These drugs interact directly with dopaminergic neurons and affect brain dopamine chemistry. The metabolism and binding of the injected radioactive scanning agents are subject to these brain chemistry perturbations. Consistent with this interpretation, the clinical parkinsonism scores in these studies were worse, not better with the dopamine agonist therapy (compared to levodopa); this is obviously opposite to the scan outcomes.

Q: Should I take pramipexole or ropinirole?

A: The evidence that pramipexole or ropinirole slows the progression of PD is highly questionable in my view. Nonetheless, you might argue that these drugs should be administered just in case they do indeed improve the progression of PD.

Pramipexole and ropinirole treat the symptoms of parkinsonism, although not nearly as effectively as levodopa therapy. They may be started as the initial treatment of PD. Hence, you might conclude that you can kill two birds with one stone, using one drug for treating both the symptoms and (hopefully) slowing progression. Levodopa could always be added later if the symptoms demanded.

Use of these dopamine agonists is also associated with a lower subsequent frequency of dyskinesias and fluctuations in response, termed wearing-off. These are primarily complications of levodopa therapy that develop after several years of treatment. Dyskinesias are involuntary movements that reflect an excessive medication effect. Levodopa-related dyskinesias and wearing-off can often be minimized by adjusting the levodopa dosage, and we will discuss this in detail in subsequent chapters.

Until recently, the dopamine agonist drugs were primarily used as add-ons to help control response fluctuations and dyskinesias. Now a school of thought advocates early administration of a dopamine agonist to reduce the subsequent risk of these problems. The likelihood is indeed reduced in clinical trials; however, whether you must start them early or whether the effect would be the same if they were simply started when needed, some years later, is controversial.

Balanced against this are some disadvantages to pramipexole and ropinirole, which can be summarized as follows.

- If used in place of carbidopa/levodopa, control of parkinsonism will not be quite as good.

- They are about five times as expensive as generic carbidopa/levodopa.

- They are complex to use, requiring multiple different-size pills during the dosage escalation. They are not tolerated if started in more than a tiny dose and it takes six to eight weeks or longer to reach therapeutic levels (see chapter 13).

- They are about three times as likely as carbidopa/levodopa to induce hallucinations (seeing things that are not there).

- Each can cause daytime sleepiness, creating the potential for automobile accidents. Although there are multiple reasons why someone with PD may be sleepy, these two drugs seem to have special propensity for contributing to this.

- They cause swelling of the legs, although this is not a major problem and is not dangerous.

As you can see, this is not a simple issue. There is uncertainty about whether these two drugs are truly advantageous if started initially in PD. Is there an early window of opportunity when these drugs must be initiated to capture unique benefits? Should we hedge our bets and start one of these drugs, despite their expense, dosing complexity, and unique side effects? There is no correct answer at this time. My own view is that the person taking the drug needs to be a party to this decision. More is said about this in the next few chapters.

Q: Should I take both pramipexole and ropinirole? If each drug has potential for slowing PD progression, perhaps both should be administered?

A: This is typically not done since these two drugs are very similar and whatever they do is likely to be through the same mechanisms. If you opt for these drugs, choose one or the other, not both.

Q: What dose of pramipexole or ropinirole should I take? If I choose one of these drugs for the potential neuroprotective effect, would a low dose be adequate?

A: Unfortunately, these studies provide no insight into the minimum dose that would capture such effects. In these clinical trials, the doses were adjusted to treat the symptoms.

People Who Are Poor Candidates for Pramipexole or Ropinirole

Pramipexole and ropinirole are probably not good medication choices for people in the following categories:

- Substantial memory problems or a history of hallucinations or delusions (bizarre thinking, paranoia, etc.)

- Over eighty years of age

- Very low blood pressure with fainting or near-fainting

- Limited income, without insurance coverage for medications

The evidence suggesting that these drugs may slow PD progression is not sufficiently compelling at present to justify prescribing them to these people. Rather, they should probably be managed with carbidopa/levodopa alone.

Coenzyme Q_{10}

Coenzyme Q_{10} is an integral component of mitochondria. In the last chapter I described how mitochondrial function is abnormal in PD. This was the rationale for investigating coenzyme Q_{10} therapy in PD.

Coenzyme Q_{10} therapy was recently investigated in a sixteen-month clinical trial, compared to placebo (sugar pill). The study was not designed to distinguish between symptomatic benefit versus an effect on PD progression. Three doses of coenzyme Q_{10} were studied and only the highest, 1200 mg daily, was beneficial, albeit modestly. Effects from the two lower doses, 300 mg and 600 mg daily, were not significantly different from placebo. Although the measured benefit was small, it suggested that this general strategy has merit. Further studies are underway, but there are many unanswered questions.

- Can this be confirmed in a larger study?

- Is the 1200 mg daily dose optimal? Would even larger doses be more effective?

- Are there any long-term dangers to this treatment, especially in higher doses?

- Finally, and perhaps most important, were the symptoms being treated, or was PD progression slowed?

COENZYME Q_{10} THERAPY AND OTHER DISORDERS

This agent has been used for years to treat people with known mitochondrial cytopathies where we are sure that the primary cause is mitochondrial dysfunction. It has not been very effective in these conditions, but used primarily because of the theoretical rationale. However, the doses previously recommended were much lower than the 1200 mg daily used in this PD trial; doses of 300 mg or less have been the previous standard treatment. Have we missed the boat in treating all mitochondrial disorders simply because we have been using too low a dose of coenzyme Q_{10}? This question should be answered in the next few years, but at this time we can only speculate.

THE SAFETY OF COENZYME Q_{10}

In this PD trial, the side effects were essentially identical to placebo over the sixteen months of the investigation. However, we have no data beyond sixteen months of treatment.

USE AND DOSAGE OF COENZYME Q_{10}

At present, there are simply too many unanswered questions about coenzyme Q_{10} treatment to recommend widespread use. This was also the view of the investigators who conducted this study. Admittedly, however, the 1200 mg dose seemed to be largely devoid of side effects over the sixteen months of the trial. Perhaps the greatest downside of this treatment is the expense; 1200 mg coenzyme Q_{10} costs $100 to $200 monthly. Furthermore, since it is not a prescription drug, pharmacy insurance plans will not cover it. Rather, it is sold over the counter at drug and health food stores. This is quite an expense for something that has only mild benefit and has not been proven to slow PD progression.

Common sense should prevail in this case. If money is no object, taking 1200 mg daily is probably a reasonable hedge on the bet that it may be doing some long-term good. It appears to be safe for at least sixteen months at a time. Further data should be forthcoming regarding longer-term use. For now, however, it seems unwise to recommend higher doses until these have been investigated.

Amantadine

Amantadine has been around for as long as levodopa therapy, a little over thirty years. Limited indirect evidence has raised speculation that it may have a favorable effect on PD progression, beyond simple symptomatic treatment. It partially blocks one of the major brain neurotransmitters, glutamate. For years, it has been speculated that excessive glutamate activity in the brain may be toxic. However, amantadine is only a weak blocker of glutamate and there is no evidence that even potent glutamate blockade changes the course of PD. One study did suggest that PD patients treated with amantadine lived longer, on the average. However, this particular study raised more questions than answers and there were alternative explanations for why those treated tended to live longer. In summary, if amantadine is prescribed as a means of slowing PD progression, this is purely on faith.

Levodopa and Longevity

We often lose sight of the fact that levodopa, our standard drug for treating the symptoms of PD, was shown to increase longevity. Mortality rates among people with PD dropped substantially when this drug became widely available around 1970. This was reported in more than a half dozen independent studies and seems irrefutable. Most likely, this was due to improved functioning (such as no longer confined to a wheelchair); however, a direct effect on PD progression cannot be excluded.

The potential for increased longevity should be a compelling argument for starting levodopa therapy early. Not only is it the most effective drug for treating the symptoms of PD, but levodopa treatment may allow you to live longer. Nothing is simple in biology and medicine, however. Some researchers have argued just the opposite, proposing that levodopa is toxic or that long-term treatment may have adverse consequences.

Why Would Anyone Think That Levodopa Therapy Is Toxic?

The issue of levodopa toxicity is the product of the oxidative stress hypothesis of PD, which we discussed in the last chapter. This theory was proposed some years ago, based on the recognition that substantia nigra dopaminergic neurons degenerate in PD. Might the presence of dopamine make these cells susceptible? Are toxic byproducts from dopamine metabolism the cause of PD?

Dopamine is broken down by more than one enzyme, but the focus has been on monoamine oxidase (MAO). MAO is one of many enzymes in the body that facilitate oxidative reactions, generating oxygen by-products. It is these oxidative by-products that have been proposed to cause cell damage. Dopamine also spontaneously oxidizes and generates these by-products. Moreover, there are substances in these substantia nigra neurons that might increase these oxidative chemical reactions, including iron plus the black pigment, melanin.

If dopamine is the bad actor, and if its oxidative by-products are dangerous to cells, are we doing harm with our treatment? Theoretically contributing to this process is anything that increases brain dopamine concentrations. Levodopa therapy, of course, is designed to do exactly that. Could levodopa administration be adding fuel to the fire?

Oxidative reactions from dopamine metabolism may well be harmless. Oxidation is ubiquitous and many oxidative chemical reactions are continuously occurring in every cell in the body. If these were excessive and uncontrolled, cells certainly would be damaged. However, because these reactions are universal and essential for life, cells have a vast array of protective mechanisms for controlling and preventing excessive oxidation. Nonetheless, this does not exclude the possibility of a role in PD.

Dopamine and levodopa toxicity has been studied by adding these substances to cells growing in culture. Scientists are able to take brain cells from animals and grow them in test tubes or petri dishes (in culture). These investigations have generated mixed results. Initial studies indicated that levodopa and dopamine were indeed toxic. However, more recent studies have found the opposite effect—that levodopa promotes longevity of cells in culture. Complicating interpretation is the fact that cells in culture are vulnerable to a variety of insults that would not affect them in their natural setting in the body. Substances that should be benign become toxic when added to these naked cells grown in glass dishes. The antioxidant vitamin C kills cells in culture; yet common sense and a wealth of experience suggest that this is not a dangerous substance.

The dilemma is that the best medicine for PD has been hypothesized to accelerate the underlying disease process. Perhaps those treated will succumb to their disease sooner. If true, this would be a cruel irony, analogous to learning that insulin accelerates diabetes. Before jumping to conclusions, let's consider the evidence.

Levodopa Is Not Toxic

Medical hypotheses are continuously being proposed and discarded; only a few stand the test of time. Levodopa has been the cornerstone of PD treatment for more than thirty years. If levodopa is toxic, this should have become apparent long before now. Evidence that has accumulated over the years argues against any substantial toxicity; let us consider the following facts.

- When levodopa was introduced years ago, scientists noted that this did not change the brain appearance under the microscope. Brains of those who had been taking levodopa therapy looked just like those from the prelevodopa era.

- The oxidative stress hypothesis has focused on the degeneration of brain cells containing dopamine; however, this ignores the fact that other neurons degenerate in PD, including those with neurotransmitters such as acetylcholine (which is quite dissimilar from dopamine). These other brain regions receive less of our attention because they are not as crucial to normal movement and behavior as the substantia nigra. Thus, if dopamine is at the core of the PD degenerative process, how does one explain the degeneration of brain areas without dopamine?

- The first brain cells affected by the PD process are probably not dopaminergic neurons. Recent evidence from neuropathologists suggests that neurons in the lower brainstem are the first to degenerate; these do not contain dopamine or any related substances. However, these have not caught anyone's attention until recently because their loss does not seem to result in prominent symptoms (unlike the substantia nigra).

- Levodopa treatment is occasionally used for other disorders and in none of these has there been evidence of damage to brain cells. This has included several reports in which brains were carefully examined after years of levodopa use.

- Two clinical trials have analyzed the before and after effects of levodopa treatment compared to placebo (sugar pill). After approximately one year of treatment, the drugs were withdrawn so that the untreated state could be analyzed and compared to the baseline. After medication withdrawal, those who had received levodopa were no worse than those who had been on placebo.

- Mice administered huge amounts of daily levodopa for many months had no evidence of toxicity, even when the brains were examined under the microscope.

- If levodopa is toxic, why the many reports of improved longevity associated with its introduction?

Although the oxidative stress theory of PD still has proponents, the hard facts from a variety of sources argue against any direct detrimental effect of levodopa on susceptible brain cells. Recently, a consensus panel of PD experts concluded that there is no compelling evidence for levodopa toxicity.

Long-Term Levodopa Therapy: Inconsistent Responses

Separate from the issue of levodopa toxicity are concerns about changes in the beneficial response to levodopa that occur over the years. The principal concern has focused on the two aspects of the levodopa response already noted:

- Dyskinesias, which are excessive involuntary movements of the body induced by levodopa

- Motor fluctuations, which reflect a transition from a very smooth beneficial response to ups and downs in the control of parkinsonism

There is no debating that these problems do occur. How frequently and when? The medical literature suggests a 40 percent likelihood of dyskinesias after about five years of levodopa treatment; thus, on the average, four people in ten will experience dyskinesias after about five years. The data is almost identical for motor fluctuations; about four people out of ten will also experience these by five years. This is not to say that affected people are disabled by these problems. These dyskinesias or motor fluctuations may be relatively mild and controlled by medication adjustments. Eventually these complications may take center stage, but there are many with PD who never experience severe problems of this type.

These levodopa dyskinesias and motor fluctuations have been a focus of PD investigators in recent years. Are there strategies for reducing the likelihood these will develop? Some have proposed that if we defer levodopa treatment, we can save the best responses for later. In other words, get by now as best you can. Does this approach have merit?

Can We Save the Best Levodopa Responses for Later?

You might infer that the longer you take levodopa, the more likely you are to develop dyskinesias and motor fluctuations. But, is the crucial factor years of treatment, or rather, how long one has had PD? After all, PD is a progressive disorder that marches along, regardless of whether you are treated or not. We could test this by enrolling people with PD into a study in which half had their levodopa treatment delayed for several years. However, this study will never be done since it would be unethical to withhold the best medication for extended periods of time. Even if our moral compass suggested otherwise, people enrolled in such a study would drop out as their parkinsonism worsened; this would make it impossible to maintain the study design and evaluate the data.

A Natural Experiment: Outcomes from the Early Levodopa Trials

Actually, thirty-five-year-old data addresses this issue. People beginning levodopa therapy when it was first introduced around 1969 often had long durations of untreated parkinsonism (i.e., not treated with levodopa). This provided a natural experiment allowing us to separate the effect of duration of PD from levodopa treatment duration.

The data from these early levodopa trials indicates that by only six months of levodopa treatment, half of these people developed dyskinesias. This contrasts with the 40 percent risk after five years of treatment in the modern era. We also evaluated the experience among our Mayo patients beginning levodopa in 1969. All but one of twenty-seven people experienced dyskinesias within the first year of treatment. Motor fluctuations were present in nearly three-fourths by two years of levodopa therapy. Again, this contrasts with the 40 percent incidence after five years of levodopa treatment in modern times. In sum, this early experience suggests that how long one has had PD is the critical factor in the development of dyskinesias and motor fluctuations. Probably it is the natural progression of PD that predisposes to these levodopa complications.

In summary, there is no good evidence that we can save our best levodopa responses. The evidence suggests this may well be fruitless, and you may be accepting a poor short-term outcome for no gain.

PART FIVE

◆ ◆ ◆

The Movement Problems of Parkinson's Disease: Medication Rationale and Choices

10

◆ ◆ ◆

Medications for Movement Problems
(Gait, Tremor, Slowness)

Although we do not have drugs that affect the underlying cause or progression of Parkinson's disease (PD), we have very good drugs for controlling many of the symptoms. The progression of PD is slow, and hence the symptomatic treatment is often gratifying for many years. Although the treatment of the symptoms is not always smooth or perfect, optimal adjustment of medications can typically keep people in the mainstream of their lives and turn back the clock on this disorder.

This symptomatic treatment capitalizes on our understanding of brain chemistry. Thus there is a rational basis for the drugs, based on scientific principles. To appreciate the treatment principles and understand the role for the medications, we will first need to review some basics about relevant brain chemistry.

Dopamine

The key region of the brain that degenerates in those with PD is the substantia nigra, as explained in chapters 2–3. This substantia nigra connects with the striatum, forming the nigrostriatal system (nigra to striatum).

In the 1960s, the chemical released by normal nigrostriatal brain cells was identified and confirmed as dopamine. This was a major breakthrough and set the stage for modern-day medical therapy of PD. When the substantia nigra degenerates in PD, dopamine levels within the striatum plummet.

Dopamine is similar in its chemical structure to adrenalin, although it serves quite different purposes. Both of these substances are found in multiple areas of our body and function as one specific means of signaling within the nervous system.

Dopamine is normally released in the striatum from this nigrostriatal connection on a relatively constant basis. In other words, the activity of this system does not change from second to second. Rather, the dopamine release seems to provide a persistent and stable modulatory effect.

What is the consequence of losing dopamine in the striatum? There are a variety of experimental means of reducing brain dopamine concentrations in animal models. The consequence is that the animal without striatal dopamine moves slowly and stiffly with a stooped posture and reduced animation. This is identical to the movement problems of someone with PD. When the experimental treatment that has lowered the animal's brain dopamine is stopped and the dopamine stores are replenished, the animal again moves normally. Such animal models illustrate the basis for medical treatment of PD, with the main focus on brain dopamine.

Impediment to Raising Brain Dopamine: The Blood–Brain Barrier

It has been known for decades that dopamine taken by mouth or administered by injection does not get into the brain. There is a natural barrier that prevents the myriad of substances that circulate in our bloodstream from entering the protected brain environment. This is called the blood–brain barrier. If it were not for this blood–brain barrier, all the products of our meals that enter our bloodstream would flood the brain (perhaps making us all psychotic). The blood–brain barrier allows only selected substances and only limited amounts to pass. Certain substances pass readily and others require special transport across this blood-brain barrier; some are absolutely blocked by this barrier. Because of dopamine's chemical structure, it cannot cross the blood–brain barrier.

Actually dopamine and other similar substances can cross the blood–brain barrier in one small region, the so-called chemoreceptive trigger zone. This is the nausea-vomiting center of the brain. This chemoreceptive trigger zone senses when certain undesirable substances are passing through the bloodstream. Somewhat paradoxically, dopamine passes into this region. If present in sufficient concentrations, dopamine stimulates the sensors there, inducing nausea and perhaps vomiting. Hence, if dopamine is given in pill form, not only will it fail to get into the brain where we want it to work, but it will make people sick.

The Role of Enzymes

In the normal state, dopamine is constantly being manufactured in appropriate brain regions. Like most natural substances in our bodies, there is a cycle in which it is continuously being made, used, and then broken down. Hence, there is a continuous cycling of dopamine. The amount produced matches the amount degraded, keeping brain dopamine levels constant. There are metabolic machines for each step in these processes. The metabolic machines are called enzymes. One given enzyme typically performs only one limited task, modifying a body chemical. It may add or delete some portion of that chemical or it may combine body chemicals. A sequence of enzymes is responsible for making almost all substances necessary for life, each enzyme performing one critical step. Enzyme systems are analogous to an automobile assembly line, where each worker on the line performs one function, ultimately resulting in the manufactured car.

The Amino Acid L-dopa (Levodopa)

Dopamine is made in our bodies from dopa, also known as levodopa or L-dopa. L-dopa is a natural substance that our body manufactures, but this also comes from our diet. To make dopamine, L-dopa is transformed by an enzyme, dopa decarboxylase. This enzyme changes one small component of L-dopa, resulting in the generation of dopamine. This enzyme is present not only in the brain but outside of it as well. Unlike dopamine, L-dopa crosses the blood-brain barrier.

L-dopa is from a class of natural body chemicals called amino acids, which serve a variety of roles in our body. Perhaps the most fundamental role is one that has nothing to do with dopamine or other brain neurotransmitters. Amino acids are the building blocks of the body's proteins. Proteins, in turn, are responsible for much of the unique structure of our body. Everything from muscle to brain to skin is made up of unique proteins that bond together with other substances to form body organs. A protein is simply a chain of amino acids strung together. There are twenty specific amino acids in our bodies, each with a unique chemical shape and property. The exact sequence of these amino acids determines the type of protein.

Dietary protein is present in high concentrations in such foods as meat, fish, poultry, and dairy products. When we eat proteins, our digestive system breaks them down into the constituent amino acids. Those amino acids are then released into the bloodstream from our intestinal system and go to various places and are used for a variety of purposes, including making new proteins.

Amino acids are also a source of metabolic energy, similar to sugar. Cells are able to transform them into metabolic fuel, yielding energy for that cell.

In the context of PD, we are less interested in how amino acids are made into proteins or burned as fuel by cells. Rather, amino acids serve a third purpose, as a precursor to certain neurotransmitters. The nigrostriatal neurotransmitter dopamine is made from the amino acid, L-dopa (levodopa). Substantia nigra neurons are able to take up L-dopa and transform it into dopamine.

Why the L in L-dopa?

Chemicals in nature are constructed with the component atoms linked together to make a three-dimensional structure. However, any three-dimensional structure may have a mirror image that is identical but oriented just opposite. Similar to gloves, which are both right- and left-handed, natural substances often have two forms, which are right and left oriented. Like many chemicals in nature, dopa has two forms, one the mirror image of the other. The type of dopa that is active in our bodies is the left-oriented form. The term "levo," which means left, is the prefix attached to dopa to indicate it is left-oriented; hence the term "levodopa," or L-dopa for short.

The other type of amino acid, dextro (for right-handed), does not have an important role in our bodies. These dextro amino acids are inert in terms of body chemistry. Body amino acids are the *L* or left-handed forms. It would be correct to simply refer to dopa, but L-dopa or levodopa is a more specific term.

Levodopa Passes the Blood–Brain Barrier

Amino acids are needed within the brain for all the purposes noted above, including manufacture of proteins, for use as fuel, and as precursors for neurotransmitters. However, their chemical structure prevents them from easily crossing the blood–brain barrier. How, then, does the brain capture adequate amounts of amino acids? It is by way of a chemical transport system. This is analogous to a train that transports coal over a bridge, across a river. Located at the blood–brain barrier are specific transport systems that recognize crucial substances in the bloodstream that are needed by the brain. They are picked up and carried across the barrier. Other substances that do not fit the mold are not picked up.

L-dopa is transported by one such transport system located at the blood–brain barrier. This transport mechanism picks up not only L-dopa, but also other amino acids of a similar type. This group of amino acids, which includes L-dopa, is called the large neutral amino acid class because of similar chemical structure. No other substances are transported by this system, including amino acids from other classes.

Levodopa as a Treatment for PD

Nearly half a century ago, research pointed toward low dopamine levels as responsible for the symptoms of PD and scientists debated strategies to restore brain dopamine. Attention focused on L-dopa, since this was known to be one step removed from dopamine and could pass across the blood–brain barrier. The early trials generated mixed results, largely because it was not very well tolerated; the initial doses were either too low to do any good or so high that nausea resulted. The nausea was because the L-dopa in the bloodstream was converted to dopamine before it crossed the blood–brain barrier. This dopamine in the circulation passed into the brain nausea center (chemoreceptive trigger zone) where the blood–brain barrier is absent.

Eventually, higher doses of L-dopa were tried. Most with PD were able to tolerate this using a strategy of low starting doses, with gradual dose escalation allowing tolerance to the nausea-inducing effect. Large clinical trials performed in the late 1960s ultimately confirmed striking success in treating the symptoms of PD with levodopa therapy. In fact, some of the outcomes bordered on the miraculous. People who had not walked for years due to PD were again mobile. Disabling tremor suddenly came under control. Some were able to leave nursing homes and return to their families. This discovery of levodopa therapy for PD was revolutionary and heralded a new era of symptomatic treatment.

Levodopa Therapy and Advancing PD

As experience with levodopa treatment continued into the 1970s it was recognized that there were shortcomings. With long-standing PD, the benefit was often found to be incomplete. Furthermore, maintenance of stable brain levodopa and dopamine levels became more problematic. With fluctuations in these levels came fluctuations in symptom control. People could be relatively normal one minute and severely parkinsonian minutes later, as the brain dopamine levels declined. If too much levodopa was administered in an attempt to control these fluctuations, dyskinesias (involuntary movements) might occur.

With the recognition of the problems came strategies for dealing with them. First, it was appreciated that levodopa dosing and timing were crucial. Second, came generations of new drugs used to supplement levodopa therapy and smooth out the responses. Levodopa remains the most effective drug we have for PD treatment and the foundation of therapy. However, it is often used together with other medications to optimize the responses.

Levodopa and Diet

Small amounts of levodopa are contained in dietary protein. Could increasing our protein intake treat PD? In a word, no. With the breakdown of dietary

protein, a variety of amino acids are generated. The blood–brain barrier transport mechanism has only a limited capacity to carry amino acids. In other
words, it is easily filled up; the cars on the train hold only so much coal. These
other amino acids may knock levodopa off the train. Levodopa cannot be
carried into the brain if competing amino acids occupy all the transport sites.
In fact, dietary protein may actually block the effects of levodopa treatment
by this mechanism.

Could PD be treated by foods that are high in levodopa and lower in other
amino acids? There are very few items in our diet with a favorable ratio of
levodopa to other amino acids. Fava beans, a staple in some southern European and Middle Eastern diets, contain proportionately high concentrations
of levodopa and are mildly beneficial as PD treatment. However, this is an
unpalatable way to treat PD for most people and not very effective when
precise doses are necessary.

Nausea Induced by Levodopa: Carbidopa

Nausea and vomiting continued to be a problem during the early years of
levodopa therapy in the early 1970s. Although this nausea is not associated
with any real damage (it does not cause ulcers or injure the stomach), it often
prevented adequate dosage. As we discussed earlier, nausea is caused by premature conversion of levodopa to dopamine outside the brain. Once dopamine is generated within the circulation, it is unable to cross the blood–brain
barrier but does pass into the brain stem nausea center (the chemoreceptive
trigger zone). The task confronting scientists back then was how to block this
premature conversion of dopa to dopamine outside the brain. Obviously, one
would not want to block the conversion of dopa to dopamine altogether or
levodopa would be ineffective for PD.

The solution was the creation of a substance that would block the conversion of L-dopa to dopamine on only the body side of the blood-brain barrier.
The enzyme dopa decarboxylase is present on both sides of the blood-brain
barrier—both within the brain and also on the body side. For levodopa therapy
to work, the brain dopa decarboxylase must be uninhibited; however, to prevent nausea, the dopa decarboxylase outside the brain must be blocked. This
was accomplished by creating a dopa decarboxylase blocking substance that
would not cross the blood–brain barrier. A number of substances were initially tried. Two such agents were subsequently identified, carbidopa and
benserazide. Neither crosses the blood–brain barrier. However, each attaches
to dopa decarboxylase and prevents dopa from also binding to it. If the dopa
doesn't attach to dopa decarboxylase, it is protected from its effects.

The combination of carbidopa and levodopa has been the mainstay of PD
treatment within the United States. The brand name of this combination

drug is Sinemet. The name Sinemet was derived from Latin, *sine emesis,* meaning without emesis (i.e., vomiting). In certain European countries and elsewhere, benserazide, rather than carbidopa, is combined with levodopa for the same effect; that brand name is Madopar. Sinemet and Madopar are essentially identical medications. Carbidopa has no advantages over benserazide and vice versa. Neither carbidopa nor benserazide appears to have any other effect apart from blocking the enzyme dopa decarboxylase. Neither has any toxicity, even when administered in relatively high doses.

Levodopa in the absence of carbidopa (or benserazide) is no longer used for PD treatment. Whenever we talk about levodopa therapy, treatment with carbidopa/levodopa is implied.

Despite carbidopa (or benserazide), nausea is still occasionally experienced by people with PD taking levodopa. Often this passes with continued use, provided that one starts with a low dose and slowly raises it. For more difficult problems with nausea, a number of strategies are available (discussed in detail in chapter 12).

Why Does Levodopa Work?

Normally, dopamine is made in the substantia nigra cells and then released in the striatum to signal other neurons in the circuit. Since these nigrostriatal cells degenerate in PD, why is levodopa effective? After all, the primary site where levodopa is converted to dopamine is lost. The brain site for generating dopamine from administered levodopa probably depends upon how long one has had PD.

In those with early PD, only 50–80 percent of the critical substantia nigra cells are lost. That means that 20–50 percent of the nigrostriatal cells are still surviving at this early stage. These surviving cells are able to increase their production and output of dopamine when bolstered by levodopa therapy. They are able to make up for what was lost. This is perhaps why those with early PD typically have very smooth and effective responses to levodopa therapy.

In those with late PD, the neurodegenerative process is slowly relentless and after a number of years, the loss of dopaminergic terminals may exceed 95 percent in some areas of the striatum. Despite this, levodopa therapy is still effective, although the smoothness of the response is lost with fluctuations in the symptoms. The clinical response fluctuates with blood levels of levodopa. At this stage, levodopa conversion primarily occurs in other cells within the striatum, which normally are not involved in dopamine generation. This includes cells that release other neurotransmitters, such as serotonin. Some of these other brain cells have enzymes capable of converting levodopa to dopamine. The supporting cells of the brain, called glia, probably also are involved in the generation of dopamine from levodopa in later-stage PD. Normally, glial cells are not directly involved in the signaling (neurotransmitter) process. Since nondopaminergic neurons and glia are not in the usual brain dopamine network, the dopamine they produce from levodopa therapy is released less smoothly and consistently. This likely plays a role in the unevenness of the levodopa response after many years.

Dopamine Agonists: Drugs That Act Like Dopamine

Scientists have developed drugs that cross the blood–brain barrier and act like dopamine. As already noted, these are called dopamine agonists.

The term "agonist" is applied to drugs that behave like the naturally occurring neurotransmitters; they stimulate the specific receptor because they chemically resemble that neurotransmitter. In the case of dopamine agonists, portions of the molecule have chemical structures that look just like dopamine and hence fool the dopamine receptors into thinking this is dopamine. They are analogous to skeleton keys. The real key opens the lock but skeleton keys have enough of the correct shape to do the same. In this analogy, the lock is the dopamine receptor and the "real key" is dopamine; the dopamine agonist is the skeleton key.

In the United States, four dopamine agonist drugs are available for treatment of PD and a few others are available in other countries. The first of these was bromocriptine (Parlodel), followed by pergolide (Permax). Within the last decade, pramipexole (Mirapex) and ropinirole (Requip) have been released for prescription use. All of these stimulate dopamine receptors to an increasing extent as one raises the dose; that is, higher doses produce a greater antiparkinsonian effect.

There is no milligram-to-milligram correspondence among these dopamine agonist drugs. In other words, 10 mg of one does not equal 10 mg of another. All four are similar in their effect when adjusted for these differences in potency. Some evidence, however, suggests that bromocriptine may be slightly less efficacious. It is the most expensive and currently is prescribed infrequently.

None of the dopamine agonist drugs is as potent as levodopa therapy. However, they do have a relatively long-lasting effect, often spanning many hours. Hence, one important role for these drugs has been as a supplement to levodopa, to smooth some of the ups and downs experienced later with levodopa treatment.

Some advocate starting one of these dopamine agonist drugs early in treatment to reduce the likelihood of the ups and downs of later levodopa treatment. Specifically, these are the motor fluctuations and dyskinesias that we just considered in the previous chapter. These tend to occur after a few years of levodopa treatment but are not a substantial problem for many people. Dopamine agonists are very useful once such problems occur. However, the crucial question is whether they should be started early in treatment to reduce the subsequent likelihood of these problems. Multiple clinical trials have shown that early dopamine agonist treatment is associated with a lower frequency of dyskinesias and motor fluctuations during the next several years. However, is it necessary to start the agonist initially to capture this benefit? Would you arrive at the same outcome if you started the agonist *after* the fluctuations or dyskinesias developed? Until the last decade, the conventional use of these dopamine agonists was exactly that; they were started when levodopa complications were noted, with concomitant adjustments of the levodopa doses. This is an effective treatment for these levodopa problems. Thus, it may not be necessary to use these drugs until dyskinesias or motor fluctuations develop; this remains a controversial issue.

A stronger argument can be made for initial therapy with a dopamine agonist in someone with young-onset PD, who has a much greater risk of experiencing dyskinesias and motor fluctuations. Young-onset PD is defined as symptoms beginning before age forty. Almost all in this age group will experience both dyskinesias and motor fluctuations by the time they have been treated with levodopa for five years. Using a dopamine agonist as their initial treatment makes sense; also those with symptoms starting a little after age 40 may also be appropriate candidates for a dopamine agonist. Regardless, if an agonist is started as the initial treatment, one can anticipate that levodopa will become necessary within a few years.

In the last chapter, we discussed evidence that two of these dopamine agonists, pramipexole and ropinirole, may slow PD progression. The jury is still out on this matter. However, this suggestive evidence makes these two drugs the obvious first choices if an agonist medication is chosen. This is not to say that pergolide and bromocriptine have no similar potential; however, neither has been studied in trials of PD progression. There are also other reasons to favor pramipexole and ropinirole, as we will subsequently discuss.

The dopamine agonist medications are all started in a very low dose. This is done to minimize nausea. The dose is then slowly increased over six to eight weeks or longer to arrive at the therapeutic range. The precise schemes for doing this are found in chapter 13. Unlike levodopa therapy, the dopamine agonist drugs do not interact with meals. In fact, to minimize nausea, each dose is usually taken after a meal. Since all four of the available dopamine agonist medications are conventionally taken three times daily, the recommendation is to take one dose after each meal.

The Most Common Mistake Involving Dopamine Agonist Medications

"I tried pramipexole (or ropinirole, pergolide, or bromocriptine) and it didn't help." I have heard this statement countless times in the clinic. A busy physician would be inclined to accept this and move on to another drug. However, one more question is necessary: How high was the dose? Most of the time, not high enough. Remember that these agonist drugs are started in a very low dose, which is too low to do any good. This is a setup for therapeutic failure because people often get stuck on these low doses. There are several reasons for this: (1) Expense: the starting doses of these drugs cost around $100 per month, despite being too low to be helpful. Some people assume that they are priced in proportion to benefit, which is not true for these low doses. (2) Complex dosing schedules: reaching the targeted dose requires six to eight weeks or longer. Moreover, multiple size pills are required to do this, switching from one size to another. Some people conclude that anything that complicated probably is not necessary. (3) Instruction cards supplied by the pharmaceutical companies: because the dose escalation schedules are long and complex, the instruction handouts from some of the drug companies only cover the first two to three weeks. Some people infer that these are the sufficient doses.

If one commits to starting one of these medications, it should be with the understanding that the dosage needs to be escalated far beyond the starting dose to capture the benefits. Also, recognize that the effect develops very gradually, making it more difficult to appreciate.

A Unique Dopamine Agonist: Apomorphine

Apomorphine is a dopamine agonist that has been used outside the United States for many years. Administration by mouth results in kidney toxicity, but it is safe when administered by injection. It is more potent than the four dopamine agonist drugs we discussed above. Injectable apomorphine has recently been approved by the United States Food and Drug Administration for rapid reversal of immobile parkinsonian states. Because of a brief effect (60–90 minutes), it won't be used for ongoing therapy, but rather saved for quick fixes (discussed in chapter 18). It is injected subcutaneously (under the skin).

Enzyme-Blocking Drugs

Dopamine and levodopa, like most other body chemicals, are constantly being manufactured and broken down. Specific enzymes mediate these breakdown processes. If the degradation of circulating levodopa or brain dopamine could be blocked, higher levels would result. These higher levels should theoretically translate into reduced symptoms of PD.

Specific enzymes convert levodopa and dopamine into inactive substances, as part of the natural sequence of biologic events. When levodopa or dopamine binds to one of these enzymes, it is chemically changed into something that is inert. Two specific brain enzymes carry on this breakdown: catechol-O-methyltransferase (COMT) and monoamine oxidase (MAO).

If these enzymes were blocked, then brain dopamine concentrations should rise and, in fact, that is the case. Hence, blocking these enzymes has been an additional strategy for treating PD. Recall that we block the enzyme, dopa decarboxylase, with carbidopa to enhance the levodopa response and prevent nausea. Similarly, these other enzymes can be blocked to reduce the breakdown of levodopa and dopamine.

Interestingly, drugs that block any of these enzymes, COMT, MAO, or dopa decarboxylase, do not substantially improve parkinsonism when given alone. However, they are effective when administered with levodopa therapy. We will now consider some of the specific drugs used for these purposes.

Catechol-O-methyltransferase (COMT) Inhibitors

Two COMT inhibitors are available as treatment for PD, entacapone (Comtan) and tolcapone (Tasmar). Entacapone does not readily cross the blood–brain barrier and its benefits derive from blocking COMT and protecting levodopa external to the brain. This results in a more sustained circulating levodopa level. Tolcapone does cross the blood–brain barrier and also blocks brain COMT, directly resulting in more sustained brain dopamine levels as well. Tolcapone is the more potent and effective of these two drugs. Each is used as a supplement to levodopa treatment.

One advantage of these drugs over the dopamine agonist medications is the ease of use. These drugs do not require dosage adjustments; the starting dose is the appropriate dose for maintenance. Entacapone enhances the levodopa effect for about four hours after administration. Hence, each dose is given with every dose of carbidopa/levodopa (unless carbidopa/levodopa is being taken at much less than four-hour intervals). Tolcapone has a longer effect and is given three times daily. Of note, these two drugs often enhance the levodopa effect enough to cause an excessive response with dyskinesias. Hence the levodopa dose may need to be reduced.

Despite better efficacy, tolcapone is not the preferred drug and this is because of side effects. Tolcapone has rarely induced severe liver problems, which in a few cases have been fatal. Although life-threatening liver toxicity with tolcapone is extremely rare, this has rendered this drug a second-line choice; if used, frequent monitoring of liver function (blood tests) is mandated. Entacapone has no known liver toxicity.

Recently a combination drug of carbidopa/levodopa and entacapone was released for prescription use under the brand name Stalevo. Its primary utility is ease of use since it combines two pills into one.

Monoamine Oxidase (MAO) Inhibitors

Brain MAO converts dopamine into an inactive substance. Blocking this enzyme raises brain dopamine levels. MAO also breaks down other substances similar to dopamine, including adrenalin (epinephrine). These adrenalin-like substances also are increased by drugs blocking MAO.

As we learned in an earlier chapter, there are two forms of MAO: MAO-A and MAO-B. There are also two types of available drugs, those that block both forms and those that block only MAO-B. Drugs that block both forms of MAO have been used for decades by psychiatrists to treat severe depression but have a potentially serious side effect spectrum. By also blocking MAO-A, they result in elevated concentrations of adrenalin-like substances in the bloodstream. If these adrenalin-like substances are markedly increased, severely elevated blood pressure may result. Clinicians have learned that special diets that are low in substances of this type allow these drugs to be used safely. However, cheating on this diet runs the risk of potentially life-threatening hypertension. These drugs are never used as treatment for PD because of this side effect, especially in conjunction with levodopa therapy.

MAO-B inhibitors, in contrast to drugs that block both MAO forms, are safe; they do not have the potential for severe high blood pressure elevations. These are used in the treatment of PD. One caveat, however, is that the MAO-B blocking drugs are safe only in conventional doses; if much higher doses are administered, they also block MAO-A and run the potential risk of severe blood pressure elevations.

Selegiline (Eldepryl) is the only currently available MAO-B inhibitor for treatment of PD. It initially went by the name "deprenyl," which is still found in the medical literature. When first introduced in the United States, there was circumstantial evidence suggesting that it might improve the long-term course of PD, as noted in the previous chapter. Multiple clinical studies have investigated this proposition and have largely failed to confirm it. Most clinicians now believe that any benefit from selegiline is from treating the symptoms of PD.

Selegiline increases brain dopamine levels and has a mild symptomatic effect. When used alone, in the absence of levodopa treatment, the symptomatic benefit is slight at best. However, improvement of parkinsonism does occur when added to levodopa therapy, although this benefit is still never marked.

Anticholinergic Medications

Dopamine is only one of several neurotransmitters released within the striatum to signal the next neuron in the sequence. Acetylcholine is another such neurotransmitter. Cells within the striatum that release acetylcholine are spared in PD. These are called cholinergic cells. In the normal situation, it appears that acetylcholine tends to counterbalance the effect of dopamine within the striatum. In other words, they tend to have opposite effects in this particular brain circuit. When dopamine is lost in PD, these cholinergic cells become more prominent in their effect and the previous balance is lost. Hence, you might expect that blocking acetylcholine would improve the symptoms of PD. As it turns out, this is the case.

Well before the advent of levodopa therapy, medications that block the effects of acetylcholine were used in the treatment of PD. These are called anticholinergic drugs. Prior to levodopa, they were largely all that was available for treatment. They have only limited benefit and now are used infrequently. Nonetheless, they do have roles in certain specific situations.

Anticholinergic medications improve only limited aspects of parkinsonism. They benefit tremor and to some extent the stiffness (rigidity). They also improve the cramp-like symptoms of dystonia that may also occur in PD (see below). They do not benefit other symptoms, such as slowness, walking problems, loss of arm swing, or facial animation. Hence, when prescribed, it is for treatment of tremor or dystonia. However, rarely are they more effective than other available drugs for these symptoms (e.g., levodopa). Occasionally they are also used for ancillary symptoms: excessive salivation or inappropriate urges to urinate; these drugs dry out the mouth and suppress the need to urinate.

Several anticholinergic drugs are available for treatment of PD, including trihexyphenidyl (Artane) and benztropine (Cogentin). Many drugs used for other purposes also have anticholinergic properties. One example is amitriptyline, an antidepressant that is also used for inducing sleep or suppressing urinary urges. Also, drugs directed at controlling urinary urgency and frequency have prominent anticholinergic properties, including oxybutynin (Ditropan) and tolterodine (Detrol). Drugs for urinary symptoms are discussed in more detail in chapter 27.

These anticholinergic drugs would be prescribed more often if it were not for the side effects. None are serious or life-threatening but are frequent and often troublesome. These include mild memory impairment, constipation, reduced ability to urinate, visual blurring, and dry mouth.

Drugs That Block Glutamate

Brain cells that release glutamate as the neurotransmitter are widespread in motor control systems. They are called glutamatergic neurons. There are intimate interactions of glutamatergic neurons with the nigrostriatal system. Animal models demonstrate that drugs blocking the effect of glutamate improve parkinsonism. However, the drugs that have been tested for this purpose have limiting side effects and are not available for prescription use.

Amantadine is a medication that has been used in the treatment of PD for more than thirty years. It is mildly helpful in reducing parkinsonian symptoms.

Until recently, the reason for the parkinsonian benefit was not fully under-stood. Now it is recognized as a mild blocker of glutamate. (Not all glutamate receptors are blocked by amantadine, but only a certain subclass.) Glutamate inhibition is thought to mediate the benefit of amantadine.

The primary role for amantadine at present is in the treatment of levodopa-induced dyskinesias, which are reduced by amantadine. Dyskinesias are invol-untary movements representing an excessive effect from levodopa treatment, which we will discuss below. However, sometimes reducing the levodopa dose enough to control the dyskinesias results in loss of the benefit. Amantadine is sometimes used in that setting where a certain dose of levodopa is necessary to control parkinsonism but which also causes dyskinesias.

Uneven Response to Medication: Dyskinesias, Dystonia, and Motor Fluctuations

Carbidopa/levodopa is the most effective medication for PD symptoms and the foundation of treatment. After several years or longer, the responses be-come less consistent with fluctuations in the benefit. As we just mentioned, involuntary movements representing excessive levodopa responses also occur, termed dyskinesias. Dyskinesias need to be distinguished from dystonias, which are abnormal postures or cramp-like states. They have a different origin than dyskinesias and usually indicate underdosing of levodopa. In this introductory treatment chapter, we would be remiss if we didn't discuss these problems in more detail since strategies for dealing with these are fundamental to treatment.

Dyskinesias

The term "dyskinesias" may be correctly used in a very general sense to imply any of a variety of involuntary movements. In the context of PD, however, the term "dyskinesias" has a very specific meaning. It refers to the choreiform move-ments that occur in response to an excessive medication effect. "Choreiform" implies flowing, dancing-like movements that are involuntary and purposeless. In this book, I use the term "dyskinesias" in this narrow sense to refer to these choreiform movements provoked by medications.

Often the person who has these dyskinesias is unaware of them. In fact they are often more bothersome to family or friends. They are painless and, if not severe, do not interfere with most activities. If marked, however, they can be both embarrassing and disabling. When pronounced, a person with dyskinesias seemingly cannot sit still. The arms or legs may be in constant motion and occasionally the head and face. Since levodopa is the most potent of the antiparkinsonian drugs, these dyskinetic movements are largely levodopa-induced. Although dopamine agonist drugs by themselves can provoke dyskinesias, this is very uncommon. However, they can exacerbate dyskinesias provoked by levodopa treatment.

Conceptually, these medication-induced dyskinesias are on the opposite end of the spectrum from the slowness that is typical of PD. The term for this slowness is "bradykinesia" (brady = slow; kinesia = movement). On a kinesia spectrum, too little movement reflects a low brain dopamine state; on the other end of the spectrum, too much movement reflects excessive brain dopamine (typically from levodopa). Thus, if we administer too much levodopa, dyskinesias result and the dose must be lowered to abolish them.

Dyskinesias rarely develop early in the course of PD but often surface after several years. By five years of levodopa therapy, about 40 percent of people will experience at least some dyskinesias. When they do occur, simply reducing the levodopa dose (or the dose of another medication) will abolish them. However, it is not always that simple. There is a distinct minority of people who have no happy medium between optimal control of their parkinsonism and dyskinesias. Usually this is after many years of treatment, but occasionally earlier. As soon as the levodopa dose is lowered and the dyskinesias go away, adequate control of the parkinsonism is lost. This subgroup of people require special measures and this will be addressed in subsequent treatment chapters.

Medication-induced dyskinesias are more common among younger people with PD. Among those whose PD symptoms started before age 40, at least mild dyskinesias are experienced by almost all after five years of levodopa treatment. Prevention of dyskinesias has been a frequent topic of discussion among those who treat PD. Dopamine agonist medications are less likely to induce dyskinesias. Should one start a dopamine agonist instead of levodopa therapy? Should one defer levodopa or keep the doses low? Do such strategies change the likelihood of dyskinesias appearing years later? If so, at what expense? The downside is that dopamine agonist therapy and low-dose levodopa may be inadequate to treat the symptoms of PD.

Since age seems to play a prominent role in the risk of dyskinesias, this is often used as a determining factor in medication choice. "Young-onset" PD (under 40) probably deserves an initial trial of a dopamine agonist drug, saving levodopa for later. If this is sufficient to control the symptoms, then the risk of dyskinesias will be very low for as long as levodopa treatment can be deferred. However, most people cannot adequately control their parkinsonism on dopamine agonist therapy indefinitely; they will require levodopa within a few years in most cases. Thus, as a long-term strategy, this has limitations.

In contrast, when PD starts later in life, it is reasonable to start with levodopa treatment, since this is the most effective drug and the one most likely to keep people mobile and active. The controversy relates to where you draw the line between "early" and "later" in life. Should we use the dopamine agonists first only among those whose PD symptoms started before age 40? Should we extend that to age 50? Or 55? This topic is discussed in more detail in subsequent chapters.

Dystonia

Dystonia is a specific type of involuntary movement. Sometimes this is lumped together with dyskinesias; however, this is conceptually incorrect. We will use these terms separately in this book. They are actually two opposite problems and best not confused.

Dystonia represents a muscle contraction state. Muscles that should be relaxed are tensed and tight. Sometimes it feels like a cramp and may be painful. However, dystonia differs from typical cramps in a couple of ways. First, it tends to be sustained, whereas the usual cramps we all experience resolve when we stretch the muscle. Second, dystonia typically twists, turns, or contorts some part of your body. PD-related dystonias are often experienced in the lower limbs, such as sustained toe curling or extension, foot in-turning, and calf cramp-like states.

Dystonias of this type are rarely medication side effects (in contrast to the choreiform dyskinesias described previously). Rather, they are features of the underlying parkinsonism and typically reflect an untreated or undertreated state. These may develop several hours after a dose of levodopa, when the effect has worn off. Thus, they are often experienced during the night or early morning, many hours after the last levodopa dose. They may also be seen throughout the day when someone is underdosed or untreated.

Those who have prominent dyskinesias from levodopa treatment display flowing, dancing movements of their limbs, trunk, or neck, head, and face. These are the typical "choreiform" dyskinesias we described earlier. When these are seen, the keen observer may also notice that there may also be some sustained muscle contractions, such as an arm involuntarily pulled backward (typically painless). Strictly speaking, one should call this dystonia. However, if it is keeping company with the rapidly flowing, dancing movements, then it likely is a side effect from the medication, as opposed to an underdosed state. Thus, it should be included in the medication-related dyskinesia category. Table 10.1 summarizes the distinction between these two forms of involuntary movements: medication-induced dyskinesias and dystonia.

Dystonia may be seen apart from PD as an independent condition. There are a variety of primary dystonic conditions that have nothing to do with PD. Hence, if someone has dystonia, this does not usually imply that he or she has PD.

Motor Fluctuations

The term "motor fluctuations" does not imply an involuntary movement. It refers to waxing and waning of the beneficial effect from PD medications, primarily levodopa. This does not develop early in PD but becomes apparent

Table 10.1.   Distinguishing Levodopa-Induced Dyskinesias from Parkinson's Disease-Related Dystonia

	Levodopa-Induced Dyskinesias*	Dystonia
Appearance	Predominantly chorea: rapidly flowing, dancing, involuntary movements**	Sustained muscle contraction causing twisting, turning, or contortion; for example, toes curled or turned up; foot turned in
Relationship to levodopa	Caused by this	Usually relieved by this
Relation to timing of levodopa	Starts within 30 minutes to 2 hours after a dose of levodopa; resolves within a few hours or less	Tends to start several hours after last levodopa dose (time of wearing off); if no or insufficient levodopa, may be present continuously
Morning, before medications	Absent, unless levodopa during the night	Often present if no levodopa during the night
Pain	No (extremely rare)	Yes (often)
Treatment	Lower the levodopa dose	Raise the levodopa dose or give more frequent doses

*Although primarily caused by levodopa, the dopamine agonist drugs may also induce dyskinesias. Any supplemental drugs added to levodopa will potentially increase dyskinesia severity.

**Dyskinesias resulting from levodopa are predominantly chorea; however, there may be a superimposed abnormal sustained posture of an arm or leg; strictly speaking, this is categorized as dystonia; however, the main feature is chorea. If there is prominent chorea, then the movements are almost certainly due to levodopa and related medications.

after several years. Similar to the incidence of dyskinesias, motor fluctuations occur in about 40 percent of people by five years of levodopa treatment. The incidence continues to slowly increase thereafter.

For some people, these motor fluctuations are not of any consequence. At the other extreme, some experience striking transitions between near normality and prominent parkinsonism. They may be in good shape one minute but parkinsonian several minutes later. These people must keep a close eye on their carbidopa/levodopa dosing schedule so that they maintain a consistent effect and avoid downtime; however, even with meticulous attention to this schedule, there may still be gaps in their coverage. This occurs to variable degrees, and for a distinct minority of people, this is a substantial problem.

Motor fluctuations relate to the way the brain responds to levodopa, which changes over the course of PD. During the early years of PD, levodopa administration produces a very sustained response. Thus, on a given daily dose, it takes about a week to achieve the full effect; if the dose is changed, it will take about another week for the effect to become fully established. If the person misses a dose, no change occurs (provided that not too many are missed). In other words, the response during the first several years of PD is not linked to each individual dose of levodopa. If levodopa treatment is stopped, conversely, it will take a week or so to return to baseline. This cumulative effect from levodopa treatment is termed the long-duration response.

After some years, the beneficial response to levodopa tends to become time-locked to each dose. Although people retain some of their long-duration levodopa effect, part of the benefit comes in the form of a short-duration response. Thus people will become parkinsonian if they have not taken their medication for several hours. Once taken, the parkinsonism will abate for several hours and then this effect will wear off; this requires another dose to recapture the effect. The term "wearing-off" is commonly used in PD circles and refers to this process.

This short-duration response may further shorten over the course of years. Some people may eventually need to take their carbidopa/levodopa at very brief intervals to maintain consistent coverage, perhaps every two hours or so.

There is a language of PD that is used to characterize the dynamics of this process. As already noted, the term "motor fluctuations" reflects the coming and going of the levodopa effect. This occurs if the interval between levodopa doses exceeds the short-duration levodopa response. We then say that the effect has "worn off." This is referred to as an "off-state," and people may comment that they are "off." Conversely, when the medication is working and the parkinsonism is controlled, we call this the "on-state"; people say they are "on." These are universal terms used in parkinsonian circles.

What Causes Motor Fluctuations?

These motor fluctuations and dyskinesias do not represent some type of toxic effect from the medications. Instead, they likely represent the interaction of chronic levodopa treatment with the natural progression of PD. Probably the primary cause is a reduced capacity to store dopamine within brain dopaminergic terminals (i.e., dopamine generated from levodopa). Early in PD, there are still sufficient remaining dopaminergic terminals within the striatum to store and release dopamine in a natural fashion. The progressive loss of this nigrostriatal system, however, requires other cells to subsequently participate. Thus nondopaminergic cells eventually become responsible for generating, storing, and releasing dopamine and are much less efficient. Instead of a natural, steady release and subsequent clearance of dopamine from the synapse, boluses of dopamine now bombard the receptor; they presumably stimulate excessively (and induce dyskinesias) and then quickly dissipate, resulting in loss of the effect (wearing-off). These nondopaminergic cells are simply not designed to slowly and continuously release dopamine or to appropriately remove the excess from the synapse. The ultimate consequences are motor fluctuations and dyskinesias. This process is exacerbated by the pulsatile and uneven stimulation of the dopamine receptors, which we know enhances the sensitivity and lability of these brain circuits.

Table 10.2. Medications for the Symptomatic Treatment of Parkinson's Disease

Class of Medication	Mechanism of Action	Available Medications
Dopamine precursor	Replenishes brain dopamine	Levodopa (carbidopa/levodopa)*
Dopamine agonist	Synthetic form of dopamine	Bromocriptine (Parlodel) Pergolide (Permax) Pramipexole (Mirapex) Ropinirole (Requip)
Unique dopamine agonist	Same, but administered only by injection	Apomorphine
Catechol-O-methyltransferase (COMT) inhibitor	Blocks an enzyme that breaks down levodopa and dopamine	Entacapone (Comtan)** Tolcapone (Tasmar)** Carbidopa/levodopa—Entacapone (Stalevo)
Monoamine oxidase B (MAO-B) inhibitor	Blocks an enzyme that breaks down brain dopamine	Selegiline (Eldepryl)***
Anticholinergic	Blocks some of the effects of the brain neurotransmitter acetylcholine	Trihexyphenidyl (Artane) Benztropine (Cogentin) Other drugs also with anticholinergic effect
Antiglutamate (glutamate antagonist)	Blocks some of the effects of the brain neurotransmitter, glutamate	Amantadine

*In Europe, benserazide/levodopa.

**Entacapone only works on circulating levodopa, partially preventing its breakdown; tolcapone also blocks COMT in the brain and partially prevents brain dopamine breakdown.

***Older name for this is deprenyl.

Supplementary Medications for Motor Fluctuations

Motor fluctuations can be managed by levodopa adjustments. However, it was especially for this problem that most of the other drugs discussed above were developed (see table 10.2). The dopamine agonist medications are the most effective supplements to levodopa for this purpose. They have a longer duration of action than the short-duration levodopa effects. Typically, these are slowly introduced, and when the dosage moves into the therapeutic range, the levodopa dosage is lowered.

The COMT inhibitor drugs (see table 10.2) were also introduced for the purpose of prolonging the levodopa responses. They are easier to use than the dopamine agonist drugs but not quite as effective. The currently available MAO-B inhibitor, selegiline, is only mildly helpful in smoothing out the levodopa response.

Exactly when a supplementary medication should be added to counter levodopa motor fluctuations is a little arbitrary. Often it is easiest and quickest to adjust the levodopa dosing schedule. We will discuss these different medication strategies in detail in subsequent chapters.

Supplementary Medications for Dyskinesias

The primary strategy for eliminating or reducing dyskinesias is reduction of the levodopa dosage. Amantadine is the only supplementary drug that has consistent efficacy in reducing dyskinesias; however, the benefit is only partial. More is said about treatment of dyskinesias in chapters 17–18.

11

♦ ♦ ♦

Starting Treatment of Movement Problems: Which Drug and When?

Now we are ready to address practical issues. If you have read the previous chapters, you should have a good background for the subject of this chapter.

Who Needs to Be Treated?

Having Parkinson's disease (PD) does not mean you must start on a medication. If we had drugs that slowed the progression of PD, then beginning them at the first sign of parkinsonism would obviously be important. Although some drugs have been touted to slow PD progression (such as pramipexole and ropinirole), compelling proof is lacking. Your symptoms determine when to start a medication for PD. If the symptoms don't bother you, medications can be deferred. Sooner or later a medication will become necessary, but this can be put off until the symptoms get in the way.

When to start medical therapy and how aggressively to treat depends on the individual circumstances; there is no one-size-fits-all approach. Treatment decisions should be based on the following premise: the goal of medical treatment is to keep those with PD in the mainstream of life. Occupational, social, and recreational pursuits are each important and should factor into the decision. Hence it is not simply the severity of the symptoms but how they affect your life. Consider two people each with the same problem: parkinsonism primarily limited to a resting tremor in one hand.

- Mrs. Jones is a trial lawyer. She is concerned that juries are focusing on that tremor, distracting them from her arguments. She is worried that they interpret this as a sign of nervousness and insecurity.
- Mr. Smith is a semiretired farmer (farmers never completely retire). His farm work is not compromised. His buddies, whom he meets at the coffee shop in town each morning, are interested in discussing farm politics; his tremor is ignored.

Mrs. Jones deserves treatment; she is worried about her law practice. Mr. Smith, with the same symptoms, is not bothered and treatment can appropriately be deferred. On the other hand, if Mr. Smith became self-conscious about his tremor and avoided going out, treatment would be appropriate.

Should We Save the Best Drugs for Later?

Medications are most effective during the first several years of PD. This is not to say that they are not effective later on. They often can keep people in the mainstream of life for many years. However, after a number of years, the effect is typically not as complete. Moreover, dyskinesias and motor fluctuations may develop, as noted in the previous two chapters. Even then, however, the wheels do not fall off the wagon. Although management becomes

Table 11.1. Motor Complications That May Develop After Years of Levodopa Treatment

Problem	Description	Levodopa and Dopamine Agonist Treatment Strategies to Reduce or Eliminate*
Dyskinesias	Involuntary movements, reflecting an excessive medication effect	1. Reduce the levodopa dose (always effective, but may result in recurrence of parkinsonism in some cases). 2. Add a dopamine agonist drug and lower the dose of levodopa.
Motor fluctuations	The beneficial effect becomes tied to each dose of carbidopa/ levodopa.	1. Adjust the interval between levodopa doses to match the duration of each response. 2. Add a dopamine agonist drug.

*These and other strategies are described in detail in subsequent chapters.

more complicated, the medication strategies often reverse many of these set-backs, as summarized in table 11.1.

Why are the medications less completely and consistently effective after many years? As explained in the previous chapter, this is primarily due to disease progression rather than being a function of the number of years someone has taken these drugs.

Older guidelines for treating PD often suggested that the best drugs, especially levodopa therapy, should be deferred until absolutely necessary. However, there is now increasing recognition that the slow progression of PD continues, regardless of whether we treat conservatively or aggressively early in the course. If we choose to suffer now, hoping to capture the best responses later, we may have done this for naught; we probably have lost an opportunity.

How Aggressive Should We Be When Starting Treatment?

The drugs that we could start for parkinsonism have quite different efficacies. Should we start with a minimally effective drug first and work toward the more potent? How aggressive we decide to be varies with the circumstances. Remember that the treatment goal is to keep people within the mainstream of their lives. If you are only marginally affected by parkinsonism, it is not crucial that we select a potent medication. However, if you are seriously challenged by parkinsonism, you will want the drug that works best.

The element of time and your own sense of urgency are also factors in selecting a drug. If we start with a low-potency drug and this proves insufficient, then another drug can be initiated. In some cases this is not a problem, but it may be in others. Consider several examples.

- How about our trial lawyer, Mrs. Jones? If she has a big case coming to trial in a month, time may be crucial to her. She needs to control her tremor and do this quickly. We may not have the luxury of using a lower potency drug, taking the time to adjust it, and then find out that another medication is necessary.

- Consider elderly Mr. Brown, who never sees doctors and doesn't particularly trust them. He came to the clinic only because his family insisted. The insightful physician knows that a low-potency drug will perhaps be discontinued and Mr. Brown may go another three years before he sees the doctor again.

- Finally, there is Mrs. Johnson, who lives in a rural area, far from her doctor and with limited transportation. Her physician recognizes that there will be few opportunities for interaction. Hence, a simpler more effective treatment strategy may be preferable.

Social and occupational circumstances influence medical treatment of PD. Fiddling with lower-potency drugs may not be expedient or practical in some circumstances.

What Are Our Choices?

Several drugs could appropriately be started as symptomatic treatment for PD and these are listed in table 11.2. It is from this list that we must choose a medication, but which one? Levodopa (carbidopa/levodopa) is the most potent, as we have discussed in previous chapters. Some physicians would favor the dopamine agonist drugs, pramipexole or ropinirole, because of the studies suggesting that they may influence the progression of PD and forestall levodopa complications (see chapters 9–10). Amantadine, selegiline, and the anticholinergic drugs (trihexyphenidyl and benztropine) are substantially less effective, but are simple to use. Note that we have not listed coenzyme Q_{10} in table 11.2 since the treatment evidence is preliminary; this may change in the future.

Which Drug to Start?

Table 11.2 gives us a lot of choices. Let's take a logical approach and narrow this down. First, let's cross the anticholinergic drugs off our list. Their benefit is usually limited and they have substantial side effects, including constipation, dry mouth, visual blurring, and memory deficits. If your physician chooses one of these as initial treatment, be aware of these potential side effects, so that if they develop, they do not become confused with the symptoms of PD.

Second, there is a very limited role for amantadine or selegiline as the first symptomatic treatment. Their advantage is that they are easy to use and the dosage adjustments are minimal, as shown in table 11.3. However, the improvement of symptoms is modest, at best, and they are usually insufficient beyond a year or two. As we discussed in chapter 9, indirect evidence raises speculation that they might slow the progression of PD, but this is without proof. Amantadine or selegiline is an acceptable choice for people with minimal PD symptoms, and this was my practice in years past; however, I no longer prescribe these as initial treatment since their benefits are marginal. Hence, we will also cross these drugs off our list, except for occasional people with very mild symptoms who wish to start a simple treatment.

We will also cross off our list two of the dopamine agonist drugs, pergolide and bromocriptine. They may be appropriate later in treatment but not as initial treatment of PD. Although they are approximately as effective in treating PD symptoms as pramipexole and ropinirole, they come in a distinct second for three reasons. First, preliminary evidence suggests that pramipexole

Table 11.2. Initial Symptomatic Treatment of PD (Available Drugs)*

Class of Drug	Brand Name	Effectiveness Against Parkinsonism	Duration Required to Escalate to Therapeutic Dose
Levodopa			
Carbidopa/levodopa	Sinemet	Marked	3–5 weeks
Dopamine agonist			
Bromocriptine	Parlodel	Moderate	4–8 weeks
Pergolide	Permax	Moderate	4–8 weeks
Pramipexole	Mirapex	Moderate	4–8 weeks
Ropinirole	Requip	Moderate	4–8 weeks
Glutamate blocker			
Amantadine	—	Mild	Immediate to a few weeks
MAO-B blocker			
Selegiline	Eldepryl	Mild	Immediate
Anticholinergics**			
Trihexyphenidyl	Artane	Mild	1–3 weeks
Benztropine	Cogentin	Mild	1–3 weeks

*The role for the nonprescription agent, coenzyme Q_{10}, has yet to be determined and, hence, isn't included here.

**These are primarily helpful for tremor and dystonia. Side effects limit utility as initial therapy. Several other anticholinergic drugs are also available.

Table 11.3. Initial Therapy with Minor Drugs

Medication	Tablet Size	Starting Dose	Adjustments	Side Effects
Selegiline (Eldepryl)	5 mg	One tablet each morning*	None necessary	Insomnia (hence administered in the morning)
Amantadine	100 mg	One tablet daily	May increase to 1 tablet 3 times daily	Purple or reddish discoloration of legs (not serious)

*Conventionally the dosage is one tablet in the morning and a second at noon; however, the primary effect of blocking MAO-B is fully present with a single tablet once daily. Rarely do people note any difference in their symptoms if switched between one and two selegiline tablets daily.

and ropinirole may have a favorable effect on PD progression. Although this is far from proven, this places them in an advantageous position over pergolide and bromocriptine. Pergolide and bromocriptine have never been studied in clinical trials of PD progression and if they had, perhaps similar results might have been reported. However, the current evidence rests with pramipexole and ropinirole.

Second, in rare cases, pergolide and bromocriptine have caused inflammation and scarring of the lungs, heart (heart lining and valves), and back of the abdomen (affecting drainage of urine from kidney to bladder). Exactly how often this occurs is not precisely known. Until recently, the risk was thought to be very low, on the order of one person in a hundred (1 percent). Recent preliminary evidence among people taking pergolide suggests that heart valve damage may be substantially more frequent.

Third, pergolide and bromocriptine are much more expensive than pramipexole and ropinirole, without any advantages.

In summary, we are left with pramipexole, ropinirole, and carbidopa/levodopa as appropriate choices for starting treatment of PD.

Levodopa Versus Pramipexole or Ropinirole as Initial Treatment

Levodopa (carbidopa/levodopa) is the most potent and effective drug for PD. Even if we begin with pramipexole or ropinirole, few with PD can go without levodopa therapy after a few years. Why not just start with levodopa? Moreover, carbidopa/levodopa is easier to use (much less complex dosing schedule) and much less expensive. Arguments for pramipexole and ropinirole as first treatment are twofold: (1) They may slow disease progression (controversial) and (2) a lower frequency of dyskinesias and motor fluctuations several years hence, compared to levodopa. We have already considered the evidence that these drugs may slow the progression of PD in chapter 9, so we won't repeat that discussion. Whether this actually occurs is anyone's guess, and, even if true, the effect was rather modest.

What about the second argument that initial pramipexole or ropinirole treatment results in fewer dyskinesias and motor fluctuations after several years? We discussed this controversy in the last chapter, but let's be certain that you know the relevant facts. Clinical evidence is indeed clear that about 40 percent of people will begin to experience these problems after approximately five years of levodopa treatment; this is in contrast to about 5 percent or less with the dopamine agonists as initial therapy. Now let's place this in a broader perspective.

- This very low frequency of dyskinesias and motor fluctuations is true only if the dopamine agonist drug is administered alone; if combined with levodopa therapy, the incidence markedly rises, although not quite as high as with carbidopa/levodopa alone.

- Pramipexole or ropinirole therapy alone is usually adequate for a couple of years; a minority can get by for three to four years. In clinical trials, the vast majority require levodopa treatment by five years.

- For many people, these dyskinesias and fluctuations are mild and inconsequential, or easily corrected by medication adjustments. The five-year, 40 percent incidence statistic (cited above) relates to the first occurrence, regardless of severity or persistence. The risk of truly troublesome problems, or those that cannot be controlled with medication adjustments, is much lower.

- Control of PD symptoms is less satisfactory with the combination of dopamine agonist plus levodopa, compared to levodopa alone. Thus, although the risk of dyskinesias or motor fluctuations is less with this combination of drugs, they not as effective in treating parkinsonism in clinical trials.

- There is no evidence that the dopamine agonist must be started initially to capture this lower frequency of dyskinesias or motor fluctuations. The outcomes might be the same if levodopa was the initial drug, and the agonist added later (after these problems developed).

Thus dyskinesias and motor fluctuations are not a major problem during the first five years of levodopa treatment in most people. On the other hand, dopamine agonist therapy alone is rarely sufficient beyond four to five years. The combination of these therapies is associated with a lower frequency of dyskinesias and fluctuations, but not necessarily requiring that the agonist be the first drug.

The Influence of Age on Dyskinesias and Motor Fluctuations

Parkinsonism starting prior to age 40 is categorized as "young-onset" PD. This is uncommon, but this group of people has been carefully studied. They have different patterns of progression and response to medications. They are more likely to experience a sustained response to levodopa for many years but also are much more likely to develop levodopa-related dyskinesias and motor fluctuations. In fact, studies have revealed that almost all with young-onset PD will experience at least some degree of dyskinesias and motor fluctuations by five years of levodopa treatment.

This extremely high likelihood of early levodopa motor complications in young-onset PD dictates a different treatment strategy. In this group, a dopamine agonist drug is a sensible choice for initial treatment. Levodopa will eventually prove necessary, but some get by for a few years without motor complications by using dopamine agonist therapy alone. Admittedly, not all will find dopamine agonists sufficient. Adherence to the dictum of keeping you in the mainstream of your life may not be possible with these drugs alone, or side effects may limit their use. Hence, levodopa treatment may be appropriate early in the course if the agonist drugs are failing.

If dyskinesias and motor fluctuations are common among those less than forty treated with levodopa, what about those slightly older? Is there a sharp cut-off at forty? Will someone whose symptoms start at forty-one respond to levodopa very differently than someone with symptoms that begin at thirty-nine years? Common sense and clinical experience argue against any sharp demarcation. The categorization is arbitrary and simply reflects the way that investigators choose to group people in clinical studies. Rather, there is a gradual shift in the way people respond to levodopa as the age of onset increases beyond forty. However, no published studies have evaluated risks of levodopa motor complications by age groupings beyond forty years.

As already noted, the likelihood of dyskinesias or motor fluctuations is about 40 percent after five years of levodopa treatment. This figure was derived from multiple studies that included people with PD of all ages and is an average. Since more than 80 percent of people with PD develop their first symptoms after sixty, this figure is probably most representative of those in this age group, with onset after sixty. Presumably those who first develop parkinsonism between ages forty and sixty have an intermediate likelihood of dyskinesias and motor fluctuations early in treatment. In other words, their risk is not as high as those with onset before forty years, but probably higher than the cited 40 percent after five years of levodopa.

As we age, medications are more likely to cause side effects and this is also true for PD drugs (the sole exception is the predisposition to dyskinesias and motor fluctuations among young people). Hence, it is often wisest to keep our medication choices simpler during the senior years. Because of this and because of lower risks of dyskinesias and motor fluctuations among seniors, carbidopa/levodopa is often a better choice. Few would quarrel with carbidopa/levodopa as initial treatment for those seventy and beyond. In selected seniors, a dopamine agonist may be added later in certain circumstances.

Summary: Influence of Age on Initial Medication Choices

Focusing solely on age, dopamine agonist drugs are a reasonable first choice for those whose PD started before forty. Conversely, carbidopa/levodopa is a reasonable starting drug for those over seventy. In between these ages, the choice is based on your interpretation of the arguments we have made for carbidopa/levodopa versus dopamine agonist treatment. However, we aren't done with our comparisons. Let's consider side effects in more detail.

Unique Side Effects of Pramipexole and Ropinirole

Because levodopa and dopamine agonist drugs both work through dopamine systems, they share many of the same side effects. However, recent head-to-head comparisons of carbidopa/levodopa versus pramipexole or ropinirole revealed notable differences. First, the likelihood of hallucinations appears to be about three times as likely with either pramipexole or ropinirole. People prone to hallucinations or delusions (e.g., paranoia) are poor candidates for these two drugs. Also, those with thinking and memory difficulty are predisposed to hallucinations and these medications may not be a good choice for them either. Drowsiness is also more common with pramipexole and ropinirole treatment. Daytime sleepiness is common among those with PD, even in the absence of medications. However, pramipexole and ropinirole may cause or exacerbate this more frequently than any of the other drugs for PD. Cases of "sleep attacks" resulting in automobile accidents have been reported with these two drugs. Compulsive gambling has been a reported side effect from pramipexole therapy and I have encountered several people where this was clearly the case. Finally, swelling of the legs is more common with these agonist drugs, but this is not a serious problem.

Carbidopa/levodopa, pramipexole, and ropinirole all share potential to lower the blood pressure in the standing position (so-called orthostatic hypotension). If this is likely to be problematic, it is much easier to manage both this and the parkinsonism with carbidopa/levodopa alone. A low blood pressure on standing is common and must be considered before starting any treatment for PD; we will give this more attention later in this chapter.

Pramipexole Versus Ropinirole

To this point, we have narrowed our choices down to three drugs: carbidopa/levodopa, pramipexole, and ropinirole. However, two of these are almost identical, pramipexole and ropinirole; there is very little to recommend one over the other. Pramipexole, however, has a slight edge in that it is less complex to use. The escalation from the initial starting dose to the target dose can be done more simply with pramipexole. Pramipexole tablets, but not ropinirole, are scored in the middle; hence, the pramipexole dosage scheme requires fewer pill sizes to advance to the target dose. The dosing schedules for these two drugs are shown in chapter 13. If you have considered all the facts and have decided to go with a dopamine agonist medication, either pramipexole or ropinirole would be a reasonable choice.

Totaling Up the Differences: Carbidopa/Levodopa Versus Pramipexole or Ropinirole

We've considered a variety of issues that influence our treatment decision. If you think this is a little confusing, you're not alone; physicians are confronted with the same issues and debate the merits. To simplify, the primary arguments for each are listed in table 11.4. Take a look at these and we will now try to help you finalize your choice.

Table 11.4. Choice of the Initial Treatment of PD: Comparisons

Advantages of Carbidopa/Levodopa	Advantages of Pramipexole, Ropinirole
• More effective • Simpler to use • Cheaper • Lower likelihood of hallucinations • Lower likelihood of daytime sleepiness	• May slow progression (unproven) • Lower likelihood of dyskinesias • Lower likelihood of motor fluctuations

The Final Verdict: Which Drug to Choose?

Medications for PD may be deferred if people are functioning well in their personal life, including the workplace. When symptoms become significant and demand treatment, the primary decision is whether to start carbidopa/levodopa or a dopamine agonist drug. We are now going to go over the factors that weigh in on this decision. These are summarized in table 11.5.

Age is perhaps the most important consideration in choice of drug. We simplified this by constructing concrete guidelines: those under age forty should probably start pramipexole or ropinirole; carbidopa/levodopa is the best choice for those over seventy. However, what about those in between? To make that decision, we must factor in all the pluses and minuses as well as situational factors that we have discussed. In my practice, I discuss this with the patient in my office (and family, if they are present); I like them to be a party to the decision. Sometimes I think people get a little confused and overwhelmed by the myriad of facts that I present during such an office visit; this is a lot to assimilate in a short time. However, that's why I wrote this book—so that the arguments can be reviewed and given thoughtful consideration at your leisure.

Table 11.5.　Which Drug to Start First for Treatment of Parkinsonism

Category	Preferable Drug
Age (years)	
Less than 40	Pramipexole or ropinirole
40–60	?
60–70	Often carbidopa/levodopa
Older than 70	Carbidopa/levodopa
Prone to hallucinations, paranoia, delusions	Carbidopa/levodopa
Prominent thinking and memory problems	Carbidopa/levodopa
Excessive daytime sleepiness	Probably carbidopa/levodopa
Low standing blood pressure (systolic below 100)	Carbidopa/levodopa
Imperative to control parkinsonism as completely and quickly as possible	Carbidopa/levodopa
Limited income and must pay for medications	Carbidopa/levodopa

In my office practice, the medication choice varies with the age group but also reflects my own biases based on my cumulative experience. Once we have reviewed the pros and cons of the medication alternatives, the breakdown of medication choices for those I treat is approximately as follows.

- The vast majority of people over sixty are started on carbidopa/levodopa (assuming they are in agreement, following our discussion).

- Those between fifty and sixty are slightly more likely to be started on carbidopa/levodopa.

- About half of those between forty and fifty are started on a dopamine agonist (about half choose this after hearing the arguments).

I'm a believer in the adage "a bird in the hand is worth two in the bush." Hence, if there are some important practical consequences favoring the more potent drug, carbidopa/levodopa, I encourage that over hypothetical arguments relating to long-term speculation. I tend to favor carbidopa/levodopa if there is any indecision, since this is such an effective drug and has a thirty-year track record. Bear in mind that the advantages of early dopamine agonist drug treatment are not proven and you must accept some of this on faith. Personally, I like people helping me make the choice, since they will be taking the medication and experiencing the benefits or side effects.

Age is not the only issue in choosing the initial treatment. Let's consider some of the other practical factors entering into the equation about your choice of drug. How severe is the parkinsonism? If the problems are quite troublesome, this weighs in favor of the more potent levodopa treatment. What is the time frame we have for treatment? If occupation or other factors demand rapid and effective treatment, levodopa is preferable. Consider our trial lawyer, Mrs. Jones. If the biggest court trial of her life starts in one month and she positively must be at the top of her game, a dopamine agonist (pramipexole or ropinirole) is not a good choice for two reasons.

- It takes five to eight weeks to raise the agonist dose to appropriate levels using conventional dosing strategies. Levodopa adjustment takes about half as long.

- The agonists are not as potent as levodopa and the control of symptoms may be incomplete. Levodopa could then be added, but that would be too late for her needs.

Will subsequent physician consultations be possible? The agonist drugs require more fine-tuning than carbidopa/levodopa. This will entail two or more additional visits to a physician. Carbidopa/levodopa is much easier to use. If given good instructions, most people will arrive at the appropriate dose and require only one follow-up visit.

My personal strategy is outlined in table 11.6.

The Final Caveat: The Potential for Low Blood Pressure

Before you start any drug, remind your doctor to check your blood pressure in the standing position. Then repeat this after the medication is started and when the dose is raised. Why? People with PD are prone to orthostatic hypotension (orthostatic = standing; hypotension = low blood pressure) for two reasons. (1) PD affects the autonomic nervous system, which controls blood pressure and predisposes to this problem (see chapter 3). (2) Carbidopa/levodopa and dopamine agonist therapy exacerbate orthostatic hypotension.

If the blood pressure is too low, you will experience light-headedness or fatigue; if extremely low, you may faint. Orthostatic hypotension is often missed because blood pressure is usually checked only in the sitting position, where it may be normal. Furthermore, if checked many hours after the last dose of carbidopa/levodopa, pramipexole, or ropinirole, it may be missed; these low pressures are usually present for no more than a few hours after each medication dose.

How Low Is Too Low?

As a general rule of thumb, if the standing systolic blood pressure is at least 90, people will feel fine (the systolic blood pressure is the upper number in

Table 11.6. My Personal Strategy for Choosing the Initial Medication: Carbidopa/Levodopa Versus Dopamine Agonist
(Pramipexole* or Ropinirole)

Age	Medication Choice	Considerations
Any age, but with history of hallucinations, paranoia, major thinking or memory deficits, excessive sleepiness, or very low blood pressure	Carbidopa/ levodopa	Dopamine agonists are much more likely to aggravate these problems. Low blood pressure (orthostatic hypotension) is often hard to manage with any of these drugs, but is more complicated with the dopamine agonists.
Less than 40 years	Dopamine agonist	
Over 70 years	Carbidopa/ levodopa	
Between 40 and 60	Dopamine agonist or carbidopa/ levodopa	A dopamine agonist is started if all 6 criteria are satisfied: 1. Person accepts "on faith" that initial agonist therapy may confer long-term benefit.** 2. Parkinsonism is no worse than moderately severe. 3. No urgency to treat. 4. Able to return to physician. 5. Money is not an issue. 6. The person being treated is satisfied with a less potent drug. Otherwise carbidopa/levodopa is the initial choice.
From 60 to 70 years	Usually carbidopa/ levodopa	I discuss the arguments for dopamine agonist therapy but usually opt for carbidopa/ levodopa if that person has no strong convictions about this.

*Pramipexole is easier to initiate and adjust than ropinirole. The tablets are scored in the middle and can easily be broken in half to assist with medication adjustments. Complete escalation to the therapeutic dose can be made with fewer pill sizes and less complexity than with ropinirole. They are essentially identical in potency and side effects (after adjusting for differences in mg).

**The long-term benefits are potentially twofold: (1) slowed progression of PD (unproven); (2) lesser likelihood of later dyskinesias and motor fluctuations (which may be just as effectively treated if the dopamine agonist is started later, only after these problems develop).

blood pressure readings, such as 120 in 120/80); systolic readings below 90 tend to result in symptoms. Recognizing that carbidopa/levodopa or the dopamine agonist will lower the blood pressure, we obviously want a slightly higher reading before starting these drugs, to allow for this drop. I like to see the standing systolic blood pressure over 100 before medications are begun, which gives us a little wiggle room.

What If My Standing Systolic Blood Pressure Is Less Than 100?

If your standing blood pressure is below 100, then you should review all your medications with your physician to determine if another prescription drug is contributing; if so, perhaps this could be discontinued. Sometimes, people are maintained on medications they no longer need, such as water pills (diuretics), blood pressure medications, and so on. Drugs that are common offenders are listed in chapter 21. If a medication cannot be eliminated to raise your systolic blood pressure over 100, the strategy I then employ is as follows.

- My choice of initial medication for PD treatment is carbidopa/levodopa. Both levodopa and the dopamine agonists lower blood pressure; however, there is proportionately better control of parkinsonism with levodopa. If pramipexole or ropinirole are started, levodopa will be necessary within a few years and the blood pressure will be extremely hard to control with the combination of drugs.

- The *standing* blood pressure should be checked frequently, including a couple of hours after carbidopa/levodopa doses. Carbidopa/levodopa will tend to lower it for a few hours following a dose, with a return to baseline after that. Probably the lowest blood pressures will be found after breakfast and this is a good time to check it (assuming you took your carbidopa/levodopa an hour before breakfast).

- Increase your salt intake and drink a lot of fluids (perhaps 6 to 8 tall glasses daily).

- If your systolic blood pressures are frequently less than 90 (standing), then review chapter 21 on dizziness, which discusses additional measures for maintaining an adequate blood pressure.

If you are one of those people with a low blood pressure and are about to start treatment for PD, invest in a good blood pressure testing device. It will prove invaluable. If you are unfamiliar and do not know how to use it, the nurse in your doctor's office should be happy to instruct you.

For most people with PD, a low standing blood pressure is not a problem and may never be an issue. However, orthostatic hypotension occurs sufficiently frequently in PD to place it high on our checklist. It is usually wise to stay one step ahead of trouble, so don't forget to have this checked.

Now What?

If you are ready to start treatment for PD, this chapter should have allowed you to make your medication decision. Those choosing levodopa treatment should read chapter12; those opting for a dopamine agonist, chapter 13.

A few people may decide to start with one of the two minor drugs, selegiline or amantadine. Some may even decide to start one of these and also carbidopa/ levodopa or a dopamine agonist. One important rule of thumb: do not start two medications at the same time. Start one drug first, let the dust settle, and only then start the other.

PART SIX

Beginning Treatment of Parkinson's Disease: Medication Guidelines

12

◆ ◆ ◆

Starting Levodopa Treatment

If you have Parkinson's disease (PD) and are about to start levodopa therapy, plan on being pleasantly surprised. The improvement is often striking. Levodopa treatment is effective, relatively easy to start, and does not have any potentially serious side effects. No blood test monitoring is necessary, since it does not damage internal organs such as liver or kidneys. There is no one-size-fits-all dose, however. Treatment begins with a low dose, which is slowly raised, guided by the response. In this chapter, we will learn exactly how to do this, what to look for, and why we do what we do.

Carbidopa

All preparations of levodopa used today in the United States contain carbidopa. To recap, carbidopa administered with levodopa protects levodopa until it can get into the brain. One benefit is that much lower doses of levodopa are necessary. However, the major advantage is that it prevents nausea caused by dopamine in the bloodstream. Levodopa is always prescribed in combination with carbidopa (or in Europe, with a similar drug, benserazide); hence, when we discuss levodopa therapy, we are really talking about carbidopa/levodopa therapy.

Types of Levodopa: Immediate-Release and Controlled-Release Forms

Carbidopa/levodopa comes in two major forms, regular carbidopa/levodopa and the sustained-release form. The brand name for these drugs is Sinemet and the sustained-release formulation is Sinemet CR (controlled release). The regular carbidopa/levodopa is also called immediate release, to distinguish it from the controlled-release formulation. These drugs do not come in injectable forms; they are all pills. Because "carbidopa/levodopa" is hard to remember and pronounce, many people simply refer to it as Sinemet.

When the *sustained-release* formulation is filled by your pharmacist, one of three names will be on the label:

- Sinemet CR (brand name)

- Carbidopa/levodopa SR (sustained-release, generic)

- Carbidopa/levodopa ER (extended-release, generic)

These are all essentially the same product. The pharmacist filling the prescription for the *immediate-release* formulation will record one of two names on the label:

- Carbidopa/levodopa (generic)

- Sinemet (brand name)

There are three formulations of immediate-release carbidopa/levodopa: 25-100, 10-100, and 25-250; these are shown in table 12.1. The first number (25 or 10) is the amount of carbidopa in each pill, in milligrams (mg). The second number, 100 or 250, is the mg amount of the active ingredient, levodopa. Two formulations of the CR are available: 25-100 and 50-200.

If the physician writes "carbidopa/levodopa" on the prescription, it will be filled with the immediate-release formulation. To obtain the sustained-release formulation, this must be specifically indicated. Most prescription drug plans will encourage or require these to be filled as the generic. This does not appear to compromise the activity of these drugs.

Newest Formulation: Orally Disintegrating Carbidopa/Levodopa (Parcopa)

As this book was going to press, the United States Food and Drug Administration approved a third form of carbidopa/levodopa, a rapidly disintegrating tablet. This tablet dissolves when placed on your tongue and is then swallowed with your saliva (it is not absorbed through your tongue or mouth). The brand name for this form is Parcopa. It appears to work in your body very similar to immediate-release carbidopa/levodopa, based on the information available from

Table 12.1. Carbidopa/Levodopa Formulations

Formulation of Carbidopa/Levodopa	Brand Name	Generic Name	Tablet Sizes	Size Used for Initial Therapy
Immediate-release	Sinemet	Carbidopa/levodopa	25-100 (yellow) 10-100 (blue) 25-250 (blue)	25-100
Sustained-release (SR) or controlled-release (CR)	Sinemet CR	Carbidopa/levodopa SR or Carbidopa/levodopa ER*	25-100 (pink; if generic, gray) 50-200 (tan or peach-colored; if generic, gray)	25-100
Orally disintegrating	Parcopa		25-100 (yellow) 10-100 (blue) 25-250 (blue)	25-100

*ER = extended release

the pharmaceutical company. The advantage is that water is not necessary when taking this; hence, it is more convenient.

Parcopa comes in the same concentrations and ratios of carbidopa and levodopa as the standard immediate-release forms: 25-100, 10-100, and 25-250. The pill colors are also the same, with the 25-100 tablets yellow, and the 10-100 and 25-250 tablets blue. It appears that these can be used interchangeably with the immediate-release pills of the same milligram size. These pills rapidly dissolve if they get wet, so they must be kept in dry containers; when taking them from the pill vial, be sure your hands are dry. They have a minty flavor.

The precise role for this new orally disintegrating formulation has yet to be established; there has not yet been widespread experience among physicians. Hence there will be little further discussion of Parcopa in this book. At the time of this writing, I would start treatment with the conventional forms of carbidopa/ levodopa (immediate-release or controlled-release), since there is broad experience with these. You can later switch to the orally disintegrating form after you establish the optimum dose. If you anticipate doing that, do not start levodopa treatment with the sustained-release form. Although the milligram amounts are comparable between the immediate-release and the orally disintegrating forms, these differ from the controlled-release form (see below).

Immediate-Release Compared to Controlled-Release Forms

Immediate-release (regular) carbidopa/levodopa will get into the system about twice as fast as the controlled-release formulation. Blood levels peak within thirty to forty-five minutes after immediate-release carbidopa/levodopa and then decline after a couple of hours. Sinemet CR blood levels persist for about an hour longer than the immediate-release formulation.

Immediate-release and controlled-release carbidopa/levodopa are not precisely interchangeable. There is not a mg to mg correspondence of Sinemet CR to the regular carbidopa/levodopa. The primary reason relates to levodopa absorption. Levodopa from Sinemet CR is not fully released into the bloodstream; about 30 percent is lost in the gut. This contrasts with immediate-release carbidopa/levodopa, which is about 99 percent absorbed. Thus 200 mg of levodopa given as Sinemet CR is not equal to 200 mg of levodopa in the immediate-release formulation; it equates to about 140 mg of immediate-release levodopa.

Cost

Generic drugs are generally cheaper than brand name medications and this is especially true for levodopa therapy. Also, the sustained-release and the new orally disintegrating formulations of carbidopa/levodopa are more expensive

Table 12.2. Cost of Carbidopa/Levodopa Therapy*

Formulation of Carbidopa/Levodopa	Typical Dose, Tablets per Day**	Cost per 100 Tablets	Cost per Month for Typical Daily Dose*
Immediate-release			
25-100 generic	6	$ 26	$ 47
10-100 generic	6	24	43
25-250 generic	2.5	30	23
25-100 brand name Sinemet	6	107	193
10-100 brand name Sinemet	6	95	171
25-250 brand name Sinemet	2.5	135	101
Sustained-release			
25-100 generic	8	$107	$257
50-200 generic	4	203	244
25-100 brand name Sinemet CR	8	120	288
50-200 brand name Sinemet CR	4	226	271
Orally disintegrating			
10-100 brand name Parcopa	6	$ 90	$162
25-100 brand name Parcopa	6	100	180
25-250 brand name Parcopa	2.5	130	98

*Retail prices, community pharmacy (2004).

**To allow comparisons, we will assume that the person initiating levodopa therapy will settle on the equivalent of 6 tablets of immediate-release 25-100 carbidopa/levodopa daily (starting with a lower dose and increasing to the optimum level). In milligrams of levodopa, this is approximately equal to 2 1/2 tablets of 25-250 per day. The sustained-release formulations are only about 70 percent absorbed and an equivalent dose is approximately eight 25-100 CR tablets daily.

than the regular formulation (immediate-release). The prices the consumer might pay from a large community pharmacy are shown in table 12.2; the comparisons are based on daily doses that are approximately equivalent in potency. Clearly, from an expense standpoint, use of the generic immediate-release formulation is a substantial cost savings compared to the alternatives.

Which Formulation Is Best for Starting Treatment?

Either the CR or the immediate-release formulation may be used to begin treatment. Which is preferable as initial therapy? Some physicians advocated the CR formulation when it was first introduced. It was assumed that the slower release and more persistent blood levels should more closely approximate the natural state. Subsequently, two large (five-year) clinical trials compared these two formulations. The outcomes were the same, regardless of which form of levodopa therapy was being administered; most people did well. Thus, there appeared to be no long-term advantage to one formulation over the other.

From a practical standpoint, the immediate-release formulation is probably the better choice for initial treatment, and it is my choice. There are three reasons for choosing immediate-release carbidopa/levodopa. First, immediate-release carbidopa/levodopa has predictable interactions with food. In previous chapters, we saw that meals (protein) reduce the amount of levodopa that crosses the blood–brain barrier. Specifically, dietary protein is digested into the component amino acids, which then compete for transport into the brain with levodopa (also an amino acid). This is not a problem if the immediate-release carbidopa/levodopa dose is taken an hour before each meal. That gives it enough time to get into the brain before the dietary protein is digested. On the other hand, the controlled-release formulation has complex interactions with meals. Levodopa in the CR formulation:

- Does not get out of the gut and into the bloodstream as well if taken *without* food, but
- Does not cross the blood–brain barrier well if taken *with* food

Hence meals produce two opposite effects on the CR formulation; how to administer with respect to meals is unclear. Moreover, the CR formulation takes up to two hours for the levodopa to be fully released and pass into the brain; thus, if empty-stomach dosing is desired, you need to wait two hours before eating. With the immediate-release formulation, the initial dosing strategy is straightforward: take each dose one hour before each meal.

Second, immediate-release carbidopa/levodopa is completely absorbed. With the CR formulation the absorption is incomplete, with about 30 percent lost in the gut. Third, immediate-release carbidopa/levodopa is less expensive.

The complex interactions with food and the incomplete absorption of the controlled-release formulation are not a problem for many patients. Levodopa is a sufficiently potent medication that it usually works out, even if things are not done ideally. A minority of people, however, will not respond as well as they should, despite what should be adequate doses of the CR formulation. The physician is then left to ponder whether the CR formulation is responsible. Hence, it is simpler to start with the immediate-release formulation.

My Recommendation: Go with Immediate-Release Carbidopa/Levodopa

In this book, the immediate-release formulation is the preferred form of levodopa therapy. Some might view this as arbitrary, but sticking with one formulation will avoid subsequent confusion. Later in the course of PD and also later in this book, the problems and solutions will get a little complicated. If you are using the immediate-release formulation, the treatment strategies will be simpler and more straightforward. This is not to say that starting therapy with the CR formulation is inappropriate. In fact, we provide a dosing schedule in supplement 12.3 at the end of this chapter for those who wish to start with CR. Parenthetically, whenever we say "carbidopa/levodopa" we will be referring to the immediate-release formulation.

Starting Treatment with the 25-100 Immediate-Release Carbidopa/Levodopa Pill

Initiating levodopa therapy will turn out to be a very gratifying experience for most people with PD. Symptoms that had been limiting lifestyle often subside as the medication is slowly increased. For some, abandoned sports and activities may again become possible.

We will start treatment with the 25-100 formulation of carbidopa/levodopa (the yellow pill). This form has more carbidopa than the 10-100 form; the additional carbidopa helps prevent nausea.

The 10-100 form is now infrequently prescribed. This and the 25-250 were the original formulations that were released in the mid-1970s. The 25-100 was subsequently introduced to reduce the incidence of nausea. The others are acceptable, but the 25-100 drug has become the convention.

HOW SHOULD I TAKE THIS MEDICINE? HOW MUCH? HOW OFTEN?

The general plan is to start with a low carbidopa/levodopa dose and gradually raise it. Increments are made on a weekly basis, guided by your response.

Start with a single 25-100 immediate-release tablet three times daily. Many with PD don't respond to this low dose so don't be discouraged if you fail to experience an initial benefit. This dose is just the beginning. It may take up to a few weeks before we have stabilized your dosing schedule. The entire dosing scheme is outlined at the end of this chapter in supplement 12.1 (consider photocopying); take a look at this now and then read on. This scheme is not complex, but questions often arise as people start treatment.

Some physicians advise beginning treatment with 1/2 tablet (25-100), three times daily. This is not unreasonable; however, in my experience, most people tolerate full tablet doses and this 1/2 tablet dosage is too low to provide substantial benefit. Hence, starting with a full 25-100 tablet (3 times daily) shortens the dose escalation scheme. The only exception is the person who experiences nausea, and we discuss this later in this chapter.

SHOULD I TAKE THIS WITH MEALS?

No. Each dose should be taken on an empty stomach. The easiest way to do this is to have a set pattern. Take each of your three doses about one hour before meals. It takes about an hour for the carbidopa/levodopa pill to get dissolved in your stomach, pass into the intestines, enter the bloodstream, and ultimately pass into the brain cells. We want this to happen before dietary protein from meals can interfere. Bear in mind that, if you eat, it takes at least two hours for the food to clear. Hence, if you forget to take your pills before you eat, it takes a couple of hours for this deleterious food effect to pass.

Some people worry that their medicine doses should be equally spaced over the course of the day, say every eight hours; however, this is not necessary when you start carbidopa/levodopa. In early PD, the only important timing factor is to keep the doses separate from meals. After a number of years, the time between doses may become crucial but we won't worry about that now.

I ONLY EAT TWO MEALS A DAY; WHAT NOW?

If you only eat two meals daily, take a carbidopa/levodopa dose an hour before each of those two meals. Take the other dose in between these meals or later in the day, at a time when your stomach is empty.

MAY I TAKE CARBIDOPA/LEVODOPA WITH MY OTHER MEDICINES?

This is okay to do except for iron pills. Iron can bind levodopa and prevent it from being absorbed. Hence don't take it with vitamin pills if they also contain iron.

WHAT IF THIS MAKES ME NAUSEATED?

If the first few doses induce nausea, reduce to 1/2 tablet doses (still three times daily). If the nausea is then tolerable, stick with it. It will likely pass over the next few days to weeks as you continue to take it. You may take the pill with dry bread or soda crackers to help counter nausea (these do not contain substantial protein). Continue with these 1/2 tablet doses (three times daily); if the nausea has resolved within one to two weeks, then increase back to one full tablet three times daily. If you tolerate that, continue on, as we will describe. Starting with lower doses and increasing more slowly is one strategy for countering nausea.

If the nausea is more persistent and troublesome, a focused strategy is necessary. This is described later in the chapter. Recall that the nausea is not dangerous; ulcers and other serious stomach problems do not result. The nausea is mediated by the brain nausea center, stimulated by levodopa treatment, rather than from stomach irritation.

WHEN SHOULD I INCREASE THE DOSE?

You may not notice benefit the first day you start this. It takes about a week for the cumulative effect of a given dose of levodopa to become fully established. Actually, recent studies have suggested that this cumulative effect may accrue over two to three weeks in some cases; however, most of the effect is present after a week. This is important: increase your doses weekly if the current dose does not result in marked improvement. You may choose to stick with a certain dose for longer than a week and that is just fine. For example, if you think you're turning the corner on parkinsonism and want to see how things go for a couple of weeks or longer, no problem. You can raise it again after that if you decide that you need better coverage.

WHAT DO YOU MEAN BY "MARKED IMPROVEMENT"?

We anticipate that all or nearly all of the symptoms of parkinsonism will improve quite substantially. This includes not only how you feel, but how you function in your activities of daily living. Set your goals high; we are going for a home run, not settling for a single. We may not achieve this in every case, but often the improvement is striking. Expect improvement in not only the classic PD symptoms, such as tremor, slowness, walking problems, and stiffness, but also the subjective symptoms, such as restlessness (akathisia), nervousness, and fatigue. The strategy is to continue increasing the dose until there has been very prominent improvement or until we reach a ceiling dose (see below). If the improvement has not been appreciable, we shouldn't accept this until we have raised the dosage high enough to be sure we have given it our best shot.

HOW MUCH SHOULD I RAISE THE DOSE?

For most people, 1 tablet three times daily will not be sufficient. However, stick with this for a week and then go up if you're not markedly improved. Raise the dose from 1 to 1 1/2 tablets three times daily if not markedly improved. This first increment is still a conservative dose.

WHAT THEN?

You probably are starting to grasp the general principles (detailed in supplement 12.1 at the end of this chapter). We continue to increase by adding 1/2 tablet to all three doses on a weekly basis.

Thus we will go from 1 1/2 tablets three times daily to 2 tablets three times per day and then 2 1/2 tablets three times daily. The quickest we want to raise the doses is weekly (to give each dose a chance to work), but you may go more slowly if you wish.

WHAT IS THE MAXIMUM DOSE?

Carbidopa/levodopa does not become dangerous when the dosage is raised beyond certain levels. It doesn't have any life-threatening side effects and there is no absolute maximum dose based on toxicity. However, experience has taught us that benefits increase up to a point and higher doses will probably just add side effects. For most people starting carbidopa/levodopa, a dose between 1 and 2 1/2 tablets, three times daily (on an empty stomach), will capture the optimum benefit.

ARE THERE EVER EXCEPTIONS?

Yes, and if you are still poorly controlled after escalating your carbidopa/levodopa dose to 2 1/2 tablets three times daily, you may go a little higher. We don't want to miss any opportunities; but almost no one benefits from individual carbidopa/levodopa doses higher than 3 1/2 tablets.

This dictum relates to the immediate-release formulation (not CR) taken on an empty stomach. Also, we are talking about individual doses, not total daily doses. This does not mean that the maximum amount you can ever take per day is 10 1/2 tablets (three times 3 1/2 tablets). Later in the course of PD, more frequent dosing may be necessary, and, consequently, the total number may exceed 10 1/2 tablets daily.

WHAT DOSE SHOULD I SETTLE ON AFTER I'VE DONE ALL THIS?

Ultimately, use the dose that works the best. If this is a higher dose, such as 2 1/2 tablets three times daily, that is perfectly fine. However, if several doses all produce the same effect, settle on the lowest of those doses; that is, if the benefits are identical, there is no reason to take more than is useful.

WHAT IF I EXPERIENCE NO BENEFIT, DESPITE RAISING THE DOSES?

If there is absolutely no benefit, despite going up to 3 tablets, or even 3 1/2 tablets three times daily, double-check the following:

- Am I taking this on an empty stomach, one hour before meals (not 15 minutes before)?
- Are my pills yellow? All the 25-100 immediate-release carbidopa/levodopa tablets are yellow, whether generic or name brand. The 25-100 CR tablets, which are lower potency, are pink or gray.
- Am I taking any medications that might block the effects of levodopa? Review chapter 6 for a list of drugs that might do this. Also, avoid taking with iron pills.

If none of these explains the lack of effect, we may be out of luck. Fortunately, this is the exception rather than the rule.

IF CARBIDOPA/LEVODOPA FAILS DESPITE HIGH DOSES, COULD THIS BE DUE TO MALABSORPTION?

Gastrointestinal problems that prevent levodopa absorption are extremely rare. When this is the cause, it should be apparent; either people have a known gastrointestinal disease or they have symptoms to suggest this, such as diarrhea, weight loss, abdominal discomfort, and so on. If you think this is a possibility, consult a gastroenterologist.

CAN I HAVE MY BLOOD LEVELS OF LEVODOPA CHECKED?

Levodopa can be measured in the bloodstream, but this is not done on a routine basis. Hence, the decisions about whether the levodopa dose is adequate must be based on your response.

HOW DO I KNOW IF I AM GETTING TOO MUCH?

The side effects from levodopa are all up front and apparent. There is no potential for any serious liver or kidney toxicity, as can occur with some other drugs. As we discussed, no blood monitoring is necessary to assess toxicity. More is said about potential side effects later in this chapter.

WHAT ABOUT CARBIDOPA?

Carbidopa, which is the other component of carbidopa/levodopa, is not an important factor in our dosing decisions. For all intents and purposes, consider the role of carbidopa as an agent to prevent levodopa-induced nausea. If you are not experiencing nausea, then your dose of carbidopa is adequate. You can raise the dose of carbidopa, but that won't affect the control of your PD symptoms. In fact, as you raise the levodopa dose to improve control of parkinsonism, you will be receiving more carbidopa (since the carbidopa is tied to levodopa in these pills). This extra carbidopa is doing neither harm nor good. Thus my advice: ignore carbidopa if you are not nauseated.

CAN YOU OVERDOSE ON CARBIDOPA?

There is no precedent for this and side effects do not occur with even high doses. In other words, there is no maximum dose of carbidopa. If nausea is a problem, however, we then want to raise the carbidopa dosage.

CARBIDOPA/LEVODOPA MAKES ME NAUSEATED; NOW WHAT?

Earlier, we mentioned that mild nausea from levodopa therapy usually goes away with continued use. Hence, just sticking with it is the appropriate strategy. For a small minority, however, nausea is more troublesome, some-times including vomiting. For this group of people, other measures are neces-sary. There are three relatively simple things that can be done, which are usually effective.

1. The carbidopa/levodopa may be taken with nonprotein food. Although the nausea does not originate from the stomach (it is due to stimulation of the brain nausea center), having something in the stomach may be helpful. Dry bread (no butter) or crackers may be tried.

2. Extra carbidopa may be administered. Plain carbidopa without levodopa is available by prescription. It comes in only one size, 25 mg tablets, and goes by the brand name Lodosyn. Take 1 Lodosyn tablet before each dose of carbidopa/levodopa. If you take it fifteen to thirty minutes before, it may be even more effective, since the carbidopa will have a chance to get into the system before the levodopa enters. If 1 Lodosyn tablet is insufficient, take 2 tablets before each dose of carbidopa/ levodopa. When filling this prescription for supplementary carbidopa (Lodosyn), the pharmacist should be reminded that it is for plain carbidopa, since this could easily be misinterpreted to be the much more commonly prescribed carbidopa/levodopa. Supplementary carbidopa is often effective. Sometimes this is all that is necessary.

3. The levodopa (actually carbidopa/levodopa) may be started in very low doses and increased more slowly. In this setting, I would start with 1/4 of a 25-100 carbidopa/levodopa tablet three times daily. Increase weekly by raising all three doses by 1/4 tablet increments. The brain nausea center typically gets used to the levodopa when it is introduced in tiny amounts and only slowly escalated. The downside of this scheme is that it takes about two to three months to arrive at the optimal levodopa dose.

These strategies for dealing with troublesome nausea are outlined in supple-ment 12.2 at the end of this chapter; you may choose to photocopy that scheme for easy access.

If nausea is a problem, explore whether there are other factors besides levodopa. Did the nausea precede levodopa? Are there other medications taken around the same time as the levodopa that are also nausea-provoking? If so, take these other drugs separately; if the other drug is not critical, perhaps put it on hold. Also, are any other medications for PD also being administered? Supplementary medications, such as selegiline (Eldepryl) or entacapone (Comtan), enhance both the good and the bad effects from levodopa, includ-ing nausea. If nausea is a problem, these should be stopped; they can be restarted later when the nausea settles down.

IF I'M NAUSEATED FROM LEVODOPA, WHY NOT SWITCH TO A DOPAMINE AGONIST DRUG?

Unfortunately dopamine agonists (pramipexole, ropinirole, pergolide, bromocriptine) also cause nausea. They may be tolerated in very low doses in those prone to nausea, but when raised to levels sufficient to improve parkinsonism, they are equally likely as levodopa to cause nausea.

IF I START SUPPLEMENTARY CARBIDOPA (LODOSYN), DO I NEED TO CONTINUE THIS FOREVER?

Supplementary carbidopa typically allows regular carbidopa/levodopa to be tolerated. With time, however, the body usually gets used to the levodopa and the nausea diminishes. Hence, it may eventually be possible to stop the supplementary carbidopa (Lodosyn). Usually I recommend that people stick with it for a few months and then try omitting an occasional dose of the supplementary carbidopa. If this is tolerated, they can skip more and more doses and perhaps eventually stop it altogether.

WHY NOT SIMPLY USE ONE OF THE ANTINAUSEA DRUGS?

Most of the available prescription drugs for nausea block dopamine within the brain. Obviously, this could be detrimental for those with PD; it could worsen parkinsonism and prevent levodopa from working. The two most commonly prescribed drugs for nausea are metoclopramide (Reglan) and prochlorperazine (Compazine). They both block brain dopamine and should *not* be used by those with PD. Two other drugs used to treat nausea also block dopamine although less potently, promethazine (Phenergan) and thiethylperazine (Torecan); they should also be avoided.

One exception to this admonition about antinausea drugs is the prescription medication, trimethobenzamide (Tigan); this drug is compatible with PD. However, it is not very potent at treating levodopa-induced nausea. It can be tried using a 250 mg tablet or 300 mg capsule taken orally, an hour before each carbidopa/levodopa dose. Alternatively, the 200 mg rectal suppository can be administered. In my own practice, I usually do not resort to this drug, except in the rare individual where other measures are inadequate.

Outside the United States, the potent antinausea medication domperidone (Motilium) is available by prescription. Domperidone is compatible with PD. This drug blocks dopamine but cannot cross the blood–brain barrier, so it spares the critical dopaminergic systems in the basal ganglia. However, the one area where the blood–brain barrier is porous is in the brain's nausea center, where domperidone can enter. Outside the United States, it is routinely used to treat nausea in those with PD. Unfortunately the company that developed this drug, Janssen Pharmaceuticals, has not recognized a large enough market in the United States to justify the expense of obtaining FDA (Food and Drug Administration) approval. Some of the antinausea drugs used in cancer chemotherapy are also tolerated by those with PD, but are too expensive for routine daily use (ondansetron, brand name Zofran; dolasetron, brand name Anzemet; granisetron, brand name Kytril).

SHOULD I WORRY THAT THE NAUSEA IS A SIGN OF A MORE SERIOUS PROBLEM?

If the nausea is due to levodopa therapy, it is not worrisome. However, if you were experiencing nausea before starting your PD medications, there is probably some other cause. Bear in mind that levodopa should not be causing stomach pain, only nausea. If you have true pain, your physician should look into this.

CAN CARBIDOPA/LEVODOPA HELP MY SLEEP?

Insomnia can be a manifestation of parkinsonism. If insomnia started around the same time as your other parkinsonian symptoms, it might be a manifestation of PD. The initial levodopa dosing schedule, described above, may adequately treat this and restore your sleep. If not, you could try adding a fourth dose of carbidopa/levodopa a little before bedtime (the same size dose that you take earlier in the day). Try this for a week. If you do not improve, you can discontinue this additional dose; but often this will work. There are, however, other reasons one might have insomnia, so a response is not guaranteed. For more on this, see chapter 20.

WHAT IF I WANT TO START WITH THE CR FORMULATION?

It is not unreasonable to initiate levodopa treatment with the controlled-release formulation. If this is chosen after considering the pros and cons, you can follow the initiation and escalation strategy outlined in supplement 12.3 at the end of this chapter. This scheme in supplement 12.3 is similar to what was described for immediate-release carbidopa/levodopa.

Typically, Sinemet CR is started with a twice-daily dosing scheme. Conceivably, immediate-release carbidopa/levodopa could just as effectively be given twice daily as well; however, the conventional dosing scheme with the immediate-release formulation is three times per day.

Sinemet CR is initiated with the 25-100 formulation, beginning with 1 tablet twice per day. It is unclear how to best administer this in relation to meals. Since it takes up to two hours to reach stable brain levels, you could argue that it should be taken two hours before a meal. This would allow the levodopa to get onboard before dietary protein, which can reduce passage across the blood–brain barrier. On the other hand, the CR formulation dissolves better and passes into the bloodstream more effectively if there is food in the stomach. My own sense is that it is more effective if administered a couple of hours before meals, taken with at least 6–8 ounces of fluids; however, this has not been adequately studied.

The dose is raised by adding 1/2 or 1 tablet to each dose weekly. If nausea occurs, the 1/2 tablet increments are preferable. If tolerated, it is quicker to go up by full tablet (25-100) increments. Breaking the tablet in half slightly reduces the sustained-release property, but this is probably not significant. However, it should not be chewed or crushed since this will abolish the sustained-release effect.

For people starting levodopa therapy, the dosage necessary to control parkinsonism is between one and four 25-100 Sinemet CR tablets twice daily. Many will find that the most effective dose is closer to 4 tablets twice daily. For those who are insufficiently controlled on 4 tablets twice a day, the dose can be increased to 4 tablets three times per day. Higher doses can be tried if necessary, but in that case, it would be wise to switch to the immediate-release formulation since there may be absorption problems with the sustained-release tablets.

Note that we are talking about dose adjustments in people *starting* levodopa therapy. More levodopa *per day* may become necessary after some years of parkinsonism because the response to each dose may be brief, lasting only a few hours or less. Hence more frequent dosing is then required.

Sustained-release carbidopa/levodopa comes in two sizes, 25-100 and 50-200. Once the dose has been established it may be more convenient to switch to the 50-200 size (two 25-100 tablets equals one 50-200 tablet). Sustained-release carbidopa/levodopa is also available as a generic preparation. There has not been good published data to compare generic to brand name Sinemet CR; my experience has been that the generic forms seem to work satisfactorily.

I'VE RAISED THE DOSE OF SINEMET CR TO THE MAX AND I'M STILL NOT DOING AS WELL AS I SHOULD; NOW WHAT?

Our strategy is to slowly raise the CR dose until control of parkinsonism is achieved, up to 400 mg (four 25-100 tablets) three times daily. If you have done this and still are doing poorly, there are two possible explanations:

- You don't have Parkinson's disease but rather a parkinsonism-plus disorder, as described in chapter 6.

- You are getting insufficient levodopa into your system as a consequence of the sustained-release properties. As already explained, there is incomplete release of levodopa from the sustained-release drug, and there are complex interactions with meals that could be a factor.

Of these two possibilities, only the second lends itself to treatment. Inadequate absorption may occur with the sustained-release formulation (Sinemet CR). To address this, we need to switch to the regular, immediate-release form of carbidopa/levodopa. This formulation has a predictable response; if you still fail to respond despite following the guidelines given for the immediate-release formulation, then we know it's not the fault of the pill.

HOW DO I SWITCH FROM THESE HIGH DOSES OF SUSTAINED-RELEASE TO THE IMMEDIATE-RELEASE DRUG?

If you are experiencing an inadequate response despite 400 mg doses of levodopa as the sustained-release preparation, then you should switch to immediate-release carbidopa/levodopa. You may do this overnight, finishing with the sustained-release formulation one day and starting the immediate-release drug the next morning in its place. Remember that only about 70 percent of the CR dose is absorbed; immediate-release carbidopa/levodopa is essentially completely absorbed. Hence we need to adjust the dose accordingly when making this transition. Let's assume you are now taking:

- Sustained-release carbidopa/levodopa (Sinemet CR) in a dose of 400 mg levodopa three times daily (two 50-200 tablets or four 25-100 tablets three times daily).

An appropriate transition would be approximately 70 percent of this dose:

- Immediate-release 25-100 carbidopa/levodopa in a dose of 2 1/2 tablets, three times daily. Note that 70 percent of 400 mg is 280 mg; this rounds out to 250 mg, which translates into 2 1/2 tablets of the 25-100 immediate-release formulation.

If no side effects, maintain this dose for a week to let the dust settle. If you are satisfied with the response, stick with this dose. You may lower the dose by 1/2 tablet reductions if side effects, or if you think that a lower dose might work as well. On the other hand, if you still don't appreciate a good benefit despite this transition to immediate-release carbidopa/levodopa, go back and reread the earlier sections in this chapter that describe what to do in that case.

SINEMET CR MAKES ME NAUSEATED; NOW WHAT?

We can use the same treatment principles described above for the immediate-release formulation to counter nausea. This includes supplementary carbidopa (Lodosyn), plus starting with a lower levodopa dose and escalating more slowly. The specifics are outlined in supplement 12.4.

THE NEWEST FORMULATION OF LEVODOPA, STALEVO; SHOULD I START WITH THIS?

In mid-2003, the FDA approved a multi-ingredient drug that combines carbidopa/levodopa with entacapone. The brand name for this is Stalevo. Should this be the drug of choice for starting levodopa treatment? After all, it's the latest drug on the market. Some may advocate this, but I suggest not. It has a role later in the course of PD; however, early in the course, simple is often better. Let's consider the facts.

Entacapone, which is the added ingredient in Stalevo, blocks an enzyme that metabolizes levodopa. This enzyme, catechol-O-methyltransferase, normally converts levodopa into an inactive form. By adding entacapone to carbidopa/levodopa, levodopa is protected in the bloodstream (it is not metabolized as readily). Consequently, the elimination of levodopa from the bloodstream is partially blocked and it stays around longer. Theoretically, this should be favorable. It works like a slow-release form of carbidopa/levodopa, not unlike Sinemet CR in some respects.

So what's the downside? There is no major risk to using this as the initial medication. However, there are several reasons to keep your life simple and stick with plain carbidopa/levodopa.

- Adding entacapone to carbidopa/levodopa enhances not only the beneficial effects, but also the side effects; this might result in side effects that would not have occurred with plain carbidopa/levodopa.

- Dosage adjustments are simpler with plain carbidopa/levodopa.

- Generic carbidopa/levodopa is much cheaper.

Probably the primary reason for sticking with plain carbidopa/levodopa is that early in the course, the entacapone effect isn't necessary.

Side Effects from Levodopa Therapy

We have already heard about nausea, which is the most common side effect. Rarely, however, does it prevent someone from achieving the appropriate levodopa dose to meet their needs, especially with the strategies outlined above. Other problems that may occur when *starting* levodopa treatment are low blood pressure (in the standing position) and, rarely, dyskinesias or hallucinations. These deserve further discussion.

LOW BLOOD PRESSURE (ORTHOSTATIC HYPOTENSION)

I explained in the last chapter that PD predisposes to a drop in blood pressure when you're standing or walking (orthostatic hypotension). Carbidopa/levodopa exacerbates this problem, as do most of the other drugs for PD. This may not be recognized, since blood pressure is conventionally checked when sitting. Very low blood pressure is associated with light-headedness and fatigue; if severe, fainting may occur. As outlined in the last chapter, symptoms may occur when the *systolic* blood pressure drops below 90 (systolic is the upper number in blood pressure readings, such as 90 in 90/60).

Because of this potential for orthostatic hypotension, it is imperative that the *standing* blood pressure be checked before starting levodopa (or a dopamine agonist). If your standing systolic blood pressure is over 100, you could start carbidopa/levodopa. If the systolic reading is below 100, you should take measures to elevate the blood pressure, as noted in the last chapter. This includes reviewing your medication list with your physician to determine if other drugs may be contributing to the low blood pressures (see chapter 21 for a list of such medications). Increased salt in your diet will also help, along with adequate fluids (6–8 glasses daily). If these simple measures are not adequate, read chapter 21 for additional strategies for raising your blood pressure, such as taking salt tablets.

HALLUCINATIONS

Hallucinations imply seeing something that is not there. They may be provoked by levodopa treatment, as well as the other medications used to treat PD. In fact, the dopamine agonist drugs are much more likely to cause these. Fortunately, hallucinations are rare among those starting carbidopa/levodopa; the likelihood during the first five years of levodopa therapy is about one in twenty.

When hallucinations develop during levodopa initiation, another offending drug is often being taken as well. If hallucinations develop when you start carbidopa/levodopa, review your list of drugs (see chapter 24). Whereas carbidopa/levodopa alone might be tolerated, sometimes another drug being taken concurrently might provoke hallucinations. For example, any of the other PD drugs markedly add to the hallucination potential when used with carbidopa/levodopa, including selegiline, amantadine, a dopamine agonist, or an anticholinergic medication.

Hallucinations occurring early in treatment are typically not very troublesome. This may manifest as seeing bugs on the refrigerator or some inanimate object moving. More troublesome hallucinations may occur later in PD and have complex causes. Hallucinations and related problems are discussed in more detail in chapter 24.

DYSKINESIAS

Dyskinesias were described and discussed in the last two chapters. These are the involuntary body movements due to an excessive levodopa effect. Levodopa-induced dyskinesias are rare early in the course of PD. The likelihood that you will experience these during the first year of levodopa treatment is less than one in ten. Thus, don't expect to encounter these as we initiate carbidopa/levodopa. We are discussing these now because people sometimes think they are experiencing these levodopa dyskinesias when, in fact, there is another explanation.

Levodopa dyskinesias become more frequent after some years of PD. By five years of levodopa treatment, about four of every ten people treated with levodopa will experience at least a slight degree of these dyskinesias.

The involuntary dancing movements provoked by levodopa are time-locked to each levodopa dose. They start thirty to sixty minutes after the dose and persist for a half hour to four hours, then resolve. With Sinemet CR, dyskinesias begin one to two hours after a dose.

Getting rid of these dyskinesias is easy: lower each levodopa dose by a small amount. The decrements should be 1/4 to 1/2 tablet, each dose; if the dyskinesias persist, the doses can be lowered again. Thus, if they developed on a dose of 2 1/2 tablets three times daily, then lower each dose to 2 or 2 1/4 tablets (still three times daily). If still present, continue to lower the dosage by 1/4 tablet decrements until they no longer are provoked.

Sometimes dose reductions that abolish dyskinesias result in inadequate control of parkinsonism. Early in the course of PD, however, this is rarely a problem. We specifically address more troublesome dyskinesias in chapters 27 and 32.

ARE ALL INVOLUNTARY MOVEMENTS DUE TO LEVODOPA?

One good way to confuse your doctor and end up with the wrong treatment is to misinterpret other symptoms for levodopa dyskinesias. If you tell your physician that you have been experiencing dyskinesias, when these symptoms were actually dystonia, akathisia, or tremor, your doctor's advice will be dead wrong. To avoid misleading your physician, we need to distinguish these other types of movement problems. These are problems that often require more levodopa, not less.

DYSTONIA VERSUS LEVODOPA DYSKINESIAS

Dystonia is an involuntary posture. This is due to a sustained contraction of muscles, which may affect any part of the body. People with PD may experience dystonia in a variety of forms with the most common being:

- Curling or arching of the toes
- In-turning of the foot
- Calf cramping

Dystonia is sometimes painful, relating to the cramp-like state. These forms of dystonia are typically due to PD and not caused by carbidopa/levodopa. They typically resolve with adequate levodopa treatment.

In contrast to dystonia, levodopa-induced dyskinesias are dancing, flowing movements, which are painless. The person with levodopa-induced dyskinesias appears unable to sit still or stand in one place. Although those with levodopa-induced dyskinesias may seem to be posturing from time to time, the predominant movements are flowing, writhing, and wiggling. This may affect one hand or foot, one side of the body, or the whole body. The neurologist's term for these dancing movements is chorea.

Table 12.3. Distinguishing Dyskinesias Caused by Levodopa from Dystonia due to PD*

	Levodopa-Induced Dyskinesias	Dystonia Due to PD
Character	Flowing, dancing movements; appears unable to sit still. Normal movements may appear exaggerated (e.g., increased arm swing).	An abnormal posture; a sustained muscle contraction. Examples include curling of toes or a foot turned in.
Where?	One limb, one side of the body or entire body; may include face.	Often one or both lower limbs, especially toes, feet, or calf; also involuntary eye closure (blepharospasm)
Subjective sensation	Dyskinetic limbs do not feel tense.	Sometimes painful, cramp-like, or tense feeling in muscle. May feel restless but does not appear restless to onlookers.
Present before levodopa therapy was first started?	No.	Sometimes.
Present before the first dose of levodopa of the day?	No (unless carbidopa/levodopa taken during the night).	Often this is when they are worst; however, may come on at other times.
Present all the time?	No.	Sometimes, if the levodopa dose is insufficient.
Comes on within one hour of starting levodopa?	Yes (or within two hours after Sinemet CR).	No; may go away at that time if dose of levodopa is sufficient.
Begins more than three hours after each dose of levodopa?	No.	Sometimes (if levodopa takes this away, it may recur when the levodopa effect has worn off).
Present more than six hours after the last dose of levodopa?	No.	Yes.
Starts when getting close to the time of the next levodopa dose?	No (rare exceptions, as discussed in chapter 17).	Sometimes.

*These guidelines relate to immediate-release carbidopa/levodopa. Since sustained-release carbidopa/levodopa (Sinemet CR) takes about an hour longer to kick in and lasts about an hour longer, the times in this table need to be adjusted accordingly.

One additional way of determining whether involuntary movements are due to levodopa is to observe when they occur. Typical levodopa-induced dyskinesias start thirty to sixty minutes after each dose and are gone within a few hours. In contrast, dystonia due to PD may be persistent throughout the day or have no relationship to your carbidopa/levodopa doses. Alternatively, dystonia may also resolve after a levodopa dose and return several hours later. Dystonia is often present upon awakening in the morning (no levodopa overnight). In contrast, levodopa-induced dyskinesias are never present before the first carbidopa/levodopa dose in the morning, unless a dose was taken in the middle of the night. Finally, if the dystonic movements were present before starting levodopa treatment, obviously levodopa is not the culprit. Characteristics that separate levodopa dyskinesias from the dystonia due to PD are summarized in table 12.3.

AKATHISIA VERSUS LEVODOPA DYSKINESIAS

People with PD often experience an inner tension or restlessness. This is termed akathisia. This tends to be relieved by levodopa, which is opposite to levodopa-induced dyskinesias. The same levodopa dose that may provoke dyskinesias relieves the akathisia. Thus, people with levodopa dyskinesias experience relief when the dyskinesias are present, even though they may appear restless to those observing them. Akathisia is a primary symptom of PD, rather than due to the medications. It is described in a variety of ways, including a feeling of anxiety, inner tension, or inner tremor. Dystonia and akathisia may occur together.

TREMOR VERSUS LEVODOPA-INDUCED DYSKINESIAS

Levodopa-induced dyskinesias also must be differentiated from the tremor of PD. Recall that we defined tremor as a to-and-fro movement. It is rhythmical, back and forth, with the same movement repeating itself over and over. This contrasts with the somewhat chaotic movements typical of levodopa-induced dyskinesias. These dyskinesias are not stereotyped repetitive movements; rather, they are random and largely unpatterned.

Tremor is not due to the drugs used to treat PD. The only exception is very rare cases where brief tremor occurs just as a levodopa dose is kicking in; this lasts minutes and is not persistent.

MUST I TREAT DYSKINESIAS?

Levodopa dyskinesias are not harmful and do not demand medication changes. If you experience these but do not find these bothersome, you do not necessarily need to change anything. On the other hand, dyskinesias are often more troubling to family, especially spouses, who may encourage treatment.

INITIAL LEVODOPA PROVOKES DYSKINESIAS AND
DOSAGE INSUFFICIENT TO CONTROL PARKINSONISM:
WHAT TO DO

About seven out of one hundred people starting carbidopa/levodopa will experience dyskinesias within the first year. Even when they do occur, simply lowering the dose should control these. However, rare individuals find that when the levodopa dose is reduced enough to abolish dyskinesias, control of parkinsonism is lost. What to do? There are strategies for treating this, which capitalize on two facts.

- Levodopa-induced dyskinesias are time-locked to each dose; they last for no more than a few hours and are then gone. Dyskinesias do not reflect the cumulative dose of levodopa over the course of the day.

- Early in PD, the *beneficial* effect is cumulative; it will slowly accrue over about a week. In other words, the antiparkinsonian effect is not time-locked to each dose, but builds up over days. This has been called the long-duration response. To capture the beneficial effect, the doses can be taken at any time (as long as not with food).

This is one of the few situations where we focus on the total daily levodopa dose. It takes about 300 to 800 mg of levodopa per day (with carbidopa) to capture a good "long-duration response." But remember that we are focusing on someone early in the treatment course. Later in PD, these doses of levodopa may not be sufficient.

There are two ways you might deal with this problem of dyskinesias: (1) frequent low doses and (2) nighttime dosing.

- *Frequent low doses.* Lower doses of levodopa don't provoke dyskinesias. Only when the dose has been raised sufficiently high do they occur. In other words, there is a dose-threshold for dyskinesias. Doses below the threshold do not cause dyskinesias and doses above do. One approach is to use only low doses of levodopa that are below the dyskinesia threshold. You will need to try several doses over several days to identify a dose that consistently comes up short of causing dyskinesias. You can then take that dose every few hours. If you don't take the doses too close together, the risk of dyskinesias will dissipate before the next dose is taken. On the other hand, if you take the doses too close together, the effects will overlap and provoke dyskinesias. You will need to experiment to learn how your body is responding and, specifically, the optimum dose and dosing interval. Work in as many doses a day as you can.

- *Nighttime dosing.* When you are asleep, dyskinesias don't occur, regardless of the levodopa dose. Thus, if you can take your carbidopa/levodopa and get to sleep, you will sleep through the time of dyskinesias. Hence, another strategy for dealing with these dyskinesias is to take your carbidopa/levodopa doses at bedtime and during the night. If you normally get up to go to the bathroom during the night, you can work in doses then, provided that you can get back to sleep. For example, you might take a dose of carbidopa/levodopa at bedtime and two other doses during trips to the washroom.

These two strategies are not mutually exclusive. You may choose to employ both. The idea is to work in a total daily dose as high as possible up to about 800 mg daily. You can experiment with this to arrive at a dosing scheme that is practical and meets your needs.

Let's consider Mr. Jones, who has this problem. He found that one 25-100 carbidopa/levodopa tablet provokes dyskinesias, yet does not adequately control his parkinsonism. Using the strategies that we just described, he could do the following. First, he needs to find the dyskinesia threshold if he is to use carbidopa/levodopa during the daytime. To do this, he should reduce the dosage to 3/4 of tablet, or if necessary, to 1/2 tablet. If a 3/4 tablet doesn't cause dyskinesias, he can then take that dose every four to six hours, choosing a dosing interval that does not allow the effects to overlap. Thus he can work in three to four doses during the waking day. If he sleeps well, he can use the nighttime dosing scheme as well. With this, he can use a larger dose, since he will sleep through the time of dyskinesias. He might be able to work his way up to two 25-100 tablets at bedtime. If he is able to do this once again during the night and get back to sleep, this would add another 2 tablets to his total. Now let's see how much he is taking of the 25-100 tablets:

Three doses of 3/4 of a tablet during the daytime = 225 mg levodopa

Two doses of 2 tablets at bedtime and during the night = 400 mg levodopa

This total of 625 mg of levodopa puts him within the range we specified of 300 to 800 mg daily. Some people may require up to 800 mg daily for the best effect, but he is pretty close. He could try working in another dose during the night on a trial basis to see if that captured an even better effect. If he gets the timing right, he should be able to avoid dyskinesias.

When Carbidopa/Levodopa Is the Second Drug Started

Some people begin treatment of their parkinsonism with a dopamine agonist medication and later wish to add carbidopa/levodopa. The dopamine agonist drugs (pramipexole, ropinirole, pergolide, and bromocriptine) are not as potent and, sooner or later, must be supplemented with carbidopa/levodopa.

The first step is to check your dopamine agonist dose to be certain that you have raised it well into the therapeutic range. When these agonist drugs are first started (see the next chapter), the initial doses are too low to be beneficial. It is only after a number of weeks of dose escalation that they become effective. A common mistake is to remain on a lower dose and assume that the drug isn't effective. Thus, before adding carbidopa/levodopa, it makes sense to optimize the agonist drug dosage first. Unless you are having trouble tolerating the dopamine agonist, follow the guidelines in the next chapter for reaching the target dose of this medication. If the response is still inadequate, then it's time to begin carbidopa/levodopa.

The guidelines for initiating carbidopa/levodopa that we provided earlier in this chapter are also appropriate for those already taking a dopamine agonist. However, because you're already taking the agonist medication, you may not need to raise the carbidopa/levodopa dose as high. Our guidelines stipulate that if you achieve good control of the parkinsonian symptoms, you don't need to raise the levodopa dose higher.

When adding carbidopa/levodopa, don't change your dopamine agonist dose. Start with one 25-100 carbidopa/levodopa immediate-release tablet one hour before each of three meals, as outlined in supplement 12.1. Although carbidopa/levodopa should be taken on an empty stomach, the dopamine agonist medication is usually taken with meals; however, if you are not nauseated, you may take the agonist drug at the same time as your carbidopa/levodopa, one hour before meals. Follow through with the weekly escalation schedule we described earlier in this chapter (also see supplement 12.1). Advance the carbidopa/levodopa dose until you capture the optimum benefit.

If the combination of agonist drug and carbidopa/levodopa results in dyskinesias, then adjust your carbidopa/levodopa dose to capture the effect that works best for you. Higher levodopa doses increase dyskinesias; reducing the levodopa dose will abolish dyskinesias. Hallucinations are another matter. If they occur, then reductions of the dopamine agonist drug are usually necessary. If severe, then the agonist drug may need to be tapered off. This is discussed in more detail in chapter 24. In other words, reduce your levodopa doses to counter dyskinesias but reduce the dopamine agonist to counter hallucinations.

Levodopa Failures

CARBIDOPA/LEVODOPA FAILED TO HELP DESPITE THESE GUIDELINES; NOW WHAT?

If you have not benefited from carbidopa/levodopa, despite raising the doses and taking it on an empty stomach, you probably do not have PD. Rather, you may have one of the conditions we discussed in chapter 6. Before reaching that conclusion, review your medication list for any of the parkinsonism-inducing drugs listed in chapter 6.

Should you continue to take carbidopa/levodopa? It is not harmful to stay on it, but why pay the money and take pills when they don't help? If it failed to help despite an adequate trial, you may discontinue it.

HOW SHOULD I GET OFF THE CARBIDOPA/LEVODOPA?

The wisest strategy for discontinuing carbidopa/levodopa is to do it slowly. A slow reduction in dose allows you to assess any possible benefit one last time. As you lower the dose step by step, any deterioration will become apparent. If so, then you can stick with any given dose.

There are a variety of ways you could taper off carbidopa/levodopa. However, the easiest strategy is to simply reverse what we did to raise the dose. Just do that in reverse. In other words, reduce all your carbidopa/levodopa doses by 1/2 tablet every week until you are down to zero.

I FAILED TO IMPROVE WITH CARBIDOPA/LEVODOPA; WILL ANY OTHER DRUGS HELP ME?

If you did everything according to the book, and if there is no response to adequate doses of carbidopa/levodopa, then the options are rather limited. What about the dopamine agonist medications, which include pramipexole (Mirapex), ropinirole (Requip), pergolide (Permax), and bromocriptine (Parlodel)? Unfortunately, they are unlikely to provide benefit if you failed to improve with levodopa therapy. Why? These dopamine agonist medications also work through brain dopamine systems. If carbidopa/levodopa, the most potent and effective dopamine-replenishing drug fails, then why should less potent drugs work? It's okay to try them, but the likelihood of success is not very great. Usually I don't prescribe them in this setting, given their expense, potential side effects, and the very low expectation of benefit.

When levodopa fails, sometimes minor drugs are tried and particularly those that do not work via brain dopamine systems. This includes amantadine, anticholinergic medications, coenzyme $Q_{10,}$ and the beta-blockers (propranolol and nadolol).

Amantadine has been used for many years to treat parkinsonism. However, it isn't very potent and with all the other excellent drugs available for PD, it has lost favor. It is helpful in treating dyskinesias that complicate levodopa therapy, as we will see in chapter 18; its current primary use is for that purpose.

Amantadine's primary site of action in the brain appears to be in neurotransmitter systems other than dopamine. It is a mild blocker of the brain neurotransmitter glutamate, which is released by brain circuits linked to the basal ganglia. The usual starting dose is a single 100 mg tablet twice daily. After a week it can be raised to three times daily. The dose could be pushed as high as five tablets a day. If it does not provide benefit, taper it off. Common side effects include leg swelling, redness or other discoloration. This is not worrisome and is not necessarily a sign that the dose should be lowered (as long as it doesn't bother you). Occasionally, it will cause confusion or hallucinations.

There are a variety of *anticholinergic drugs*, but the two most commonly used in this setting are trihexyphenidyl (Artane) and benztropine (Cogentin). They are unlikely to help the slowness or walking problems of parkinsonism, but are appropriately used as treatment for tremor. They might also help the stiffness. If you decide to try one of these drugs, review chapters 14 and 18 for guidelines, but beware of the side effects from this class of medications, as discussed in those chapters.

The clinical experience with *coenzyme Q_{10}* for treating parkinsonism is limited. Hence it's unclear whether it will benefit those who do not respond to levodopa therapy. In the single clinical study that demonstrated benefit in PD, the effective dose was 1200 mg daily (300 mg four times per day). Someone not responding to levodopa could try this on faith, recognizing, however, that it is expensive ($100 to $200 monthly) and that insurance plans will not reimburse for this.

Propranolol (Inderal) and *nadolol (Corgard)* are from a class of drugs called beta-blockers. They block parts of the adrenalin response. They have been used to treat all types of tremor. They may be helpful for tremor treatment in someone who has failed levodopa; however, they will not benefit other aspects of parkinsonism. They can lower the blood pressure, so this must be watched. Details regarding other side effects and dosing are found in chapter 14.

Supplement 12.1. (Photocopy for easy reference)

Initial Dosage Schedule, Immediate-Release Carbidopa/ Levodopa, 25-100 (Standard Sinemet)

Start with a low dose and increase weekly if you are tolerating the carbidopa/levodopa. Your parkinsonian symptoms will guide us (walking difficulties, tremor, slowness, stiffness, etc.). When you find a dose that works well, stick with it. If several doses are equally effective, then settle on the lowest of the equally potent doses.

Carbidopa/levodopa should be taken on an empty stomach, such as one hour before each meal. *If you skip a meal, take that dose whenever it is convenient.*

If you feel faint standing on your feet, check your standing-up blood pressure, which may be lowered by carbidopa/levodopa. If the systolic blood pressure is less than 90, then this needs attention.

Week 1: Start with one 25-100 carbidopa/levodopa (yellow) tablet, three times per day (1 hour before each meal). If nausea:

- Reduce to 1/2 tablet three times daily.

- If you tolerate this, raise the dose back to 1 tablet, three times daily after a week. If still okay, continue on. If nausea is a problem, refer to supplement 12.2.

Week 2: Increase to 1 1/2 tablets carbidopa/levodopa, three times per day, unless markedly improved.

Week 3: Increase to 2 tablets, three times daily, unless markedly improved.

Week 4: Increase to 2 1/2 tablets, three times per day, unless markedly improved. Most people starting carbidopa/levodopa don't need to go higher than 2 1/2 tablets three times daily. Those who have not experienced substantial benefit should try going a little higher.

Weeks 5–6: Raise to 3 tablets, three times per day for a week. Ultimately you can go up to 3 1/2 tablets three times daily.

Final Recommendation: Stick with the most effective dose. If several doses are equally effective, choose the lowest.

Supplement 12.2. (Photocopy for easy reference)

Initial Dosage Schedule for People with Nausea

Start low and go slow with immediate-release carbidopa/levodopa (25-100), supplemented with extra carbidopa (Lodosyn). Raise the carbidopa/levodopa doses until your parkinsonism is markedly improved (walking difficulties, tremor, slowness, stiffness, etc.). Note that the initial doses are too low to expect benefit.

It may not be necessary to continue Lodosyn indefinitely, since the nausea may subside with continued carbidopa/levodopa use.

If you feel faint standing on your feet, check your standing-up blood pressure, which may be reduced by carbidopa/levodopa. If the systolic blood pressure is less than 90, then this needs attention.

Take one to two 25 mg Lodosyn (carbidopa) tablets before each carbidopa/levodopa dose. (Don't take more than 2 Lodosyn tablets with each dose.) You should take the carbidopa/levodopa an hour before meals, but you may take it with dry bread or crackers.

Week 1: Start with 1/4 of a 25-100 standard (yellow) carbidopa/levodopa (25-100) tablet, three times per day (one hour before each meal).

Week 2: Increase to 1/2 tablet, three times per day.

Week 3: Increase to 3/4 tablet, three times per day.

Week 4: Increase to 1 carbidopa/levodopa tablet, three times per day.

Week 5 Through the Next Several Weeks: Add 1/4 to 1/2 tablet of 25-100 carbidopa/levodopa to all three doses on a weekly basis, guided by the response. You may slowly raise the dosage up to as high as 2 1/2 tablets three times daily. For most people, this dose is sufficient. Settle on the most effective dose. If several doses are equally effective, choose the lowest.

Supplement 12.3. (Photocopy for easy reference)

Initial Dosage Schedule, Controlled-Release Carbidopa/ Levodopa, 25-100 (Sinemet CR)

Increase weekly if tolerated. Your parkinsonian symptoms will guide us (walking difficulties, tremor, slowness, stiffness, etc.). You may continue to increase the dose until these symptoms are markedly improved and you are satisfied. When you find a dose that works well, stick with it.

The CR formulation may work better when taken on an empty stomach, about two hours before each of two meals. *Take it with plenty of fluids and you may take it with dry bread or crackers.*

If you feel faint on your feet, check your standing-up blood pressure, which may be reduced by levodopa therapy. If the systolic blood pressure is less than 90, then this needs attention.

Week 1: Start with one 25-100 CR carbidopa/levodopa tablet, twice daily. If nausea:

- Reduce to 1/2 tablet twice daily.

- If you tolerate this, raise the dose back to 1 tablet twice daily after a week. If still okay, continue on. If nausea is a problem, refer to supplement 12.4.

Week 2: Unless markedly improved, increase the dosage to 2 tablets, twice daily.

Week 3: If your symptoms are still troublesome, increase the dosage to 3 tablets, twice daily.

Week 4: If still there is not substantial improvement, increase again to 4 tablets, twice daily.

Final Recommendation: Stick with the most effective dose. If several doses are equally effective, choose the lowest. You may be able to simplify your regimen by substituting one 50-200 Sinemet CR tablet for two 25-100 tablets.

For those who have not experienced substantial benefit, raise the dose to 4 tablets three times daily. If you fail to respond to this, switch to the immediate-release carbidopa/levodopa (see Chapter 12).

Supplement 12.4.   (Photocopy for easy reference)

Initial Schedule for CR (Controlled-Release) Carbidopa/ Levodopa When Nausea

Start low and go slow with CR carbidopa/levodopa (25-100), supplemented with extra carbidopa (Lodosyn). Raise carbidopa/levodopa doses until your parkinsonism is markedly improved (walking difficulties, tremor, slowness, stiffness, etc.). Note that the initial doses are too low to expect benefit.

Take one to two 25 mg Lodosyn (carbidopa) tablets before each CR (controlled-release) carbidopa/levodopa dose. (Don't take more than 2 Lodosyn tablets with each dose.) For the best response, take the CR carbidopa/levodopa about two hours before meals, but you may take it with dry bread or crackers. Take with plenty of fluids.

Week 1: Start with 1/2 CR carbidopa/levodopa (25-100) tablet, twice daily (2 hours before meals). The pill is pink (brand name Sinemet CR) or gray (generic).

Week 2: Increase to 1 carbidopa/levodopa CR tablet, twice daily.

Week 3: Increase to 1 1/2 carbidopa/levodopa CR tablets, twice daily.

Week 4: Increase to 2 carbidopa/levodopa CR tablets, twice daily.

Week 5 Through the Next Several Weeks: Increase weekly: add 1/2 carbidopa/levodopa CR tablet to both daily doses, guided by the response. You can slowly raise the dosage up to as high as 4 CR tablets twice daily.

Settle on the most effective dose. If several doses are equally effective, choose the lowest. For convenience, you may substitute one 50-200 CR tablet for two of the 25-100 tablets.

Continue supplementary carbidopa (Lodosyn) as long as you experience nausea.

13

◆ ◆ ◆

Starting Dopamine Agonist Treatment

In chapter 12, we considered principles and guidelines for starting carbidopa/ levodopa. Now we examine the use of dopamine agonist medications. As you read this chapter, you will recognize that many of the same principles that were discussed in this previous chapter also apply to dopamine agonist therapy. Dopamine agonists are used to treat Parkinson's disease (PD) in two situations: (1) as the initial medication and (2) added to carbidopa/levodopa later in the course to help counter motor fluctuations. We will address both uses in this chapter, since the dosage guidelines are similar. In subsequent chapters we will look at levodopa-related motor fluctuations in more detail; when they demand dopamine agonist treatment, we will refer back to the guidelines in this chapter.

Background: Dopamine Agonist Drugs

As you have already learned, dopamine agonist medications are like synthetic forms of dopamine. They go directly to the brain and stimulate dopamine receptors. They are not as effective as levodopa, but are more potent than any of the other drugs used to treat PD.

In the United States, four dopamine agonist medications are available for prescription use. Bromocriptine (Parlodel) was introduced over twenty years ago, followed by pergolide (Permax) and, more recently, pramipexole (Mirapex) and ropinirole (Requip). Table 13.1 summarizes information about these four drugs.

Table 13.1.   Dopamine Agonist Medications

Generic Name	Brand Name	Tablet or Capsule Sizes, in Milligrams (mg)	Typical Total Daily Dose (mg)*
Bromocriptine	Parlodel	2.5, 5	30
Pergolide	Permax	0.05, 0.25, 1.0	3
Pramipexole	Mirapex	0.125, 0.25, 0.5, 1.0, 1.5	4.5
Ropinirole	Requip	0.25, 0.5, 1, 2, 4, 5	12–15

* The total daily amount is taken in three separate doses; e.g., bromocriptine is typically taken in a dose of 10 mg three times daily (total daily dose of 30 mg). The doses shown are approximately equivalent in potency and would be sufficient to provide a prominent antiparkinsonian effect. These drugs are started in very low doses and only gradually increased to these levels.

These agonist medications are not equivalent on a milligram (mg) basis. In other words, 1 mg of a given agonist drug does not have the same potency as 1 mg of another. Comparisons require adjustment for potency. For example, experience has taught us that 3 mg of pergolide daily is approximately the same potency as 4.5 mg of pramipexole per day. Similarly, these are about as potent as 12–15 mg of ropinirole or 30 mg bromocriptine per day, as shown in table 13.1. The larger the dose of any of these agonist drugs, the more effective; however, the larger doses have greater potential for side effects. This balance between benefit and side effects is what determines the "typical doses" shown in table 13.1.

Each of these four drugs is taken in three doses per day, usually with each of three meals. Mealtime dosing is recommended initially to reduce the potential for nausea; however, if you don't experience nausea, you may take these on an empty stomach. Contrast this to carbidopa/levodopa, which may not get absorbed if taken with meals.

Why Choose a Dopamine Agonist for Initial Treatment of PD?

A dopamine agonist medication may be used as the first drug in the treatment of PD. The primary reason for starting therapy with an agonist drug is the lesser risk of dyskinesias or response fluctuations within two to five years, compared to carbidopa/levodopa. However, these less potent dopamine agonists do not by themselves adequately control parkinsonism for very long. They are only sufficient for a few years or less. Subsequently, when a dopamine agonist medication is combined with carbidopa/levodopa, then the risks of dyskinesias and response fluctuations increase substantially, although not quite as much as with carbidopa/levodopa alone.

There is no debate that the agonist drugs reduce levodopa motor complications when added to carbidopa/levodopa therapy. However, there is no proof they must be started first to capture these benefits. Moreover, these motor complications may not be highly troublesome and many manage these adequately with simple carbidopa/levodopa adjustments.

A dopamine agonist is a reasonable first drug for people with a high likelihood of developing dyskinesias and fluctuating responses. These problems are most likely among those with young-onset parkinsonism, defined as parkinsonism developing prior to forty. Thus starting treatment with a dopamine agonist drug in this select group of young people makes good sense. Even for those slightly older a dopamine agonist may be a reasonable choice as first drug. Among those much older, however, the risk of dyskinesias and response fluctuations is lower and the comparative benefits of carbidopa/levodopa take precedence. Thus my strategy is to start carbidopa/levodopa, rather than an agonist, in those sixty and over.

In chapter 9, I summarized the brain imaging evidence that the dopamine agonist drugs may slow the progression of PD. As noted, interpretation of these findings is complicated and the results are controversial. Moreover, head-to-head clinical comparisons of long-term dopamine agonist versus levodopa therapy favors levodopa. Parkinsonian scores are better after several years of carbidopa/levodopa compared to dopamine agonists, even when the agonist is later combined with levodopa. If dopamine agonists slowed PD progression, the results should be just the opposite.

When Is a Dopamine Agonist a Poor Choice?

Carbidopa/levodopa is a better choice among people with hallucinations, paranoia, or cognitive impairment (thinking, memory problems). The dopamine agonist drugs are much more likely to cause hallucinations, and people who are experiencing cognitive problems are vulnerable. If the memory and thinking problems are slight, then these drugs would still be acceptable. However, they are best avoided if the problems are substantial.

Both dopamine agonists and levodopa therapy can lower blood pressure in the standing position (orthostatic hypotension). This is usually not a problem among those starting treatment for PD. The exceptions, however, are the occasional people who start with a very low blood pressure, such as 90/60. When you start this low, there is not much room for further blood pressure reduction. With low blood pressure, overall management will be much simpler with carbidopa/levodopa. A dopamine agonist could be used, however, if another medication is responsible for the low blood pressure and if it can be discontinued (see chapter 21 for more details). To put this into concrete terms, if your *systolic* blood pressure is less than 100, then carbidopa/levodopa may be a better choice ("systolic" refers to the upper blood pressure number, such as 120 in 120/80).

The two oldest of the dopamine agonists, bromocriptine and pergolide, are from a unique class of drugs called ergots, with potential for constricting blood vessels. In most people, this is not a problem. However, pergolide and bromocriptine are not good choices in those with certain types of circulatory problems, most notably angina (chest pain due to impaired circulation to the heart) and Raynaud's syndrome (cold-induced impaired circulation to the hands). They are also poor choices for those with chronic lung or heart valve disease, since they can cause similar problems that may be difficult to distinguish. More about these ergot side effects is discussed below. Pramipexole and ropinirole are from a different drug class and do not affect circulation, heart, or lungs.

Drug Costs

Therapeutic doses of dopamine agonist drugs are much more expensive than generic carbidopa/levodopa. Even the starting doses of the agonist medications are costly, despite the fact that these initial doses are too low to be beneficial. The retail prices for carbidopa/levodopa and the agonist drugs purchased at a typical large community pharmacy are shown in table 13.2.

Therapeutic doses of pramipexole (Mirapex) and ropinirole (Requip) are priced similarly, although the initial starting dosage of pramipexole is less costly. These two are the least expensive of the dopamine agonist class of drugs. The monthly expense of pergolide is almost twice that of pramipexole and ropinirole, whereas generic bromocriptine is nearly three times higher, as shown in table 13.2. As we will see later, bromocriptine seems to have no advantage over the other three drugs, and the high price makes this medication a last choice for dopamine agonist treatment.

Generic carbidopa/levodopa is relatively inexpensive, as shown in table 13.2. Unfortunately, no similar inexpensive generic formulations are available for the dopamine agonist drugs (bromocriptine and pergolide are available as generics, but they are not cheap). If price is an important factor, this weighs in favor of carbidopa/levodopa.

One strategy for minimizing the expense of the dopamine agonist drugs is to use a larger pill broken in half to make a smaller dose. For example, the conventional starting dose for pramipexole is one 0.125 mg tablet three times daily. As shown in table 13.2, this will cost approximately $3.54 per day. However, if the next larger tablet (0.25 mg) is broken in half to generate a 0.125 mg size (1/2 of 0.25 mg = 0.125), then the expense is reduced by a dollar a day ($2.24). This is possible with pramipexole and pergolide since they can be easily broken. Ropinirole tablets are small, not scored in the middle, and not easily broken; hence, this strategy doesn't work well with ropinirole.

Table 13.2. Cost of Dopamine Agonist Therapy*

Medications and Doses	Cost per 100 Tablets	Cost per Day, Starting Dose**	Monthly Cost for Typical Therapeutic Dose***
Pramipexole (Mirapex)			
0.125 mg	$118	$3.54	
0.25 mg	149	2.24****	
0.5 mg	260		
1 mg	260		
1.5 mg	260		$234
Ropinirole (Requip)			
0.25 mg	149	4.47	
0.5 mg	149		
1 mg	149		
2 mg	152		
4 mg	262		
5 mg	262		236
Pergolide (Permax)			
0.05 mg	142	4.26	
0.25 mg	232		
1 mg	463		417
Bromocriptine (Parlodel)			
2.5 mg generic	245	3.68	
5 mg generic	341		614
2.5 mg brand name Parlodel	348	5.22	
5 mg brand name Parlodel	529		952
Comparison: carbidopa/levodopa 25/100 (immediate-release generic)	$ 26	$0.78	$ 47

*Retail prices, community pharmacy (2004).

**By convention, pergolide and bromocriptine are started with less than three doses daily. To allow comparisons, we have converted their starting doses to three times daily.

*** For this comparison we have used the therapeutic daily doses shown in table 13.1. For carbidopa/levodopa, a dose of six 25-100 tablets daily is given for comparison.

****Using 1/2 tablet of 0.25 mg pramipexole, instead of a whole 0.125 mg tablet.

Choosing an Agonist

Once the decision has been made to start a dopamine agonist drug, we then must decide which of the four to start. This is not easy, since none of these stands out as being substantially more effective than the others. In a perfect world, there would be comparative trials, pitting each drug against the others. However, very few trials of this type have been conducted. Such trials are expensive and federal funding agencies have typically not underwritten the cost. On the other hand, pharmaceutical companies have been loath to organize such studies, comparing their drug versus another. What if the competitor's drug came out on top? Although head-to-head studies of these agonist drugs have been few, several have compared bromocriptine to one of the others. In the aggregate, bromocriptine seems to come in second when compared to the other three drugs in this class, albeit a close second.

As already noted, bromocriptine and pergolide are from the ergot class of drugs. Because of this chemical structure, they also have additional side effects not shared by pramipexole or ropinirole. Specifically, they may rarely cause inflammation and scarring in the lungs, heart valves, or in the region of the kidneys. They may also induce spasm of blood vessels, such as heart arteries, in those predisposed. This is discussed in more detail later in this chapter. Pergolide and bromocriptine are also considerably more expensive than the other drugs in this class (pramipexole and ropinirole). In fact, I no longer prescribe bromocriptine (although I will renew the prescription if someone is doing well on stable bromocriptine doses). Bromocriptine's expense, slightly lower efficacy, and the risk for ergot side effects is dissuasive. Hence, we are going to cross bromocriptine off our list. I will provide bromocriptine dosing guidelines in this chapter for the occasional individual living in countries abroad where other newer drugs are unavailable. Also, pergolide has received some recent bad publicity, with preliminary evidence suggesting that it causes heart valve damage more often than previously suspected. Thus, pergolide is a distant third choice behind pramipexole and ropinirole.

Pramipexole Versus Ropinirole

Pramipexole and ropinirole are similar drugs and are priced comparably. I usually choose pramipexole, however, because it is simpler to use. Each of these dopamine agonist drugs is started in a very low dose and then the dose is slowly escalated to the therapeutic range over six to eight weeks or longer. Pramipexole tablets are scored; this allows fewer pills of different sizes to be used in the dosage escalation. Does this seem to be a trivial reason for making this choice? Perhaps, but after you see the dosing schedules for each of these agents later in this chapter you may tend to agree. These dosing escalation schedules are complex and require multiple steps. Although this may be relatively easy for physicians, I can assure you that the patients in my office don't quite see it that way.

How Many Times a Day Should I Take One of These Agonist Drugs? May I Take Them with Food?

The conventional way of administering the dopamine agonists is with meals, three times daily. They can be taken on an empty stomach but tend to cause nausea; they are better tolerated with meals. These drugs do not cause irritation of the stomach or ulcers. The nausea is mediated through the brain nausea center. Hence, if nausea occurs, it is not a danger sign.

Multiple Steps to an Effective Dose

All four agonist drugs require graduated dosage escalation over many weeks to achieve a dose that relieves symptoms. Hence patience is necessary; do not expect any dramatic improvement with any of these drugs during the first few weeks of treatment. How rapidly one increases the dose primarily relates to how it is tolerated. Often side effects are minimized if one goes up slowly.

The dosing schedules provided below for each of the four dopamine agonist drugs are precisely structured. You are given a starting dose and then very specific dosing instructions for the ensuing weeks, guiding you to the target dose. However, don't interpret this to mean that you must precisely comply with this regimen. These schedules are fairly arbitrary and minor variations are acceptable, if you tolerate them. For example, if you are tolerating a drug and wish to advance the dose a day or two early, that should be okay. The general principle is to start with a very low dose and raise it gradually over several weeks until there is a favorable effect.

Target Doses

In these dopamine agonist dosage schedules, we slowly raise the amounts until we reach our target doses, shown in table 13.3. The "targets" I have chosen are doses that are usually quite effective, and yet tolerated by most people. They are a bit arbitrary and your physician might have slightly different targets; that is okay. These specific target doses are:

- Pramipexole, 4.5 mg daily
- Ropinirole, 12–15 mg daily
- Pergolide, 3.0 mg daily
- Bromocriptine, 30 mg daily

Table 13.3.   Dopamine Agonist Drugs: How High May I Go?

Drug	Typical Daily Targeted Dose, Milligrams (mg) per Day*	Acceptable Higher Dose (If Tolerated), in mg per Day*	Absolute Highest Daily Dose (mg per Day)*
Bromocriptine (Parlodel)	30	40–50	60
Pergolide (Permax)	3	5	6
Pramipexole (Mirapex)	4.5	6	9
Ropinirole (Requip)	12–15	21	27

*Usually divided into three doses taken with meals.

Some physicians might choose slightly lower doses; however, I prefer setting the targets high enough so that we have a reasonable likelihood of benefit. The most common cause of dopamine agonist failure is too low a dose.

What if a lower dose works well? Fine, stick with that dose. Common sense dictates that we don't change what is working well. There is no reason to go higher if we achieve our goals with a lower dose.

May I Go Higher Than the Target Dose?

Again, these target doses are somewhat arbitrary. What works for one person may not work for another. If you are at the targeted dose and still not doing as well as you would like, you may go higher. However, only do this if you are not experiencing any substantial side effects. No blood tests are necessary.

If a dopamine agonist raised to the target dose proves insufficient, you may alternatively add carbidopa/levodopa. This is my practice; I prefer starting carbidopa/levodopa at that time, rather than pushing the dopamine agonist much higher than the target dose. We discuss below how to do this.

What Is the Highest Agonist Dose?

Higher and higher doses will capture more benefit. However, if we go too high, sooner or later, side effects will occur. Table 13.3 shows what would be acceptable higher doses. You may push the doses into this range if no side effects appear. If you do that and experience no further benefit, then you should probably reduce the dosage back to the target values.

Table 13.3 also defines the absolute limits of doses. There are exceptional cases where there are few other options; in those cases we may push the doses to these levels. Again, however, we do this only if there are no substantial side effects. It is rare that I have people raise their agonist drug much higher than the targeted doses.

Would It Be Helpful to Switch to a Different Dopamine Agonist Drug?

Changing from one dopamine agonist to another primarily makes sense for reasons of side effects. The four dopamine agonists are fairly similar in potency, provided that the dose can be increased to the targeted level. If you have raised one of these drugs to the target range and perhaps beyond, there is not a high likelihood that switching to another will better control your parkinsonism. There are occasional cases where this does occur, but usually this switch is done in only exceptional circumstances.

What If You Are Taking Carbidopa/Levodopa and Wish to Add a Dopamine Agonist?

We have already considered the use of a dopamine agonist drug as initial therapy for PD. These drugs are also added to carbidopa/levodopa to smooth out fluctuations in the response, which develop after several years. In fact, this has been the primary role of these drugs over the years. The guidelines in this chapter also cover this supplementary use of dopamine agonist drugs. The dosing strategies are the same whether the agonist is started as the first therapy, or added years later to levodopa treatment. The primary difference is that levodopa adjustments may also be necessary when the agonist is added. The specific strategy is discussed in chapter 18.

What If I Experience Side Effects As I'm Raising the Agonist Drug Doses?

The most common side effects of these drugs include the following (in no particular order):

- Nausea
- Low blood pressure (may result in fainting)
- Hallucinations
- Swelling (legs)
- Sleepiness
- Dyskinesias

If one of these develops but is trivial, it is okay to continue with the dosage escalation. Common sense should dictate what you do. Don't raise the dose if the side effects are substantial. Here are some general guidelines that pertain to the side effects listed above.

Nausea can sometimes be circumvented by raising the doses more slowly than shown in the dosage schedules. Your body will tend to acclimate to this side effect. As with levodopa, there is no danger of ulcers; the nausea is mediated via brain nausea centers, rather than resulting from a direct effect on the stomach. Unlike levodopa therapy, dopamine agonist drugs may be taken with food and in fact the doses are taken after eating. Having a full stomach aids tolerability.

Low blood pressure is only a problem if it results in symptoms, such as faints, near faints, or chronic lightheadedness. It is wise to occasionally check your standing-up blood pressure before starting agonist treatment and then periodically while the dose is being raised. Focus on the systolic blood pressure (the upper number, such as 120 in the reading of 120/80). If it is less than 90, then this is in the troublesome range. In that case, do not raise the drug dose any higher. This needs to be addressed by your physician, and the general guidelines for treating this are found in chapter 21. Remember that we are talking about the blood pressure in the standing position. Your blood pressure can be normal while sitting but very low when standing. Hence, the conventional seated blood pressure may miss important readings.

Hallucinations signal that the agonist drug will probably not be tolerated, at least at the dose being administered. If hallucinations are minimal (not bothersome or disruptive), it is okay to continue with the same dose, but higher doses are asking for trouble. If you are taking quite a high dose of the agonist, you may lower it back to levels that did not induce hallucinations. If the agonist dose is still in the low range (i.e., insufficient to produce much benefit), you should taper this drug off. You can do this by using the dosage schedules shown and going in reverse. Carbidopa/levodopa as the sole therapy would be a better choice in that case.

Swelling of the legs may occur with these drugs but it is not dangerous. It is reasonable to continue with the dosage escalation in spite of this. There may be other causes for leg swelling than the agonist medication, such as heart failure or a blood clot in the leg vein (in that latter case, the swelling is predominantly in one leg, which is also tender when squeezed). Hence it is wise to discuss this with your doctor to make certain there is not some other cause. Elevating your legs when sedentary is an effective means of reducing leg swelling. Elevate them high to allow gravity to pull the fluid out of your legs. How high? When seated, your feet should be at about your chest level.

Sleepiness caused by the agonist drug may prevent raising the dose. Certainly one concern is falling asleep while driving a car. The two newer agonist drugs, pramipexole and ropinirole, have been especially associated with falling asleep while driving. If you sense this problem is developing, do not raise the dose higher, and lower it if you continue to drive. Do not drive until this sleepiness has resolved. Bear in mind, however, that those with PD are often sleepy for other reasons, including poor sleep at night. Before blaming your agonist drug, you may wish to read chapter 20.

Dyskinesias may be provoked by higher dopamine agonist drug doses, as explained in previous chapters. Let's address separately dyskinesias provoked by dopamine agonists when taken alone versus with carbidopa/levodopa.

- Dyskinesias are rare when dopamine agonists are taken without carbidopa/levodopa. If they occur, they are usually mild and do not affect functioning or cause embarrassment. You can raise the dose higher, recognizing that if dyskinesias worsen, the agonist dose can then be lowered.

- Dyskinesias are more common when a dopamine agonist is added to carbidopa/levodopa. They don't develop with the lower doses but once the agonist has been raised to near the target dose, the likelihood increases. If these dyskinetic movements are slight, perhaps nothing needs to be done. However, if they become troublesome, then reduce the dose of carbidopa/levodopa (not the agonist). If you are using the carbidopa/levodopa 25-100 tablets, lower the doses by 1/4 to 1/2 tablet decrements until they are controlled. Once you have done that, you may raise the dopamine agonist doses again, if that seems appropriate. Dopamine agonists may be added even when someone is already experiencing dyskinesias from carbidopa/levodopa alone. The idea is to raise the agonist until the dyskinesias worsen, then lower the carbidopa/levodopa until they are controlled. Going up with the agonist and down with levodopa may provide better brain dopamine balance.

The dopamine agonist drugs, primarily pramipexole, have also rarely been linked to pathologic gambling. Prototypic is a middle-aged businessman I recently saw in the clinic who previously had enjoyed an occasional trip to the casino, never betting heavily. With pramipexole treatment, he began to experience euphoria when gambling. He couldn't pull himself away and would gamble all night. Gambling became an obsession. When he mortgaged his business to underwrite his gambling, his family pressured him to seek medical attention. It was clear from his history that his gambling compulsions started shortly after initiating therapeutic doses of pramipexole. When this was recognized and pramipexole discontinued, he became his old self.

Unique Side Effects from Pergolide and Bromocriptine

We have already alluded to certain unique side effects from pergolide or bromocriptine related to their ergot chemical structure. Most notably, this includes inflammatory reactions with scarring in certain internal organs. These don't occur immediately, but after months or even years of medication administration. Typically this is not a widespread process, but primarily involves one organ or area of the body. Three organ systems may be affected.

- *Lungs and lining around the lungs* (pleura). The primary symptom is shortness of breath. If this is suspected, appropriate tests include a chest X ray, breathing tests, and perhaps a lung scan.

- *Heart*. This includes the outside lining of the heart (pericarditis), as well as the valves (generating a heart murmur). If severe, heart failure might occur. The symptoms include shortness of breath and swelling. The workup typically includes an echocardiogram (an ultrasound of the heart) and consultation with a cardiologist.

- *Kidneys*. This occurs from inflammation and scarring in the back of the abdomen, constricting the drainage system carrying urine from the kidneys to the bladder (ureters). If kidney function starts to decline, this possibility should be considered. Appropriate tests include imaging studies, such as an intravenous pyelogram (also called excretory urogram); this visualizes dye passing from the kidneys to the bladder.

These complications have been uncommonly reported, diagnosed in about 1 percent of people taking therapeutic doses of these drugs. However, recent studies in people taking pergolide suggest that damage to heart valves may occur much more frequently; one may infer that the same may occur with bromocriptine. This is sufficiently troublesome to discourage many physicians from prescribing these two drugs. If they are used, an echocardiogram should be performed yearly to assess potential heart valve damage. Also, because of the potential lung and kidney problems, a chest X ray and a blood test of kidney function (creatinine) should be done yearly if these drugs are being used.

Any damage from these processes may be permanent, although sometimes improvement or resolution does occur if the offending drug is stopped. Hence, if there is a reasonable suspicion of this condition, even if unproven, it is wise to taper off the drug (pergolide or bromocriptine). Pramipexole and ropinirole do not appear to have any potential for these types of reactions.

Ergots have a tendency to constrict blood vessels. This is not a problem in most people taking pergolide or bromocriptine. However, rare individuals will experience chest pain due to ergot-induced spasm of the blood vessels to the heart. Like angina, in general, it may occur only with exercise. If this happens to you, a general recommendation is to cut the dose in half and consult your physician. This may prevent you from continuing with the drug.

Pergolide and bromocriptine can also occasionally cause spasm of blood vessels of the hands in cold weather, called Raynaud's syndrome. People experiencing these symptoms will note that their hands turn white and go numb in the cold; with warming, they become purple, red, and tingly.

Pergolide and bromocriptine can also cause hallucinations, leg swelling, and a low standing blood pressure. These side effects, however, appear no more likely than with pramipexole or ropinirole. They appear less likely to induce daytime drowsiness than pramipexole or ropinirole.

What If I Need to Stop My Dopamine Agonist Drug?

If side effects are a problem, then you may need to discontinue your agonist drug. As is true for all the drugs used to treat Parkinson's disease, it is wiser to taper off the medication rather than stop it abruptly. When you start the agonist drug, you begin with very low doses and then gradually increase it over six to eight weeks (starting schedules are provided later in this chapter). If you are taking the doses indicated for the first two weeks of therapy, you could stop it abruptly (since it is so low already). Higher doses should be lowered gradually. To do this, you can reverse the steps in the dosing schedules. However, you do not need to go as slowly in reverse; you could lower the dose every three days or so. What if the side effect is severe and you wish to taper off more quickly? In that case, cut the dose in half and then again halve the dose every three days until you are off the drug.

What If I Can't Tolerate the Dopamine Agonist Medication?

I listed earlier six of the most common side effects experienced with all the dopamine agonist drugs. If one of the agonist drugs causes substantial problems in any of those spheres, it is likely that the other agonist agents will do likewise. The exceptions may be swelling and sleepiness, which are probably less likely with pergolide and bromocriptine. Hallucinations, low blood pressure, and nausea are probably equally likely with any of the four available dopamine agonist medications. Dyskinesias may be slightly more likely with pergolide than the other dopamine agonist drugs.

If there are substantial side effects with agonist drugs, it may signal the need to switch to carbidopa/levodopa instead (or stick with carbidopa/levodopa alone if already on this drug). The only exception is dyskinesias, which are more prominent with carbidopa/levodopa. Carbidopa/levodopa is significantly less likely to induce hallucinations or swelling. Levodopa also has a lower risk for daytime sleepiness; when this does occur, it often is due to poor nighttime sleep, which often can be remedied with levodopa doses at bedtime or during the night (see chapter 20).

Adding Levodopa Therapy When the Agonist Proves Insufficient

Imagine you have recently developed PD and are using a dopamine agonist as your first drug. You have adjusted the agonist dose to the target range, but your parkinsonian symptoms are not well controlled; the tremor is still prominent, walking remains impaired, and you still are restricting your activities. Now what? My recommendation at this juncture is simple: add levodopa therapy. Although raising the agonist drug higher than the target dose is acceptable, I favor starting levodopa in this particular situation.

The schedule for starting and adjusting carbidopa/levodopa is the same as we outlined in chapter 12, using the immediate-release 25-100 formulation. Briefly, you start with a single tablet taken one hour before each meal (three doses per day). You then raise the dose by adding 1/2 tablet to all doses weekly until you are satisfied with the response, up to about 2 1/2 tablets three times daily. Refer to chapter 12 for the specific instructions.

What to do with the dopamine agonist? My recommendation is to maintain the dopamine agonist in the current dose and simply add the carbidopa/levodopa. There are three reasons.

First, less carbidopa/levodopa is necessary if the dopamine agonist is continued. It will therefore be easier to adjust the carbidopa/levodopa to control the symptoms.

Second, tapering off the dopamine agonist drug adds another level of complexity. The agonist drug should not be stopped abruptly. Neither should it be reduced at the same time you are adjusting carbidopa/levodopa (don't change doses of two medications simultaneously or you won't be able to figure out the cause if there are problems). The agonist could be tapered off over two to three weeks before starting levodopa therapy, but this would further delay control of parkinsonian symptoms. Alternatively, it could be tapered off once the levodopa adjustments have been completed. If that were done, however, parkinsonian symptoms might worsen, requiring further adjustment of carbidopa/levodopa to make up for the loss of the agonist drug.

Third, having a dopamine agonist on board might be helpful in the long run. It takes awhile to initiate and adjust agonist drugs (6–8 weeks or longer). They are often very helpful later in Parkinson's disease when there are ups and downs in the levodopa response (so-called motor fluctuations). Hence such problems may be delayed by virtue of having the dopamine agonist treatment already in place. This may prevent some later ruffles in your parkinsonism control.

There may be situations, however, where it is wise to taper off the dopamine agonist drug before starting levodopa therapy. If it has been minimally beneficial and you must pay out of pocket for these expensive drugs, you may wish to use levodopa therapy alone. Also, if the agonist drug provoked hallucinations, it is a good idea to taper off before starting carbidopa/levodopa. The agonist medications are more likely to cause hallucinations than carbidopa/levodopa. Carbidopa/levodopa alone might not provoke hallucinations, even though they occurred with dopamine agonist treatment.

Dosing Schemes for Each of the Four Dopamine Agonist Medications

The strategies for initiating each of the four dopamine agonist drugs (pramipexole, ropinirole, pergolide, and bromocriptine) differ from one another. Following you will find guidelines for each. The supplements at the end of this chapter summarize the specific instructions. You might want to photocopy them and tack them on your bulletin board.

PRAMIPEXOLE (MIRAPEX) DOSING SCHEDULE

Printed dosing instructions are imperative when starting any of the dopamine agonist drugs; the escalation schedules are complex. The pharmaceutical company making pramipexole provides a dosing instruction sheet, which is straightforward and relatively easy to use. However, if that is not available, you can use the schedule summarized in supplement 13.1 or 13.2 at the end of this chapter. The schedule shown in supplement 13.1 is almost identical to that provided by the pharmaceutical company; I have simplified it slightly to reduce the required numbers of different tablet sizes. The schedule shown in supplement 13.2 is my own preferred scheme, which requires only two tablet sizes to arrive at the target dose.

Note that we start with a very low dose and then aim for the target dose of 1.5 mg three times daily. The starting dose of 0.125 mg daily is too low to do any good; don't expect to feel better in the first two to four weeks.

The pramipexole tablets are all white, so it is not easy to determine the dose from the appearance of the tablet. Keep them in their labeled vials so that they don't get mixed up.

Side effects may require you to go a little slower and that is okay. Some side effects resolve with time, such as nausea. Hallucinations, however, do not. If hallucinations occur, this usually warrants switching to levodopa therapy. Watch out for daytime drowsiness and do not drive a car if that occurs.

Three prescriptions must be provided if one uses the schedule shown in supplement 13.1; there are three tablet sizes required to raise the dose to the therapeutic target. The physician must write prescriptions for 0.25 mg, 0.5 mg, and 1.5 mg size tablets. The pharmaceutical company's dosing schedule requires five tablet sizes and also includes the 0.125 mg and 1.0 mg sizes. Hence, if that schedule is used, prescriptions for these tablets are also necessary. My modified scheme shown in supplement 13.2 requires prescriptions for only two tablet sizes.

Some people may find that a lower dose of pramipexole is very effective. In that case, there is no need to push the dose higher. You may stick with that dose.

Bear in mind that the cost is more a reflection of the number of tablets daily, rather than the number of milligrams per day (see table 13.2). You can save money by using one larger tablet instead of two smaller tablets, when these provide equivalent doses. For example, if you find that two 0.5 mg tablets three times daily is effective, it will be cheaper to get a prescription for the 1.0 mg tablets and take one of those three times daily. This is true for all the dopamine agonist drugs.

ROPINIROLE (REQUIP) DOSING SCHEDULE

The ropinirole initiation strategy is similar to pramipexole, only a little more complicated. There are six different ropinirole tablets. They are not scored in the middle and it is hard to break them in half. Our schedule will require all six tablets, as shown in supplement 13.3, and you will need prescriptions for all. The tablet colors are also listed in this supplement; however, these are pastel shades and it may be a little hard to distinguish these because the colors are not very distinct.

Benefits should not be expected until about the week 6 dose and the dose of 2 mg three times daily. As with pramipexole, you do not need to push the dose to the maximum. If you find that a given dose is working well, stick with that.

Occasionally, the dose is pushed even higher than the 15 mg daily shown in supplement 13.3. Doses up to 24 mg daily have been employed (maximum is 27 mg daily; see table 13.3). This is acceptable if side effects allow and if these higher doses are necessary for the best effect. To raise the dose beyond the week 10 level of 5 mg three times daily (15 mg per day), add a 1 mg tablet to all three doses each week, up to 8 mg three times daily (24 mg daily). In other words, increase weekly from 5 mg three times daily to 6 mg, then 7 mg, and then 8 mg three times daily. If this does not add any benefit, you should go back to the lower, equally-effective dose you were using before.

Although the schedule specifies increases on a weekly basis, you may go more slowly. If side effects are a problem, sometimes going slowly allows these to pass (except for hallucinations, which do not resolve unless a lower dose is used). As with pramipexole, do not drive a car if you find that ropinirole makes you sleepy.

The goal is to settle on the most effective dose. However, if several doses are equally effective, then choose the lowest of those. There is no point taking a larger dose when a smaller one works just as well.

PERGOLIDE (PERMAX) DOSING SCHEDULE

The conventional dosing schedule for pergolide, as well as bromocriptine, advances the dose at intervals of less than a week. This contrasts with pramipexole and ropinirole, where the dose is increased every week. Actually, how we raise the dose is somewhat arbitrary. We will stick with the dosing schedule traditionally employed with pergolide therapy. Unlike pramipexole and ropinirole, pergolide is conventionally started with only one dose per day, although it is quickly advanced to the three times daily dosing schedule.

Pergolide comes in three tablet sizes, 0.05 mg (cream-colored), 0.25 mg (green), and 1.0 mg (lavender). These tablets break in half fairly easily. The smallest size, 0.05 mg, is started in a dose of a single tablet per day. Initially, the dose is raised daily by adding a single 0.05 mg tablet to the total daily dose, going to 12 tablets per day (4 tablets three times daily). As shown in supplement 13.4, we switch to the larger tablet, 0.25 mg, at the start of week 3. From that point on, the doses are increased every half week. These green, 0.25 mg tablets are used until we reach the target dose of 1 mg three times daily. It is cheaper and easier to use the 1 mg tablets, once we reach that level.

Although we have set as our target 1 mg three times daily, you may have experienced an excellent response at a lower dose. In that case, stick with that. Don't take more than you need.

To reach the target dose you will need prescriptions for both the 0.05 mg and the 0.25 mg tablets to be used before arriving at the 1.0 mg size. This will require 101 tablets of the cream-colored 0.05 mg size and about 150 tablets of the 0.25 mg (green-colored) size.

As indicated in supplement 13.4, you may raise the dose higher than 3 mg daily. If you find a need for a more potent effect and tolerate higher doses, you can go as high as 2 mg three times daily. You can do this by adding a 0.25 mg tablet to all three doses weekly until you reach a more favorable level, up to 6 mg daily.

BROMOCRIPTINE (PARLODEL) DOSING SCHEDULE

Bromocriptine is much more expensive than the other three agonist drugs, without any clear advantages and some disadvantages, as discussed. Hence, it is not likely that you will be using this particular drug. Perhaps the primary exception would be if side effects precluded all of the other agonist medications and you wanted to try one more.

About twenty years ago, before the newer dopamine agonists were available, use of "low-dose" bromocriptine was in vogue. The target dose in that scheme was approximately 10–20 mg daily. This was beneficial in several clinical trials; however, the effects were not substantial in many cases. Hence, the target dose we are using here is a little higher, 30 mg daily. This is of similar potency to the target doses of the other dopamine agonist drugs. During the early years of bromocriptine use, doses up to and exceeding 100 mg daily were occasionally administered. It became clear, however, that with very high doses, side effects were common.

A variety of dosage escalation strategies have been employed for bromocriptine over the years. Some have been painfully slow and delayed before reaching the target dose, extending well beyond six months. The pharmaceutical company's schedule calls for raising the dose by 2.5 mg every two to four weeks. With that scheme, it would require twenty-four to forty-eight weeks to reach our target of 30 mg daily. This is excessively slow. The scheme we will use here is a hybrid of the various schemes that have been published over the years, but with quicker escalation than in some of the current schedules. By convention, bromocriptine is usually increased at two-week intervals, and we will stick with dose changes every two weeks. With this schedule, we will reach 30 mg daily by a little over four months, as illustrated in supplement 13.5.

To keep things simple, we will use only one tablet size, the 2.5 mg formulation. Bromocriptine also comes in a 5 mg capsule. It is cheaper to use a 5 mg capsule than two 2.5 mg tablets (see table 13.2). Hence, once the dosage escalation is completed, it makes sense to switch to the 5 mg capsule to save money.

As with the other agonist drugs, do not feel compelled to reach the target dose (30 mg), if you are doing well on a lower dose. The target dose is only an approximation of what we expect to be effective without substantial side effects, *on the average.*

The Most Common Mistake When Starting a Dopamine Agonist

The most notorious mistake made with dopamine agonist drugs is failure to raise the dose into the therapeutic range. People often get stuck on one of the initial doses of these lengthy dose escalation schedules. The doses employed in the first two to four weeks are too low to do any good. People who fail to raise the dose then conclude the agonist drug is worthless.

This problem seems most frequent with ropinirole, perhaps for a couple of reasons. First, this drug has the most complex dosage escalation schedule. To get to the targeted dose it takes about two months and five to six different tablet sizes. Few other medications for any disorder require such an extended dosing strategy. Second is the pricing scheme; the low doses are quite expensive (e.g., $134 monthly for the starting ropinirole dose; see table 13.2). People intuitively conclude that if their pharmacy bill for the drug is over $100, the dose should be therapeutic.

Thus, if a dopamine agonist drug is to be used, push the dose up to the range where some benefit can be expected. Maintaining lower doses is usually an expensive waste of time. If doses in the therapeutic range cannot be tolerated, then it is necessary to go to levodopa therapy.

What are the minimum *daily* doses of the agonist drugs that should achieve some benefit? They are approximately as follows:

Pramipexole: 2 mg

Ropinirole: 6 mg

Pergolide: 1.5 mg

Bromocriptine: 15 mg

Note that these are per day, not per dose. Doses below this range are too low to expect much help. Obviously there are occasional exceptions to every rule, and if you experience benefit from a dose below these values, it is okay to maintain that; however, do not expect this to happen.

Supplements for Quick Reference

Now that you have had a chance to digest these dopamine dosing strategies, I'm sure you're thinking that these are a bit complex. They are. Unfortunately there are no shortcuts to using these drugs. They become even more complicated when you factor in carbidopa/levodopa therapy, which may need to be adjusted or added. To make these dosing schemes work, you will need to have a set of printed instructions. The supplements at the end of this chapter provide you with specific guidelines for each of the four dopamine agonist medications. You may photocopy them and place them on your bulletin board to guide you, week by week, as you follow the directions.

Later in this book, I will detail the strategies for adding a dopamine agonist to ongoing carbidopa/levodopa therapy. You will then be referred back to this chapter for the dosage schedules.

Some Typical Questions

Q: I've been on ropinirole for a month and I'm still no better. Should I try another drug?

A: Most likely, the dose is not yet into the therapeutic range. Dopamine agonist drugs are all started at very low doses (subtherapeutic) and must be raised sufficiently high to achieve benefit. Rather than starting another drug, this person should raise the dose further.

Q: I seem to get sleepy when I drive. I have been taking pramipexole and my Parkinson's disease symptoms are better.

A: Pramipexole may be the cause of sleepiness, provided that this individual was not drowsy before starting it. There are a variety of reasons why someone with PD may experience daytime sleepiness (see chapter 20). However, if the sleepiness developed in conjunction with pramipexole, this may be the culprit. To counter this, he could lower the dose and if necessary stop it altogether. Daytime sleepiness may be tolerated in most circumstances, but not when driving a car. Are there alternatives? Among the dopamine agonist drugs, pergolide is less likely to induce sleepiness. Carbidopa/levodopa is also a good alternative if he is not already taking it.

Q: I've been short of breath recently. It never goes away. However, my Parkinson's disease is doing well on carbidopa/levodopa and pergolide.

A: Pergolide may cause a serious lung or cardiac reaction. A physician needs to determine if there are any other likely causes. If there is any reasonable suspicion that pergolide is responsible, it should be tapered off. Shortness of breath is sometimes a symptom of Parkinson's disease and resolves with the usual medications for PD (especially carbidopa/levodopa). The clue is that a dose of carbidopa/levodopa transiently abolishes the shortness of breath.

Q: I've been taking carbidopa/levodopa for many years and recently added ropinirole; now I have jerky involuntary movements. What should I do?

A: Dyskinesias are likely being described, indicative of an excessive medication response. Although levodopa therapy is notorious for causing dyskinesias, they may also develop when a dopamine agonist is added to carbidopa/levodopa. If these are a problem, reduce each of the carbidopa/levodopa doses by 1/4 to 1/2 tablet and see if the dyskinesias resolve. If not, continue to similarly reduce the carbidopa/levodopa doses until the result is satisfactory.

Supplement 13.1.

Conventional Dosage Schedule, Pramipexole (Mirapex)

See also the alternative pramipexole dosing schedule, supplement 13.2, which requires only two tablet sizes.

- Take with meals (okay to take on empty stomach if not nauseated).
- Increase weekly if tolerated until symptoms adequately controlled.
- Do not increase further if excessive drowsiness or hallucinations (also do not drive a car if these develop).
- Check your standing blood pressure occasionally to make certain not low. We want systolic blood pressures over 90.
- You will need prescriptions for three different tablets to work your way up this schedule: 0.25 mg, 0.5 mg and 1.5 mg.

Week/ Tablet Size, Milligrams (mg)	Instructions	Total Number of Tablets per Day	Total Daily Dose (mg)
1 0.25 mg	Take 1/2 tablet 3 times daily	1 1/2	0.375 mg
2 0.25 mg	Take 1 tablet 3 times daily	3	0.75 mg
3 0.5 mg	Take 1 tablet 3 times daily	3	1.5 mg
(The benefit will likely start after this point in the schedule.)			
4 0.5 mg	Take 1 1/2 tablets 3 times daily	4 1/2	2.25 mg
5 0.5 mg	Take 2 tablets 3 times daily	8	3.0 mg
6 0.5 mg & 1.5 mg	Take one 0.5 mg tablet plus one-half of a 1.5 mg tablet 3 times daily	three 0.5 mg tablets plus one and a half 1.5 mg tablets	3.75 mg
7 1.5 mg	Take 1 tablet 3 times daily	3	4.5 mg*

*This final dose usually captures the best balance between benefits and side effects. However, your physician may choose to raise the dose to 6.0 mg daily. To do this, add a 0.25 mg tablet to all three doses for a week or two; thereafter, take two 1.0 mg tablets three times daily.

Supplement 13.2.

Simplified Dosage Schedule (My Scheme), Pramipexole (Mirapex)

- Take with meals (okay to take on empty stomach if not nauseated).
- Increase weekly if tolerated until symptoms adequately controlled.
- Do not increase further if excessive drowsiness or hallucinations (also do not drive a car if these occur).
- Check your standing blood pressure occasionally to make certain it is not low. We want systolic blood pressure over 90.
- You will need prescriptions for two different tablet sizes to work your way up this schedule: 0.25 mg and 1.5 mg.

Week/ Tablet Size, Milligrams (mg)	Instructions	Total Number of Tablets per Day	Total Daily Dose (mg)
1 0.25 mg	Take 1/2 tablet 3 times daily	1 1/2	0.375 mg
2 0.25 mg	Take 1 tablet 3 times daily	3	0.75 mg
3 0.25 mg	Take 2 tablets 3 times daily	6	1.5 mg
(The benefit will likely begin at this point in the schedule.)			
4 1.5 mg	Take 1/2 tablet 3 times daily	1 1/2	2.25 mg
5 0.25 mg & 1.5 mg	Take one-half 1.5 mg tablet and one 0.25 mg tablet 3 times daily	one and a half 1.5 mg tablets plus three 0.25 mg tablets	3.0 mg
6 0.25 mg & 1.5 mg	Take one-half 1.5 mg tablet plus two 0.25 mg tablets 3 times daily	one and a half 1.5 mg tablets plus six 0.25 mg tablets	3.75 mg
7 1.5 mg	Take 1 tablet 3 times daily	3	4.5 mg*

*This final dose usually captures the best balance between benefits and side effects. However, your physician may choose to raise the dose to 6.0 mg daily. To do this, add one 0.25 mg tablet to all three doses for a week or two; thereafter, take two 0.25 mg tablets plus one 1.5 mg tablet three times daily (or two 1 mg tablets 3 times daily).

Supplement 13.3.

Dosage Schedule, Ropinirole (Requip)

- Take with meals (okay to take on empty stomach if not nauseated).
- Increase weekly if tolerated until symptoms adequately controlled.
- Do not increase further if excessive drowsiness or hallucinations (also do not drive a car if these develop).
- Check your standing blood pressure occasionally to make certain it is not low. We want systolic blood pressure over 90.
- You won't notice improvement for the first few weeks.
- You will need prescriptions for six different tablet sizes to work your way up this schedule: 0.25 mg, 0.5 mg, 1 mg, 2 mg, 4 mg, and 5 mg.

Week/ Tablet Size, Milligrams (mg)	Tablet Color	Instructions	Amount Each Dose	Total Daily Dose, (mg)
1 0.25 mg	White	Take 1 tablet 3 times daily	0.25 mg	0.75 mg
2 0.5 mg	Yellow	Take 1 tablet 3 times daily	0.5 mg	1.5 mg
3 0.25 plus 0.5 mg		Take 1 tablet of each size 3 times daily	0.75 mg	2.25 mg
4 1.0 mg	Green	Take 1 tablet 3 times daily	1.0 mg	3 mg
5 0.5 and 1.0 mg		Take 1 tablet of each size 3 times daily	1.5 mg	4.5 mg
6 2.0 mg	Pink	Take 1 tablet 3 times daily	2.0 mg	6 mg
7 0.5 and 2.0 mg		Take 1 tablet of each size 3 times daily	2.5 mg	7.5 mg
8 1.0 and 2.0 mg		Take 1 tablet of each size 3 times daily	3.0 mg	9 mg
9 4.0 mg	Brown	Take 1 tablet 3 times daily	4.0	12 mg
10 5.0 mg	Blue	Take 1 tablet 3 times daily	5.0	15 mg*

*A higher dose may be recommended by your physician, up to as high as 8 mg three times daily (24 mg daily). If instructed to do this, you may increase the dose every 1–2 weeks. Start by adding one 1.0 mg tablet to your three 5 mg doses to make 6 mg three times daily. If tolerated, you can then add another 1.0 mg tablet to all three doses to make 7 mg three times daily, and ultimately raise the dose to 8 mg three times a day.

Supplement 13.4.

Dosage Schedule, Pergolide (Permax)

- Take with meals (okay to take on empty stomach if not nauseated).
- It is started as one dose a day, then two doses daily and thereafter three doses a day.
- It is initially increased daily; after the first two weeks, it is increased every half week.
- Increase until your symptoms are adequately controlled, provided you tolerate it.
- Do not increase further if excessive drowsiness or hallucinations (also do not drive a car if these develop). Consult your physician if chest pain.
- Check your standing blood pressure occasionally to make certain it is not low. We want systolic blood pressure over 90.
- You won't notice improvement for the first 2–3 weeks.
- You will need prescriptions for three different tablet sizes to work your way up this schedule: 0.05 mg, 0.25 mg, 1.0 mg.

[Photocopy the following page for easy reference.]

Dosage Schedule, Pergolide (Permax)

Day of Therapy	Size of Tablet (mg)	Tablet Color	Tablets with Breakfast	Tablets with Lunch	Total with Supper	Total Daily Dose (mg)
Day 1	0.05	Cream	1	0	0	0.05
2	0.05	Cream	1	1	0	0.10
3	0.05	Cream	1	1	1	0.15
4	0.05	Cream	2	1	1	0.20
5	0.05	Cream	2	2	1	0.25
6	0.05	Cream	2	2	2	0.30
7	0.05	Cream	3	2	2	0.35
8	0.05	Cream	3	3	2	0.40
9	0.05	Cream	3	3	3	0.45
10	0.05	Cream	4	3	3	0.50
11	0.05	Cream	4	4	3	0.55
12–14	0.05	Cream	4	4	4	0.60

Week of Therapy	Size of Tablet (mg)	Tablet Color	Tablets with Breakfast	Tablets with Lunch	Total with Supper	Total Daily Dose (mg)
Week 3*	0.25	Green	1	1	1	0.75
3 1/2**	0.25	Green	1 1/2	1 1/2	1 1/2	1.125
4	0.25	Green	2	2	2	1.5
4 1/2	0.25	Green	2 1/2	2 1/2	2 1/2	1.875
5	0.25	Green	3	3	3	2.25
5 1/2	0.25	Green	3 1/2	3 1/2	3 1/2	2.625
6	1.0	Lavender	1	1	1	3.0***

*Beginning with day 15.

**Week 3 1/2 implies making the change midweek, such as on day 18.

***If higher doses are recommended by your physician, the dosage can be raised from 1 mg 3 times daily by adding a 0.25 mg tablet to all three doses every 1–2 weeks, up to 6 mg per day (2 mg 3 times daily). Thus the dose for the week following week 6 would be 1.25 mg 3 times daily; then 1.5 mg 3 times daily; then 1.75 mg 3 times daily; finally, 2 mg 3 times daily.

Supplement 13.5.

Dosage Schedule, Bromocriptine (Parlodel)

- Take with meals (okay to take on empty stomach if not nauseated).
- It is taken twice daily for the first two weeks and three times daily thereafter.
- It is increased every two weeks.
- Increase until your symptoms are adequately controlled, provided you tolerate it.
- Do not increase further if excessive drowsiness or hallucinations (also do not drive a car if these develop). Consult your physician if chest pain.
- Check your standing blood pressure occasionally to make certain not low. We want systolic blood pressure over 90.
- You won't notice improvement for the first 6–8 weeks.
- You will need a prescription for one size tablet, 2.5 mg. Once you have completed your dosage adjustments and arrive at a stable dose, you may substitute one 5 mg capsule for two 2.5 mg tablets (saves money).

Week	Instructions, Using the 2.5 mg Tablet	Total Daily Dose, Milligrams (mg) per Day
1–2	Take 1/2 tablet 2 times daily	2.5 mg
3–4	Take 1/2 tablet 3 times daily	3.75 mg
5–6	Take 1 tablet 3 times daily	7.5 mg
7–8	Take 1 1/2 tablets 3 times daily	11.25 mg
9–10	Take 2 tablets 3 times daily	15 mg
11–12	Take 2 1/2 tablets 3 times daily	18.75 mg
13–14	Take 3 tablets 3 times daily	22.5 mg
15–16	Take 3 1/2 tablets 3 times daily	26.25 mg
17–beyond	Take 4 tablets 3 times daily	30 mg*

*Your physician may recommend higher doses if the benefit is insufficient and if no substantial side effects. If advised to do this, continue to increase by one-half of a 2.5 mg tablet added to all doses, every other week. The dose may be raised to 40 mg per day and in rare circumstances up to 60 mg daily.

14

◆ ◆ ◆

Refractory Tremor Syndromes: "Medications Don't Help My Tremor!"

Parkinsonian tremor typically is controlled with levodopa and sometimes with dopamine agonist therapy. Usually it is not completely abolished but is markedly attenuated. In many cases, it tends to creep back at times, but is mostly quiescent and much less obtrusive. The primary exception is when stress or excitement sabotage tremor control, seemingly overriding the effect of medications. This chapter focuses on people with prominent tremor that is poorly responsive to levodopa and dopamine agonist therapy. This may occur in one of several settings:

- Inadequate medication dosing

- Breakthrough tremor (tremor comes and goes)

- Only partial tremor control (despite maximum treatment)

- "Benign tremulous parkinsonism"

- Not PD, but a variant of essential tremor

- Combination of PD and essential tremor

Inadequate Medication Dosing

Dopamine agonists often do not control the rest tremor of PD nearly as well as levodopa. Thus, if you are taking only an agonist medication, the strategy is simple: add levodopa therapy (see chapter 12).

If you are already on levodopa therapy, the first issue is whether you have followed all the guidelines in chapter 12, including:

- Using the immediate-release 25-100 formulation (the controlled-release is not fully absorbed)

- Taking it on an empty stomach (dietary protein blocks the effect)

- Pushing the dose to the maximum

Sometimes higher than usual doses of carbidopa/levodopa are required to control tremor. If your tremor isn't responding to more moderate doses, you may slowly push the dose up to 3 1/2 tablets of the 25-100 immediate-release formulation of carbidopa/levodopa three times per day (1 hour before each meal). If after a week or two on this dose the tremor persists, then read on.

Breakthrough Tremor

Some people report poor control of their tremor, when in fact this is true only part of the time. The tremor is quiescent at times but not consistently. Tremor is conspicuous, unlike bradykinesia and other aspects of parkinsonism, which blend into the background. When tremor is present, you see it, feel it, and can't easily ignore it. When it is gone, people tend to take that for granted and have a selective memory for the tremor recurrences. Obviously there is potential to mislead your physician if your tremor control is intermittent but you do not perceive it that way. Thus you need to be a good observer.

Intermittent tremor control may lend itself to further treatment. There are three possibilities to consider:

- Your levodopa dose is not quite high enough to be consistently effective

- Your levodopa effect is wearing off

- You are experiencing stress-induced tremor

Let's discuss each.

If your dose of carbidopa/levodopa is right on the margins of effectiveness, your parkinsonian symptoms may respond intermittently: sometimes it will be effective and sometimes not. If that's the case, raising the dose slightly should effectively treat this. If you suspect this is your problem, raise all your doses by 1/2 tablet (assuming you are taking the 25-100 immediate-release formulation); if still inadequately controlled, you could go up by another 1/2 tablet. If this is the problem, small increases should be sufficient.

REFRACTORY TREMOR SYNDROMES

A second explanation for intermittent tremor control is the wearing-off of the levodopa effect. In this case, each dose of carbidopa/levodopa results in tremor control for a few hours or less; the tremor recurs when it is getting close to the time for the next levodopa dose. There are a variety of strategies for dealing with this, as described in chapters 17–18. The simplest approach is to reduce the interval between doses to match the duration of the levodopa response. As you shorten the interval between doses, you will need to add an extra dose or two each day.

Tremors of any type get worse under stress. This is true for both good stress (such as watching sporting events or an emotion-provoking movie) and bad stress. When our stress levels go up, medication control of the tremor is often lost. This may be the case for even the best levodopa responders. Once the stress is over, the tremor again responds to medications, as it did before the stressor. Unfortunately intermittent loss of tremor control due to stress is nearly impossible to treat, other than to minimize life stressors as much as possible.

Only Partial Tremor Control, Despite Maximum Treatment

Sometimes PD tremor is inadequately controlled despite maximum levodopa doses, and perhaps with dopamine agonist therapy. This is not the case of tremor coming and going described above; rather, the tremor is persistent and levodopa and the agonists only take the edge off. Here two other classes of drugs are worth considering: anticholinergic medications and the beta-blockers. Unfortunately neither has a high likelihood of success in this setting but may be helpful in certain cases. However, we also need to be cognizant of their potential side effects.

Propranolol (Inderal) and nadolol (Corgard) are beta-blockers used for treating essential tremor and may be employed to dampen parkinsonian tremor. Both drugs lower blood pressure, which can be a problem in people with PD who may have a tendency to a low standing blood pressure (orthostatic hypotension). Dosing instructions are found later in this chapter. If these medications are started, monitor your blood pressure closely when standing. If you start out with a low blood pressure, you may not tolerate them.

The anticholinergic medications have been used for over a century to treat PD. They are largely ineffective for many aspects of parkinsonism but tremor may respond. If you have been unable to control your parkinsonian tremor with levodopa therapy, you might consider trying an anticholinergic medication. There are several anticholinergic drugs on the market; none seem to have any advantage over any of the others. Those most frequently used for parkinsonian tremor are trihexyphenidyl (Artane) and benztropine (Cogentin).

Trihexyphenidyl (2 mg tablet) or benztropine (1 mg tablet) can be started in a dose of half of a tablet once daily. If you tolerate this, you may then raise the dose every week. Go to 1/2 tablet twice daily, then three times daily. If you are still tolerating this, but with inadequate benefit, the dose can be pushed up to a whole tablet three times per day. This is about the highest dose that most adults will tolerate; however, if you are not experiencing side effects, it could be raised further to 1 1/2 and then 2 tablets three times per day. If no benefit, slowly taper it off. Benztropine and trihexyphenidyl are similar drugs; if you failed with one, you are unlikely to respond to the other.

These anticholinergic medications have no life-threatening side effects, but frequently cause constipation, slowed urination, dry mouth and eyes, visual blurring, and mild memory impairment. These side effects often limit the use of these drugs. They are a poor choice for anyone with substantial thinking or memory difficulties.

Finally, bear in mind that just because tremor is present does not mean that it must be treated. If it does not bother you, there is no need to aggressively add medications to control your tremor.

Benign Tremulous Parkinsonism

Very little has been published about a variant of PD that is sometimes termed benign tremulous parkinsonism. This is a condition that I occasionally see in the clinic, and it is marked by the following features:

- Prominent parkinsonian tremor
- Other aspects of parkinsonism are relatively mild
- Very slow progression (much slower than usual)
- Tremor that responds poorly to medications

This is a good news–bad news condition, although more good than bad. Those with this disorder tend to remain stable for many years and, apart from the tremor, are not very troubled. These are people I often see back yearly in the clinic and note little change from one year to the next. The bad news is that the tremor sometimes is not very treatable. However, the same medications are tried as with PD in general. Over many years, there is some deterioration, but it tends to be less troublesome and less pronounced than with typical PD.

Essential Tremor, Not PD

Sometimes essential tremor is misdiagnosed as PD. This is usually not a problem for head or voice tremor, since these are recognized as typical of essential tremor and not PD. However, misdiagnosis occurs more frequently when essential tremor involves the hands, since they are affected in both conditions. Although we considered the distinctions in chapter 6, I will briefly summarize the hallmark features of essential tremor of the hands.

- The tremor is present only when the hands are in use, for example, when holding something (eating utensil, drinking glass). It is also present when the hands are not moving but held against gravity (arms outstretched). It tends to abate when the hands are relaxed. This contrasts with the typical PD tremor, which is primarily present when the hands are in a relaxed position, such as at one's side when walking.

- There are no other neurologic signs seen in essential tremor, including no signs of parkinsonism.

So how could essential tremor get misdiagnosed as PD with tremor? There are at least a couple of ways this could easily occur.

- Some people with essential tremor also have a tremor when their hands are in a relaxed position, like the "rest tremor" of PD. This is most likely if essential tremor is long-standing.

- Over the age of seventy to eighty, we all tend to get a little stooped, walk a little more slowly with shorter steps, and so on. If these signs are present in conjunction with essential tremor, it could be mistaken for PD.

Essential tremor does not respond to carbidopa/levodopa or dopamine agonist drugs. However, we will discuss treatment of essential tremor briefly later.

Combination of PD and Essential Tremor

If someone has both PD and essential tremor, the parkinsonism should respond to levodopa treatment, whereas the essential tremor will not. Do PD and essential tremor ever occur together in the same person? There are a couple of ways this might happen.

- Both PD and essential tremor are common conditions. PD occurs in about one person in one hundred, whereas essential tremor develops in a few people out of one hundred. Occasionally both conditions occur in the same person by chance.

- There are occasional people with PD whose symptoms include a tremor very much like essential tremor. In other words, coinciding with the onset of generalized parkinsonism is a tremor identical to essential tremor. Sometimes the first symptom of PD is a tremor identical to essential tremor, which may confuse the diagnosis.

If your tremor seems to have features of essential tremor and doesn't respond to levodopa therapy or dopamine agonist drugs, read on.

Medications for Essential Tremor

There are a variety of drugs employed in the treatment of essential tremor. A detailed description of how to treat essential tremor is beyond the scope of this book. However, let's digress and consider the class of medication usually chosen as first-line treatment of essential tremor: the beta-blockers. Occasionally they are also used in the treatment of refractory parkinsonian tremor.

Beta-blockers inhibit certain of the effects of adrenalin-like substances in our body. Not all beta-blockers are useful for tremor control, however. The two that are most effective are propranolol (Inderal) and nadolol (Corgard). Generally, each is started in a low dose and gradually increased, depending on the response.

Beta-blockers should not be used in anyone with a tendency toward asthma. Also, they slow the heart rate and lower the blood pressure. If your blood pressure is already low, beta-blockers may lower it further and make you faint. If you have a very slow heart rate, your physician may also advise against this (although they are often used to treat many other heart problems). Regardless, the heart rate and blood pressure should be checked periodically after starting these medications. Occasionally, they will cause depression or lethargy; nadolol is probably less likely to do this than propranolol. Finally, if you are diabetic on insulin and prone to low blood sugar reactions, you should probably avoid these drugs; they can mask the early warnings of low blood sugar.

The beta-blockers are commonly prescribed, and physicians are familiar with their use. Guidelines for initiating therapy with these drugs for tremor are as follows.

- Propranolol: Start with 1/2 of a 40 mg tablet once to twice daily. After a couple of weeks, this can be raised to a whole tablet once to twice daily. Alternatively, the long-acting form, Inderal LA, could be started with a single morning dose of 60 mg. Higher doses of either formulation can be employed if needed and if tolerated. A typical therapeutic dose of immediate-release propranolol for tremor is 60 mg twice daily, with occasionally doses as high as 240 mg daily (in divided doses). A typical therapeutic dose of Inderal LA is 160 mg once daily, occasionally with doses twice as high as that.

- Nadolol: This long-acting drug is administered as a single daily dose taken in the morning. Start with a dose of 40 mg daily. After a couple of weeks it could be doubled, then subsequently tripled (to 120 mg daily). Occasionally, doses as high as 240 mg once daily are employed for tremor control.

Neither propranolol nor nadolol will completely control tremor of any type. The best we can do with these drugs is to reduce tremor severity by about two-thirds. The response is better when the tremor is less severe. Note that other drugs are available for treating essential tremor. If this is your problem, discuss this further with your physician.

Severe and Unresponsive Tremor: Consider Surgery

Tremor of any type (essential tremor, PD, or other) can be controlled most of the time with brain surgery, either thalamic deep brain stimulation or thalamotomy. The target of this surgery, the thalamus, was illustrated in figure 2.5 (chapter 2). This is major brain surgery and is not a trivial endeavor. However, it often is dramatically effective in abolishing or nearly abolishing severe tremor. Other PD brain surgeries, specifically pallidotomy or subthalamic nucleus deep brain stimulation, also improve tremor, but not quite as consistently as when the thalamus is the brain target. If your tremor has failed medical treatment, is disabling, and you are in otherwise good health, you may be a candidate. For more details, see chapter 33.

PART SEVEN

♦ ♦ ♦

The Early Years on Medications

15

◆ ◆ ◆

The First Few Years on Carbidopa/Levodopa Treatment

This chapter addresses the newly diagnosed person with PD who has recently started carbidopa/levodopa. Will I need to raise the dose every few months? Will I become tolerant? Will it stop working? The answer to all three questions is no. You are now on automatic pilot for the near term. This assumes, of course, that you followed the dosing scheme in chapter 12 and raised the dose sufficiently to adequately treat your problems. Once you've done that, further major changes in your medication schedule should not be necessary in the near future. Are there ever any exceptions? Actually, there are, as illustrated in this chapter.

Q: My PD problems were easy to control with a single Sinemet tablet three times a day. Now, a couple of years later, I'm slow and shaky all day long.

A: The problem here is low-dose therapy or mealtime dosing. A larger dose of carbidopa/levodopa may be necessary after several months to years if only a low dose was used in the first place. In this case, the starting dose of carbidopa/levodopa was maintained without any further escalation. This dose may need to raised, using the general scheme outlined in chapter 12.

The second possibility is that this person got careless and started taking the carbidopa/levodopa doses with meals. Remember that carbidopa/levodopa must be taken on an empty stomach for maximum effect.

Q: My parkinsonism was controlled all day long; now the symptoms come and go.

A: The problem here is wearing-off. After several years, but occasionally after a year or two, the response to carbidopa/levodopa becomes less consistent. In other words, the benefits come and go. The beneficial response becomes tied to each dose.

When levodopa therapy is first started, the benefit is cumulative and long-lasting; you can skip a dose and experience no decline. Later, usually after a number of years, the benefit becomes time-locked to each dose. Although there is still some long-lasting effect, part of the benefit wanes several hours after each carbidopa/levodopa dose. This results in recurrence of parkinsonian symptoms if the doses are spaced too far apart.

The first step in treating this is to recognize what is happening. If your parkinsonism is coming and going, pay attention to the time course. Are you better an hour or so after each dose of carbidopa/levodopa (or 2 hours after sustained-release carbidopa/levodopa)? Is there a decline when it's getting close to the time for your next dose? If so, this represents the wearing-off effect. The response to each dose is wearing off before the next dose is taken.

Usually this is a minor problem when it occurs during the first years of PD and may never be more than that. If this wearing-off effect is troublesome, the simplest strategy is to move the doses closer together so that one dose is kicking in just before the previous dose wears off. This will require adding an extra dose or two each day to provide continuous coverage. If this becomes more problematic, then a variety of additional strategies can be employed, which are addressed in detail in chapters 17–18.

Q: What about adding pramipexole (or ropinirole or pergolide) instead of increasing carbidopa/levodopa?

A: The problem here is wearing-off. Adding a dopamine agonist is an acceptable alternative to making the adjustments of levodopa therapy. Some physicians might choose this option, especially those who favor early use of a dopamine agonist with the conviction that the long-term results will be better.

My choice in the above scenarios was to make carbidopa/levodopa adjustments since the problems were relatively straightforward and the medication changes simple. Moreover, the expected improvement will be rapid; improvement typically occurs quickly with carbidopa/levodopa adjustments. In contrast, escalating a dopamine agonist to therapeutic levels takes about 6–8 weeks. Moreover, these simple adjustments of carbidopa/levodopa are much easier on the pocketbook; adding a dopamine agonist drug is not cheap.

The dopamine agonist medications are excellent choices when simple carbidopa/levodopa adjustments are not adequate. However, early in the course of PD, it's easier and quicker to fine-tune the levodopa regimen.

Q: I'm experiencing these twitchy movements of my hand. It's always moving.

A: Levodopa-induced dyskinesias are being described. The medications for PD, and primarily levodopa, can induce involuntary movements termed dyskinesias. These are fidgety-looking movements of an arm, leg, head, or trunk; any part of the body or all the body may be involved (described in more detail in chapters10–12). Bear in mind that dyskinesias are not dangerous. If they don't bother you or your family, it is okay to make no changes in your medications.

Dyskinesias are often easy to treat, especially during the first 5–8 years of PD. The basic problem is an excessive levodopa effect. Hence the strategy is to lower each dose of levodopa. Typically only a small decrement is necessary. For example, if you are taking 2 1/2 tablets of 25-100 carbidopa/levodopa (immediate-release) three times a day, you should lower the doses by 1/4 tablet decrements until the dyskinesias are gone, minimal, or tolerable. Thus you could try 2 1/4 tablets three times daily and if that still did not adequately control the dyskinesias, then 2 tablets three times a day.

The dyskinesia-inducing effect is tied to each individual dose of carbidopa/ levodopa. There is no buildup of this problem. In other words, each individual dose of carbidopa/levodopa is crucial, rather than the total daily dose. If dyskinesias occur, they will be present for a few hours or less after each carbidopa/levodopa dose and then abate until another dose is taken. That is why we worry about lowering each individual dose of carbidopa/levodopa rather than focusing on how much we are taking per day.

Sometimes it is not possible to control dyskinesias without reducing the carbidopa/ levodopa dose so low that parkinsonism recurs. If that is the case, you then need to decide whether the parkinsonism or the dyskinesias are more troublesome and adjust the doses accordingly. Dyskinesia control is addressed in chapters 17–18.

Q: I've been on carbidopa/levodopa three times a day for several years and I'm still doing well. However, for the past few months, I can't get to sleep.

A: Another dose of carbidopa/levodopa is probably needed to get to sleep. Many with PD find it hard to sleep when their parkinsonism isn't well controlled, and we examine this in detail in chapter 20. Briefly, the restlessness and discomfort of parkinsonism may prevent sleep. During the first years of PD, there is a carry-over effect from levodopa treatment that lasts around the clock (the long-duration effect). In other words, the timing of the doses isn't crucial (except to take them on an empty stomach). Later, part of the response becomes time-locked to each dose, as mentioned above (the wearing-off effect). In that circumstance, it may be hard to get to sleep or stay asleep when the last dose of carbidopa/levodopa is taken before supper; that is, the effect may have worn off by night.

In this case, the simple solution is to add a dose of carbidopa/levodopa a little before bedtime. If necessary, another dose can be taken upon awakening in the middle of the night.

Q: I get cramps at night.

A: Inadequate levodopa coverage is likely the cause. In the setting of PD, frequent cramps usually signal wearing-off of the levodopa effect (i.e., levodopa underdosage at the time they are occurring). Rather than adding a specific cramp medication, like quinine, these are better treated by adjusting the dosage of carbidopa/levodopa. These cramps could be prevented by adding another dose of carbidopa/levodopa at bedtime or during the night. If sleep is still disrupted, you may wish to review chapter 20.

Parkinsonian cramps may be typical "charley horses" with a painful contraction of calf muscles. However, they frequently involve the toes, which may painfully curl up or down. These can also develop during the day, reflecting the levodopa effect wearing off.

Q: I was doing great and suddenly control of my parkinsonism deteriorated.

A: This does not represent progression of PD. Although PD progresses, it does so very, very slowly. Any change for the worse that happens over hours, days, or weeks is not due to PD progression. Did this person inadvertently change the carbidopa/levodopa dose or timing (e.g., switching to mealtime dosing)? Was a new medication started? Has an illness or medical condition developed (e.g., pneumo-nia, urinary tract infection, thyroid disease, depression)? You should not assume that any rapidly developing problems reflect progression of PD.

Q: I never had any problems with carbidopa/levodopa until recently. Now I'm always nauseated and have a pain in my stomach.

A: The problem here is something other than carbidopa/levodopa. Nausea is common with carbidopa/levodopa therapy. However, when it occurs, it is early in the treatment or immediately after raising the dose. If you have been taking a stable dose of carbidopa/levodopa without side effects and only months later experience nausea, look for another source. Furthermore, carbidopa/levodopa does not cause stomach pain (only nausea). This person needs to see his or her doctor and consider another cause.

16

◆ ◆ ◆

The First Few Years on a
Dopamine Agonist Drug
(Pramipexole, Ropinirole, or Pergolide)

In chapter 15 you read about how things typically go during the first few years of carbidopa/levodopa treatment. What if you started a dopamine agonist rather than carbidopa/levodopa after you were first diagnosed? Will the problems be the same? Will it go as smoothly? Will the dose need to be changed? Will carbidopa/levodopa be necessary and if so, when? In this chapter we will focus on these and other questions that arise when your only drug for PD is pramipexole, ropinirole, or pergolide.

Worsening Parkinsonism

Parkinsonism tends to slowly worsen over months to years. This is never rapid but insidious. The dopamine agonist drugs are not as effective as carbidopa/levodopa and they may become inadequate after one to a few years. Sometimes a dosage change is sufficient to overcome the problem, whereas in other cases, the addition of carbidopa/levodopa may be necessary.

What sorts of problems suggest medication changes may be necessary? For the most part, these are the same problems that led to the diagnosis and initial treatment of PD: slowness, stiffness, walking problems, tremor, loss of normal animated movements (e.g., arm swing, facial animation, inflections in voice, gesturing when talking). Cramps may also signal undertreated PD. Symptoms other than those classically associated with PD may also signal undertreated PD, such as restlessness (akathisia) or extreme fatigue. These and related symptoms translate into impairment of daily living. A compromised lifestyle strongly suggests medication changes should be considered.

Q: What should I do if my parkinsonism is no longer controlled?

A: The strategy is relatively simple. (1) Consider the dopamine agonist dose. Is it at the target level mentioned in chapter 13? If not, follow the guidelines in that chapter and slowly raise the dose. (2) If the dopamine agonist dosage is at the target level, start carbidopa/levodopa. It certainly would be acceptable to push the dopamine agonist dose higher than the target dosage, but that is not the approach that I usually take; I go straight to carbidopa/levodopa when target doses of the agonist prove inadequate.

Q: Is it imperative that carbidopa/levodopa be started if the symptoms are increasing?

A: Not necessarily; if these symptoms don't bother you or interfere with your life, it is okay to defer carbidopa/levodopa.

Q: How should I start carbidopa/levodopa?

A: The details for starting carbidopa/levodopa were provided in chapter 12. Refer back to that chapter and use the same scheme. The strategy involves starting with a low carbidopa/levodopa dose and gradually raising it until symptoms are satisfactorily controlled. When you are already taking a dopamine agonist, you probably will not need to raise the levodopa dose as high as those taking no other drugs.

Q: Should I change the dose of the dopamine agonist drug when I start carbidopa/levodopa?

A: No; keep the dose the same as you slowly increase the carbidopa/levodopa dosage. Note that carbidopa/levodopa works best if taken on an empty stomach. The immediate-release formulation is conventionally taken one hour before each meal. On the other hand, the dopamine agonist drugs are typically taken with meals. As you are initiating and raising carbidopa/levodopa, continue with this scheme. However, once you have made the final adjustments, you could try taking the dopamine agonist drug on an empty stomach at the same time as the carbidopa/levodopa for convenience. This is acceptable, as long as there is no nausea. The only reason we recommend taking the dopamine agonist with meals is to reduce the risk of nausea.

Q: I'm taking less than the target dose of the agonist but experiencing side effects and can't go higher; what now?

A: Some side effects are more likely with the dopamine agonists than with carbidopa/levodopa and sometimes limit the use of the agonist drugs. These especially include daytime sleepiness, hallucinations, delusions and paranoia, as well as orthostatic hypotension (low blood pressure when standing). They may not have been present during the initial treatment with the agonist medication but appear as the dose is increased. The exception may be orthostatic hypotension, which on rare occasions is provoked by the initial dose of dopamine agonist drug. Here's what to do if these problems develop.

- *Daytime sleepiness.* This is a common problem among those with PD irrespective of medications, and there may be some other cause apart from the dopamine agonist drug. However, if sleepiness started only after you raised the dosage of pramipexole or ropinirole, it may signal that higher doses are not possible. In that case, lower the dose to a level where this is not troublesome, wait a week, and then start carbidopa/levodopa. Pergolide is less likely to cause daytime sleepiness than pramipexole or ropinirole. See chapter 20 for more discussion of this subject.

- *Hallucinations, delusions, paranoia.* Seeing things that are not there (hallucinations), bizarre beliefs (delusions), or extreme suspicions (paranoia) may be provoked by any of the medications for PD, and the dopamine agonist drugs are perhaps the most likely to do this. If these problems develop, this usually signals the need to taper off the dopamine agonist agent. Often carbidopa/levodopa can be started later without reprovoking these symptoms. However, allow a couple of weeks to elapse after stopping the dopamine agonist medication before starting carbidopa/levodopa. Chapter 24 addresses these problems in more detail.

- *Orthostatic hypotension.* As you have learned previously, those with PD are predisposed to low blood pressure when standing or walking (which may be normal when sitting). All the drugs we administer for PD aggravate this problem, and the worst offenders are the dopamine agonists and carbidopa/levodopa. If this is not resulting in symptoms and if the systolic blood pressure stays above 90, you could simply monitor the blood pressures. (Recall that the systolic blood pressure is the upper number; for example, 120 in the reading of 120/80.) However, if the blood pressures drops so low that you feel faint, or if the systolic values are often below 90, it would probably be wise to taper off the dopamine agonist when carbidopa/levodopa is due to be started. Orthostatic hypotension is difficult to treat when both a dopamine agonist and carbidopa/levodopa are used concurrently. Since sooner or later, carbidopa/levodopa will be necessary, I prefer going with carbidopa/levodopa alone when this problem arises. Chapter 21 addresses orthostatic hypotension in detail.

Other side effects may not require such drastic measures; common sense usually dictates what you do. In general, if side effects prevent escalation of the dopamine agonist dose to therapeutic levels, then the usual strategy is twofold: (1) lower the agonist dose to a level where the side effects are not troublesome. If even low doses cause side effects or if only very *low doses* are tolerated, taper it completely off and (2) wait a week or two after completing the adjustments of the dopamine agonist and then start carbidopa/levodopa.

Possible Serious Side Effects with Long-Term Pergolide or Bromocriptine Treatment

In chapter 13 I outlined certain worrisome side effects that uniquely develop with pergolide or bromocriptine use. These drugs may induce an inflammatory reaction primarily affecting the lungs or heart. Shortness of breath or other heart or lung symptoms are clues to this problem. If your physician confirms that one of these two drugs is the cause, it needs to be discontinued. This is not a problem with pramipexole or ropinirole.

Tapering Off a Dopamine Agonist

It is usually unwise to suddenly stop any of the drugs for PD, including the dopamine agonist medications. They should be slowly tapered off. The exception is with very low doses, such as those used during the first two to three weeks when they are initially introduced; in that range, the drug may be stopped abruptly. Tapering guidelines are discussed in chapter 13. In general, there is no single correct way to do this. The idea is to gradually reduce the dose; how rapidly you do this depends on the side effect that is forcing the issue. It is usually safe to cut a dose in half, and that often is a good starting point in the reduction schedule. Further reductions by half every three to four days are as rapid as is usually done.

Parkinsonism That Suddenly Worsens

Parkinson's disease progresses very, very slowly. If any rapid changes in parkinsonism develop, consider other causes. This might include medication changes or some other illness superimposed. Sometimes the symptoms of other conditions may be mistaken for parkinsonism. For example, the extreme fatigue associated with viral illness or the sudden weakness of a stroke might be initially mistaken for worsening parkinsonism. Rapid worsening should be the signal to consider other factors.

Insomnia

Insomnia is common among adults. If this has been a lifelong problem, predating parkinsonism by many years, it may have nothing to do with PD. In that case, the usual treatments for insomnia in the general population are appropriate. You should discuss that with you physician.

If insomnia started after parkinsonism developed, then PD may be the cause. Insomnia is extremely common in PD and can often be treated with PD medications. This is addressed in detail in chapter 20. However, if you are only taking a dopamine agonist drug at this juncture, the initial strategies for treating this include the following.

- Shift the time of your third agonist dose of the day to about an hour before bedtime. Thus, your first two doses would still be with meals, perhaps breakfast and lunch.

- Instead you could add a fourth dose of the dopamine agonist a little before bedtime. Use the same dose of the agonist that you are taking earlier in the day; for example, if you were taking 3 mg of ropinirole three times daily, the bedtime dose should also be 3 mg, to make a new total daily dose of 12 mg.

- You could instead take that fourth agonist dose in the middle of the night. This is appropriate if you easily fall asleep but awaken during the night, unable to return to sleep. Have it on your night stand with a glass of water ready to take.

- If you prefer, you could take a mild sleep medication at bedtime. This might include an over-the-counter drug such as Tylenol PM, which contains diphenhydramine (Benadryl). Alternatively, you could take plain diphenhydramine, also available over the counter. The appropriate dose of diphenhydramine as a sleep aid is 50 mg, although occasionally 25 mg will work. Instead, your physician might prescribe trazodone (50 mg, with the option of raising to 100 mg) or amitriptyline (25–50 mg) a little before bedtime.

Some Typical Problems

Q: I've been taking ropinirole (Requip) for a couple of years and doing okay. Recently I've started to shake and my writing is terrible. I'm taking 2 mg of ropinirole three times a day; I don't take any other medications.

A: Despite a stable dose of ropinirole, your parkinsonism is worsening. However, the dose, 6 mg daily, is considerably below the target dose for ropinirole (see chapter 13), which is 12–15 mg daily. The simplest strategy is to raise the dose according to the schedule in that chapter.

Q: I've started to slow down and shuffle when I walk; sometimes I use a cane. I'm taking 1.5 mg of pramipexole (Mirapex) three times a day but no other drugs for my Parkinson's.

A: These gait problems from parkinsonism are undoubtedly affecting activities of daily living, despite the pramipexole dose at the target level. Raising the dose of pramipexole a little higher could be tried but probably would be insufficient. My recommendation would be to start carbidopa/levodopa at this juncture, while maintaining the current dose of pramipexole.

Q: My wife is becoming paranoid. She thinks her friends are conspiring to take our money. She's never acted like this before. Her only medication is pergolide (Permax); she takes a 1 mg pill three times a day.

A: Pergolide could well be causing the paranoia. It should be tapered off. Assuming that her parkinsonism is troublesome, carbidopa/levodopa could later be started; it has a lesser risk for these types of problems.

Q: I was doing fine until two days ago. I was jogging three times a week. Now I can barely walk. Do you think I need more pramipexole?

A: Parkinson's disease does not change rapidly. Deteriorating over a week from recreational jogging to being barely able to walk must have an explanation other than simply PD. Consider other factors causing this dramatic change in ambulatory ability. This might include anything from orthopedic problems to some generalized illness. A physician needs to sort this out. More pramipexole won't help.

PART EIGHT

◆ ◆ ◆

Later Medication Inconsistency: Motor Fluctuations and Dyskinesias

17

◆ ◆ ◆

Movement Problems That Develop Later: Dyskinesias, Motor Fluctuations, and Treatment with Levodopa Adjustments

More complex movement problems often surface after several years of carbidopa/levodopa treatment. This includes excessive movements (dyskinesias) as well as fluctuations in control of parkinsonism. These may be treated by adding one of several medications, and we will cover their use later in this book; however, the quickest and most expedient solution is often adjustment of the carbidopa/levodopa dosage, which will be our focus now. This will be easiest if you are taking the immediate-release form of carbidopa/ levodopa, but the same principles apply if you are using the sustained-release (Sinemet CR) formulation.

The guidelines in this chapter are appropriate if you are taking carbidopa/ levodopa alone or with a dopamine agonist. If you are experiencing no substantial side effects from the agonist medication, we won't change the dose. In this chapter, we will focus on carbidopa/levodopa adjustments and ignore the agonist.

Questions to Ask When Things Aren't Going Well

Those with PD know when things aren't going well but don't always recognize some of the crucial clues that point to solutions. Here are several questions that will get you warmed up and focused on what is important.

- Am I a lot better during certain times of the day than others?
- Am I better an hour or two after my levodopa doses?
- Are my problems primarily when it's getting close to the time for my next dose?
- Can I walk better at some times than others?
- Does my tremor come and go?
- Do toe or foot cramps come and go?

These questions address whether there is substantial variability in your day. If there are ups and downs in your parkinsonism, this is crucial to recognize. Answering yes to these questions suggests that you are experiencing fluctuations in your levodopa response. We need to distinguish this from the person who experiences no variability in his parkinsonism.

Doing Poorly with No Variation

We will start with those who answer no to all these questions. They are simply doing badly (slow, stiff, stooped, tremulous, etc.), without any variation. There are four possibilities.

- They are underdosed on levodopa therapy.
- The parkinsonism responds only partially to medications.
- They have nonmovement symptoms requiring other drugs.
- They are not paying attention to their responses.

Let's consider each of these in detail.

UNDERDOSED

If you are slow, stiff, and walking poorly throughout the day with no let-up, you may be taking insufficient levodopa. Go back and look at the guidelines for starting carbidopa/levodopa in chapter 12. Key points to consider include the following.

- Have you raised the carbidopa/levodopa dose sufficiently to capture the maximum effect? You have not reached the maximum dose until you are up to around 2 1/2 to 3 tablets of the 25-100 immediate-release formulation at least three times daily. Some people require even a little more levodopa to capture the full effect.
- Are you using the immediate-release formulation? If there are uncertainties about your response, it usually works best to use the immediate-release, rather than the controlled-release (CR) formulation. However,

if you are on the CR formulation and wish to stick with it for now, I would push the dosage slowly up to 4 of the 25-100 CR tablets (or two of the 50-200 tablets) three times daily. If still not doing better, you should switch to the immediate-release formulation, using the conversion guidelines provided in chapter 12.

- Are you taking your doses on an empty stomach? With immediate-release carbidopa/levodopa, take each of your doses an hour before each meal; that assures us that the levodopa will have gotten to the brain before dietary protein products can compete with it. But what about those who are taking Sinemet CR? As we discussed previously, the CR formulation has complex interactions with meals. Food in the stomach helps release levodopa from the pill and into the bloodstream. On the other hand, dietary protein products in the bloodstream compete with levodopa for transport into the brain. If you are concerned this could be a problem but are wedded to the use of the CR formulation, you could do the following on a trial basis. Take each of your three doses of Sinemet CR 2 hours before each meal (it takes up to 2 hours to get the levodopa into the brain with the CR formulation). Drink at least 6 ounces of fluid with these pills. When you take each CR dose, also eat a piece of dry bread, several soda crackers, or some other nonprotein food. This will facilitate getting the levodopa out of the stomach and into the bloodstream; if the food is nonprotein, it won't inhibit it from crossing the blood–brain barrier.

PARTIAL RESPONSE TO PD MEDICATIONS

For some with PD, the response to levodopa therapy is only partial. Despite raising the dose to maximum levels, no further improvement occurs. If you have addressed the points in the above section, this could be the case, and then we don't have much more to offer. You could try adding a dopamine agonist drug, but this is unlikely to add substantial benefit if you have maxed out on carbidopa/levodopa.

NONMOVEMENT SYMPTOMS THAT REQUIRE ANOTHER MEDICATION

You might be experiencing nonmovement symptoms that require a different treatment strategy than carbidopa/levodopa. For example, if the problem is depression, an antidepressant rather than more carbidopa/levodopa would be appropriate. If you are feeling weak and lightheaded, the problem might be low blood pressure (orthostatic hypotension), which can be exacerbated by higher levodopa doses. These and other problems are addressed in subsequent chapters; you may wish to skim through the chapter headings to see if any of your problems fit.

FAILURE TO PAY ATTENTION

I frequently hear patients deny fluctuations in their response, only to observe them during the course of their office visit with me. People often have poor recognition and recall of these waxing and waning changes in their parkinsonism. They recall the bad times and forget the good ones; they remember that they couldn't walk in the shopping mall (just before their next carbidopa/levodopa dose) but forget that they walked well a couple of hours before.

When I suspect such fluctuations in the response but need to confirm it, I often observe people in the office for a few hours; this allows me to document the full levodopa response cycle. Typically we start in the morning, beginning before the first dose of medications. I observe walking and movement, then repeat these observations an hour or two after the first dose of carbidopa/levodopa. At that time, the levodopa response should be fully developed. I then repeat this over the next few hours to capture the complete cycle, documenting wearing-off of the levodopa effect. You can make the same observations at home.

The bottom line: pay close attention to your responses over time. Have your spouse help with these observations as an objective observer. Note how you are doing just before, and then 1–2 hours after a carbidopa/levodopa dose; continue to observe without taking any more pills or eating for the next few hours. If there is substantial variability, we can work with this (see below).

Variability in the Levodopa Response

If control of your parkinsonism waxes and wanes over the course of the day, a short-duration levodopa response is likely. Let's review this in more detail. Initially when levodopa treatment is started, the response is consistent and unvarying. You can be late with a dose and not skip a beat. We term this the long-duration levodopa response. It is a cumulative effect that builds up over about a week or two. With progression of the disease process, the brain cells that store and release dopamine are gradually lost. Some are left behind, but this system has a diminished capacity to store dopamine. Other cells take their place but are not as efficient at storing and releasing dopamine. Inconsistent and pulsatile dopamine release into the synapse induces secondary changes in receptor sensitivity. Dopamine levels fluctuate in the synapse and the responses are magnified by the sensitized receptors. The outcome: development of the short-duration levodopa response, where the benefit becomes tied to each carbidopa/levodopa dose. Each time a dose is taken, the response works for a few hours or less, then tails off. The long-duration effect is not lost completely but fades into the background; we almost never see it because carbidopa/levodopa is rarely stopped long enough for this to become apparent.

The first step in treating this short-duration response is to recognize it. Ask yourself how you are doing at specific times:

- The first thing in the morning before medications are taken
- Sixty to ninety minutes after each dose of carbidopa/levodopa (or 2 hours after, if you are taking Sinemet CR)
- Just before each dose of carbidopa/levodopa

These are times that reflect the highs and lows of your levodopa cycle. Construct in your mind the full levodopa response over time. How am I before I take it? How long does it take to kick in? How long does this effect last? When does the effect wear off after each dose? If you can answer these questions, you can then envision the full levodopa cycle, as illustrated in figure 17.1.

Keep in mind that the response to a dose of carbidopa/levodopa is not immediate and takes up to one hour to kick in (up to 2 hours with the sustained-release formulation). This occasionally is a source of confusion with doses later in the day; if your dosing interval is just a little too long, wearing-off may begin right *after* a dose is taken and persist until this new dose starts to work.

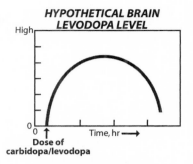

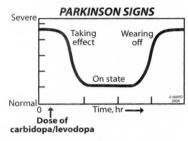

17.1 The short-duration levodopa response. Upper graph depicts the buildup and decline of levodopa (and dopamine) in the brain after a dose of carbidopa/levodopa. Parallel to this is improvement in parkinsonism, shown in the lower graph. In this hypothetical case, the initial parkinsonian symptoms are "severe" until the levodopa effect kicks in, heralding the on-state. Later, the effect wears off, linked in time with the decline of brain levodopa and dopamine concentrations.

Dyskinesias

Dyskinesias also tend to develop later in the course of PD, primarily provoked by levodopa therapy, although dopamine agonists may contribute. They may or may not occur in conjunction with short-duration responses and wearing-off. We have considered dyskinesias in previous chapters, but now we need to focus on their treatment.

The cause of dyskinesias relates to the same factors that cause short-duration levodopa responses. Early in the course of PD, the many surviving dopamine brain cells not only store and release dopamine, but also regulate the dopamine levels in the synapse. If the released amount is too great, they can suck it back up. The scientific term for sucking it back into the neuron is "reuptake"; this is illustrated in figure 17.2. Hence these dopamine brain cells tightly control the

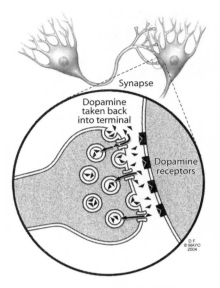

17.2 A dopaminergic terminal releases dopamine into the synapse. The released dopamine binds to receptors on the postsynaptic neuron. Excess dopamine is sucked back up into the terminal, which keeps the levels constant. This "reuptake" prevents excessive synaptic concentrations and recycles dopamine. Excessive dopamine in the synapse results in dyskinesias.

amount of dopamine at the receptor and prevent it from becoming excessive. With progression of PD and loss of these dopamine-releasing neurons, other cells substitute. However, they are not very good at regulating the dopamine levels at the receptor; they simply were not made for that purpose. After a dose of levodopa, the receptor may be flooded with dopamine without any means of keeping the levels optimal. The receptor is then overstimulated, and this secondarily makes this whole brain circuit oversensitive and irritable. The consequence is dyskinesias—excessive body movements.

WHAT DO DYSKINESIAS LOOK LIKE?

Dyskinesias induced by levodopa are dancing movements, as described in chapter 12. Neurologists refer to these dancing movements as chorea. They may be present in only one area of the body, such as a hand or an arm, or they may involve half the body, such as the arm and leg on one side. They may affect the entire body or just the head and neck. These dancing movements are the essence of levodopa-induced dyskinesias. The involved area of the body appears to be in constant motion. Sometimes the chorea is mixed with posturing (dystonia, in the language of neurologists). For example, the dancing arm (chorea) may be positioned behind the body in an inappropriate position or posture (dystonia). Dyskinetic neck movements may move the head in a chaotic fashion (chorea) but also tilted to one side (a dystonic posture).

DYSTONIA WITHOUT CHOREA

Dystonia without chorea is usually not due to an excessive levodopa effect. Although levodopa-induced dancing movements (chorea) may be accompanied by abnormal postures, these postures (dystonia) may occur alone. In that case, they are usually not from medications. Dystonic postures without dancing movements (chorea) are usually due to the parkinsonism itself. This is especially likely if these postures are painful or if the muscles feel very tense and tight. They typically signal an underdosed rather than overdosed state. Examples include dystonic curling of the toes or involuntary turning up of the toes. Painful "cramps" of the calves, sometimes with in-turning of the foot, are another typical PD dystonia; this also signals an underdosed state. In summary:

- Chorea (i.e., dancing movements) plus dystonia (i.e., posturing) = levodopa excessive effect

- Dystonia alone = parkinsonism (i.e., not medication excess, but too little levodopa effect)

- A painful cramp in someone with PD = probably dystonia due to parkinsonism (not likely a medication effect)

If you tell your doctor that you are experiencing dyskinesias, he or she will likely lower your levodopa dose. However, if the movement is simply dystonia, that would be exactly the wrong strategy.

IS RESTLESSNESS DYSKINESIA?

Restlessness is not dyskinesia. Typically restlessness represents the opposite effect. Akathisia, or inner restlessness, is a common symptom of PD and often reflects an untreated or undertreated state. Although the person with akathisia feels restless, he or she appears just the opposite to onlookers, slow and stiff. If you have PD and feel restless, you probably need additional treatment.

Ironically, those with dyskinesias typically do not feel restless, even when so severe that they can't sit still. In fact, this is when they often feel the most relaxed. This is another example of symptoms we should avoid confusing, since this could result in exactly the opposite treatment we desire. In summary:

- "I feel restless" = parkinsonism

- Moving constantly but not feeling restless = dyskinesias

Dyskinesia and akathisia sound similar but are on opposite ends of the spectrum.

DISTINGUISHING TREMORS FROM DYSKINESIAS

Patients have called and told me they were experiencing terrible dyskinesias, only to discover later in the office that they were actually experiencing tremor. Others have told me about their troublesome tremor, which later was recognized as dyskinesias. Don't mix these up or the treatment will be wrong.

Tremor is rhythmic, to and fro, always with the same recurring pattern. This stereotyped, back-and-forth pattern keeps a constant rhythm. It may appear and subside, but when present, the back-and-forth movement is apparent. Among people with PD, tremor most often affects the hand(s) but may also affect one or both legs. A knee that involuntarily goes up and down with a regular rhythm while the person is seated represents tremor. The chin is another common area of parkinsonian tremor.

Contrast this recurring, stereotyped, back-and-forth pattern of tremor to chorea. By definition, chorea is chaotic, without much pattern. The movements of chorea provoked by levodopa (dyskinesias) make that part of the body look fidgety, in fairly constant motion but without a true rhythmic, or to-and-fro, pattern.

LEVODOPA TIMING AND DYSKINESIAS

If you are wondering whether an involuntary movement represents levodopa dyskinesia, consider when it occurs. Focusing on your first morning dose of carbidopa/levodopa, ask yourself these questions:

- Is it present in the morning before the first dose of carbidopa/levodopa? If so, then you can't blame this on levodopa (assuming you didn't take a dose of carbidopa/levodopa during the night).

- Does it begin 30–75 minutes after the first morning dose of carbidopa/levodopa (or 1–2 hours after sustained-release carbidopa/levodopa)? If so, this suggests that the involuntary movement is levodopa dyskinesia.

- If it occurs after the first dose of carbidopa/levodopa in the morning, does it go away after a few hours or less? (To assess this, don't take a second dose of carbidopa/levodopa until the involuntary movement goes away.) If so, this is consistent with levodopa dyskinesias.

Early in the morning is obviously a good time to make these assessments, since the observations thus start in an unmedicated (off) state (assuming you have not taken any carbidopa/levodopa during the night).

Rarely, one of the dystonias described above is due to levodopa rather than PD. For example, involuntary, sustained eye closure can also occur from an excessive levodopa effect (dystonic eye closure, or blepharospasm). However, you should be able to figure this out based upon the timing, as just described.

DYSKINESIAS AND THE DOPAMINE AGONISTS

Dyskinesias are primarily due to an excessive effect of levodopa. However, combining a dopamine agonist drug with levodopa may contribute. When dopamine agonists are used alone, however, dyskinesias are only rarely provoked.

Doing First Things First:
Optimizing the Levodopa Schedule

As already noted, the two common problems occurring with chronic levodopa therapy are (1) short-duration responses with wearing-off and (2) dyskinesias.

Now we will consider how to adjust the carbidopa/levodopa doses to treat these problems.

WEARING-OFF EFFECTS

The wearing-off effect results from a short-duration levodopa response; the effect wears off before the next dose is taken. If you have experienced fluctuations in your response, and if they follow the simple pattern just described, the medication adjustments are straightforward. Let's break this down into the two crucial components of this levodopa cycle, which are illustrated in figure 17.1: (1) peak effect of the dose and (2) duration of the response. To effectively treat a short-duration levodopa response, we need to consider these two components separately.

THE PEAK EFFECT OF THE LEVODOPA DOSE: SUFFICIENT RESPONSE?

The maximum effect is fully developed about 60 minutes after each dose of carbidopa/levodopa (or, in the case of Sinemet CR, 2 hours after the dose). Ignore the timing of the dose and the duration of the response for now; instead, focus on the size of this dose. Ask yourself, "How am I doing an hour after each carbidopa/levodopa dose (or 2 hours if you are taking the sustained-release formulation)?" If you are doing well, then we have the correct dose. On the other hand, if you are experiencing substantial parkinsonism when the dose should be peaking, a larger dose may be necessary. How much larger? You could raise the dose by 1/4 to 1/2 tablet increments until you find the dose that works best for you. For example, if you are taking 2 tablets each dose but with an insufficient response, try 2 1/4 tablets. If still insufficient after a few trials, raise it to 2 1/2 tablets.

If you are using the sustained-release formulation, adjust the doses by 1/2 tablet increments up to as high as 4 of the 25-100 tablets, each dose. If still an inadequate peak response, switch over to the immediate-release formulation, using the guidelines in chapter 12.

"But how often should I take this?" We are going to defer that question for the moment. For the time being, keep the doses sufficiently far apart so that the effects do not overlap and accumulate. We want to determine the individual dose strength first. Once we have that sorted out, we will then focus on how often to take it.

RAISING THE DOSE

Often you can capture a better effect as you raise the doses, but there is a limit to this, as noted in chapter 12. Most people max out at about 2 1/2 tablet doses (25-100 immediate-release carbidopa/levodopa), although some people may require slightly more. It is rare that individual doses much higher than three 25-100 tablets provide any further benefit; hence, I usually recommend pushing up to 2 1/2 to 3 tablets. The primary exception relates to any doses that fall close to meals (discussed below). Also, someone who is suspected of having a gastrointestinal malabsorption syndrome may be instructed to try higher doses.

The sustained-release formulation of carbidopa/levodopa is incompletely absorbed and the ceiling dose is higher, approximately 4 of the 25-100 tablets, each dose (occasionally even slightly higher). As with immediate-release carbidopa/levodopa, there is no limit to the total number of doses per day, provided that they match your requirements.

EXCESSIVE RESPONSES (DYSKINESIAS)

If we push the individual doses too high, dyskinesias might occur. These dancing movements signal that we cannot raise the individual doses any higher

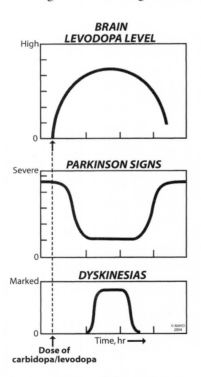

17.3 Dyskinesias follow a short-duration pattern, time-locked to each carbidopa/levodopa dose. As brain levodopa (and dopamine) concentrations peak, the levels may be excessive and result in dyskinesias. These dyskinesias abate as the concentrations later decline.

(although we may be able to raise the total daily dose if necessary; see below). Dyskinesias are not dangerous and if you feel the best when these are present, it is okay to stick with the dose that provokes these. However, if they are pronounced, they will be an impediment to your normal activities.

The concept of these dyskinesias is illustrated in figure 17.3. They coincide with the peak of the levodopa level in the brain after a carbidopa/levodopa dose. Thus, as the brain concentrations of levodopa (and dopamine) are at their highest level, and the parkinsonian symptoms improve, dyskinesias are also provoked by an excessive effect. When the levodopa level starts to decline, the dyskinesias resolve. Dyskinesias follow this time pattern. They are time-locked to each dose of carbidopa/levodopa; they do not directly reflect the total *daily* amount of levodopa. Thus they follow a short-duration pattern; there is no long-duration dyskinesia effect.

GETTING RID OF DYSKINESIAS

You can always abolish dyskinesias. You simply lower each dose of carbidopa/levodopa. As you can see in figure 17.4, this may be conceived as a matter of thresholds. The dose of carbidopa/levodopa elevates brain levodopa

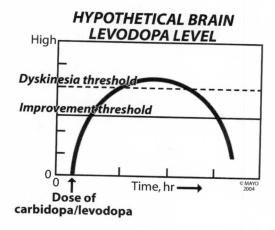

HYPOTHETICAL BRAIN LEVODOPA LEVEL

High

Dyskinesia threshold

Improvement threshold

0

0   Time, hr ⟶   © MAYO 2004

Dose of carbidopa/levodopa

17.4 Levodopa short-duration responses tend to be all or none in many cases. This is illustrated as separate thresholds for both the anti-parkinson effect (improvement) and dyskinesias. With this type of response, the levodopa dose should be adjusted so that the peak brain levodopa level exceeds the improvement threshold, but is less than the dyskinesia threshold. Some people have thresholds that are very similar, making it difficult to abolish dyskinesias without compromising control of parkinsonism.

levels. A certain minimum dose is necessary to surpass the improvement threshold, which results in improved parkinsonism. If a larger dose is administered, the brain concentrations elevate further and may then surpass the dyskinesia threshold.

Is it really this simple? Unfortunately, not in certain cases. With the reduction of levodopa to abolish dyskinesias, control of parkinsonism may also be lost. For people with this problem, the thresholds for dyskinesias and improvement are identical. This affects a sizable minority of people with PD who are left with a dilemma: accept the dyskinesias or live with the increased parkinsonism. Most choose dyskinesias, although with doses adjusted to keep these as minimal as possible. There are additional strategies for reducing dyskinesias, which we will consider in chapter 18. Also, for the rare person with severe dyskinesias complicating parkinsonism, surgical options may be considered, as discussed in chapter 33.

DYSKINESIAS ARE SHORT-DURATION EFFECTS

Dyskinesias are the consequence of each levodopa dose, not the total daily dose. The potential for provoking dyskinesias lasts for no more than a few hours after each dose of carbidopa/levodopa. It does not relate to how much levodopa you take per day but per dose. This fact has important practical implications.

- You can get rid of dyskinesias by simply not taking another levodopa dose until they go away; they will resolve in no more than a few hours.
- When you find a dose of carbidopa/levodopa that is below the dyskinesia threshold, adding doses at other times (such as during the night) will not provoke dyskinesias.

To summarize, there is no buildup of levodopa that leads to more dyskinesias with subsequent doses. The only exception occurs with controlled-release carbidopa/levodopa (Sinemet CR). Rarely people taking this formulation will experience a doubled effect in the late afternoon. It may be linked to a skipped response in the early afternoon; that is, they will note an insufficient response right after lunch and excessive response later in the afternoon following the next dose. Even less often, this occurs at other times during the day. This presumably reflects delayed release of levodopa from the pill. If this delay is sufficiently long, the effect from one dose overlaps with the next. If you are taking immediate-release carbidopa/levodopa, you don't need to worry about this.

DURATION OF THE LEVODOPA RESPONSE

Once you have determined the optimal amount of carbidopa/levodopa to take in each dose, focus on how often to take it. The general rule of thumb for those with wearing-off (a short-duration levodopa response) is: *Match the interval between doses to the duration of the response.* When you have established the dose, observe how long it takes each dose to kick in and how long that effect lasts. Then reduce the interval between doses so that the effects slightly overlap. The goal is to have the current dose kick in just before the effect from the last dose is wearing off. Remember that the response is not immediate following any given dose. It takes 30–60 minutes for immediate-release carbidopa/levodopa to start working. You need to allow for this when determining the interval between doses. If you are using the controlled-release formulation (Sinemet CR), the effect will take 1–2 hours to kick in.

DO HIGHER DOSES PROLONG THE LEVODOPA RESPONSE?

Taking a larger dose of carbidopa/levodopa to make the effect last longer doesn't work. The response may last slightly longer, but it usually is not substantially lengthened. Instead, you will likely just add to side effects, especially dyskinesias.

The only exception to this rule relates to people who have been taking a very small dose of carbidopa/levodopa that is right on the margins of a response. If your individual doses are one 25-100 immediate-release tablet or less, then increasing the dose may occasionally capture a longer response. If a 1/2 to 1 tablet increment doesn't extend the response, you can revert back to the previous dose and follow through with the strategies we have outlined. This same strategy applies to those taking the sustained-release formulation in doses of 1 1/2 of the 25-100 tablets or less.

NUMBER OF DOSES PER DAY

If you shorten the interval between your carbidopa/levodopa doses, you will need to add an extra dose or two, to keep the effect going through bedtime. There are no limits to the number of doses, provided they fit your needs.

Guided by these principles, take as many doses as you need to provide continuous coverage.

The duration of the levodopa response varies among people with fluctuations. For most, the effect lasts a few hours; however, for a few, it may be as brief as 2 hours or in rare cases, about 1 hour. Thus many daily doses may be necessary.

WHAT IS THE MAXIMUM AMOUNT OF LEVODOPA PER DAY

For those with fluctuations in their levodopa response, we have focused on the size of the individual doses and ignored the total daily dose. Should we now set some limits? In fact, there is no reason to do this. For those with fluctuating levodopa responses, ignore the total daily dose and worry only about the size of each individual dose and the dosing interval. There is no ceiling on how much you can take per day as long as you follow the principles just outlined.

SHOULD I WORRY ABOUT THE CARBIDOPA DOSE?

Carbidopa is inextricably tied to levodopa (both are in the same pill). As you raise or lower levodopa to manage your responses, you will also be changing your carbidopa dose. However, this is of no practical consequence and you may ignore it. It is only important if you are bothered by nausea from levodopa. In that case, you need all the carbidopa you can get, as explained in chapter 12.

WILL I NEED TO PROGRESSIVELY INCREASE MY LEVODOPA DOSES?

Once you have determined the dose that produces the optimum on-response, this typically will not change substantially over the next several years. In other words, if two 25-100 tablets kick in consistently, you won't need 3 tablets per dose in 2 years or 4 tablets in 5 years. Some minor adjustments of the size of each dose may be necessary, but you should not experience an ever-increasing requirement for higher and higher doses.

Although the optimum size of each carbidopa/levodopa dose typically doesn't change substantially over time, the optimum dosing interval does change. With the typical evolution of PD, the capacity of the brain to take up and store levodopa and dopamine gradually diminishes, as we discussed. The consequence is a reduction in the duration of response to each carbidopa/levodopa dose. Whereas you might initially have experienced a five-hour effect following each dose of carbidopa/levodopa, it may be down to 3 hours several years later.

If you adjust the interval between levodopa doses to match the response duration, then more doses per day will be required. Consequently, the total daily dose of carbidopa/levodopa tends to increase over the years.

Although the total daily requirement of levodopa increases over the years, this isn't a sign of medication tolerance or addiction. This isn't analogous to a person taking a narcotic drug for pain control, who needs higher and higher doses. The tolerance of narcotic drugs relates to the body's getting used to a certain drug dose. The body habituates to the narcotic dose and subsequently more is necessary to produce the same response. With levodopa, more frequent dosing is primarily reflective of the natural progression of PD. With true drug tolerance, there is usually a concerted effort to keep the dosage as low as possible. With levodopa therapy, however, drug tolerance is not truly the problem and there is no real merit in restricting the dosage.

IN SUMMARY

For those with fluctuating responses, there are two basic principles to using carbidopa/levodopa: (1) Adjust the size of the individual doses to produce the optimum response and (2) shorten the interval between doses to match the response duration, and take as many doses per day as necessary to provide continuous coverage. Don't worry about the number of doses per day or the total daily levodopa dosage as long as your parkinsonism is well controlled.

These adjustments of the levodopa dose are not the only strategies to employ in managing these levodopa complications. Supplemental drugs have a major role in treatment, as we will discuss in the next chapter, plus brain surgery is an option for those with the most resistant problems (see chapter 33). However, if simple adjustments of carbidopa/levodopa control the problem, these are an appropriate initial first step. Could we have deferred carbidopa/levodopa dosage adjustments and simply started a dopamine agonist? We could have done this and may have achieved our therapeutic goals. However, making the levodopa adjustments is quicker, cheaper, and often sufficient.

Sustained-Release Levodopa (Sinemet CR) and Wearing-off

The initial rationale for developing a sustained-release formulation was to extend the effect and counter short-duration levodopa responses. For those with wearing-off, a longer levodopa effect requiring less frequent dosing would certainly be desirable. The sustained-release pill contains a sticky matrix that binds the active ingredients, carbidopa and levodopa; this holds the active ingredients longer and, hence, the longer effect. The downside of this strategy, however, is twofold: (1) the response is delayed and (2) the release may be erratic.

If you need a quick return to your levodopa on-state, this delay of the response can be a frustration. Also, because release of levodopa from the matrix is not as consistent as with the immediate-release tablet, the results are less predictable. This is balanced against the longer levodopa response.

What is the trade-off; how much longer is the response with sustained-release carbidopa/levodopa? Actually, not that much longer, only 60–90 minutes beyond the immediate-release formulation. Because of the downside of the sustained-release formulation, only rarely do I switch to this form to treat wearing-off. Nonetheless, this is an option.

WHO MIGHT BENEFIT FROM SWITCHING TO THE SUSTAINED-RELEASE FORMULATION?

Those who fulfill two criteria are potential candidates for the sustained-release formulation: (1) *predictable* short-duration levodopa responses and (2) responses to the immediate-release formulation that last 2 1/2 hours or longer. This is not to say that everyone fulfilling these criteria should be switched to the sustained-release formulation and, again, this is not my usual strategy.

SWITCHING FROM IMMEDIATE-RELEASE TO SUSTAINED-RELEASE CARBIDOPA/LEVODOPA

The sustained-release drug does not release all of its levodopa (only about 70 percent), in contrast to the immediate-release formulation, which is fully absorbed. Thus larger doses of the sustained-release formulation will be necessary. Also complicating the transition is that the timing will be different; the sustained-release drug is taken less often. However, there are certain rules we can apply that should make this go smoothly.

For these rules to work, you must have determined the best possible immediate-release carbidopa/levodopa dosing schedule. You will use these parameters to choose the comparable Sinemet CR dose, and dosing interval. Thus, before switching, you need to know the immediate-release carbidopa/levodopa dose that produces the best on-response; you also need to know the duration of that response—the dosing interval. These parameters will be your reference points for making the transition to the sustained-release formulation.

If your immediate-release carbidopa/levodopa is adjusted as well as possible and you're ready to switch to Sinemet CR, here are the rules for making the switch. Bear in mind that we are focusing on the levodopa content of the pills; ignore carbidopa.

- The levodopa in each dose of the sustained-release formulation should be 30–50 percent higher than the immediate-release dose. The individual doses of the sustained-release drug should be 130 percent to 150 percent of the current immediate-release doses.

- Increase the interval between doses by 60–90 minutes (you can start with the longer increment, 90 minutes, and then reduce, once you have seen how long it lasts).

- By doing this, the total daily levodopa should be slightly higher than with the immediate-release formulation.

- Anticipate that the first dose of the day will often not kick in reliably and may need to be 50-100 mg higher than subsequent doses (or take 1/2 to 1 immediate-release 25-100 tablet with that first dose).

Once you have done this and experienced the responses, some further fine-tuning may be necessary.

- If your doses are not reliably kicking in, raise the levodopa in each dose by 50 milligram (mg) increments (half of a 25-100 sustained-release tablet).

- If dyskinesias are excessive, lower each levodopa dose by 50 mg decrements (half of a 25-100 sustained-release tablet).

- Further shorten the interval between doses if wearing-off is present.

- If the first dose or two still does not reliably kick in, gradually raise it even higher until it does.

Drink 6–8 ounces of fluid with your dose to help it get dissolved and working. Avoid milk or other protein drinks; all other fluids are okay. Remember to stick to the schedule. Since the sustained-release formulation is slow to kick in, you don't want to be late with the doses.

Consider the person taking 2 1/2 of the 25-100 immediate-release tablets four times daily at 3-hour intervals and experiencing a predictable response. The intent of the transition would be to take it less frequently. Following the guidelines above, let's do the levodopa arithmetic:

- The first step is to increase the levodopa by 30–50 percent. The new sustained-release dose should be 130 percent to 150 percent of the current levodopa dose. Thus 130 percent of 250 mg (2 1/2 tablets) is 325 mg, whereas 150 percent is 375 mg. We can round out the dose to fit with the available pill sizes. Sustained-release comes in 100 mg and 200 mg sizes (i.e., 25-100 and 50-200). When you round out the dose, you can decide whether to hedge up or down. Here, a 350 mg dose would be within the 130–150 percent range and translates to one 50-200 mg tablet plus 1 1/2 of the 25-100 mg tablets (200 + 150 = 350).

- Next, we increase the interval between doses by 60–90 minutes. We can go from doses at 3-hour intervals to 4 or 4 1/2 hours.

- If we have done the arithmetic correctly, the total daily dose should be "slightly higher" with the sustained-release formulation. If you take 350 mg four times daily, that would equate to 1400 mg per day. This compares to 1000 mg daily with the immediate-release formulation.

- If the first dose of the day doesn't kick in reliably, we could add 1/2 to one 25-100 immediate-release tablet to that dose, along with the 350 mg of the sustained-release formulation.

This represents our best estimate but additional fine-tuning may be necessary. With this transition, you may temporarily worsen if we have not captured your optimum sustained-release dosage. If the doses don't kick in consistently, they could be raised to 400 mg or if necessary, to 450 mg. On the other hand, if dyskinesias developed, they could be correspondingly reduced.

SLOW TO KICK IN

Sustained-release carbidopa/levodopa can be very slow to kick in. It generally takes at least an hour and often up to two hours to work. You need to factor this in when making adjustments of the levodopa-dosing interval. When deciding how far apart to schedule your doses, take into account the time it takes for the sustained-release drug to start working. Also, avoid being late with your pills.

If you are having problems with the slow kick-in, there are two strategies to consider:

- Drink plenty of fluids with each dose. You could also ingest dry bread or soda crackers to put some nonprotein food in your stomach.

- You could add a small amount of immediate-release carbidopa/levodopa with each dose of the sustained-release formulation. How much to add? Start out with 1/2 tablet of the 25-100 immediate-release pill with each sustained-release dose. If necessary, you could try a whole 25-100 immediate-release tablet. If the combined effect is too much, however, side effects may occur, most often involuntary movements (dyskinesias).

If the slow kick-in is a problem, despite trying all of these things, you have the option of switching back to the immediate-release formulation.

COMBINED SUSTAINED-RELEASE AND IMMEDIATE-RELEASE

We just mentioned taking a small amount of immediate-release carbidopa/levodopa with each dose of the sustained-release formulation. Sounds like a good idea; the immediate-release dose kicks in early and the sustained-release kicks in late. In fact, doing this for a single dose often works fine, but if you extend this strategy over the course of the day, it sometimes makes for very unpredictable and erratic responses. It's okay to try this if it seems appropriate. However, if you find yourself randomly fluctuating between dyskinetic and off states, you should then stick to one formulation.

WHO SHOULD SWITCH FROM SUSTAINED-RELEASE TO IMMEDIATE-RELEASE LEVODOPA?

Sustained-release carbidopa/levodopa is an acceptable choice when the responses are predictable and consistent. However, for those with erratic and relatively brief levodopa responses (2 hours or less), greater consistency can be obtained with the immediate-release formulation. The guidelines for switching from the sustained-release to immediate-release were detailed in chapter 12.

SLEEP AND SUSTAINED-RELEASE CARBIDOPA/LEVODOPA

In my own practice, I favor immediate-release carbidopa/levodopa to treat parkinsonism. Frequently, however, I add a dose of sustained-release carbidopa/levodopa at bedtime. Why? The answer relates to the slow kick-in. This is a disadvantage during the day but an advantage at bedtime if you require levodopa coverage throughout the night to sleep. For those who awaken 2–4 hours after falling asleep because their levodopa effect has worn off, sustained-release levodopa extends the night time coverage. If you take it just before your head hits the pillow, the delayed kick-in (up to 2 hours) is an advantage, beginning when you are asleep. Moreover, the effect will last 60–90 minutes longer than regular (immediate-release) levodopa. Typically, this strategy will allow a long stretch of sleep. We consider this and other strategies for treating insomnia in chapter 20.

Advancing PD, Short-Duration Levodopa Responses, and Meals

After many years, some with PD have difficulty sustaining a consistent response, even though they have made all the levodopa adjustments discussed above. Poor predictability of the levodopa response may be a major source of disability. Meals are perhaps the most frequent impediment to a consistent levodopa response. However, this is often unrecognized. Consider the following conversation in the doctor's office.

MR. JONES: Several times a day I lapse into an off-state, and I have no idea why.

DOCTOR: Is there any pattern; does this occur at certain times of the day?

MR. JONES: Nope, I have no idea when this is going to happen.

DOCTOR: How are you doing in the late morning and late afternoon?

MR. JONES: Usually, I'm pretty good then.

DOCTOR: How are you doing right after lunch? . . . after breakfast?

MR. JONES: Well, I guess those are bad times.

As you can see, there was a pattern, but Mr. Jones didn't appreciate it. His off-states occurred right after meals. This is a common theme among people with PD, but frequently overlooked.

During the early years of PD, what and when you eat makes no difference, as long as you avoid taking your carbidopa/levodopa with meals. With advancing PD, however, the timing and content of meals may crucially influence the control of your parkinsonism. Advancing PD results in a change in how your body responds to carbidopa/levodopa, as already noted. Early in the course, the levodopa response builds up over days (the long-duration response) and skipping a dose is inconsequential (as long as you don't skip too many doses). With advancing PD, the medication effect becomes linked to each carbidopa/levodopa dose (the short-duration response); your last dose and how long ago you took it determine how you are doing. Furthermore, any factor that even partially inhibits levodopa from getting to the brain will potentially prevent it from kicking in; the consequence is an off-state with immobility, tremor, walking difficulties, and so on. Obviously we want nothing to sabotage the effect of levodopa, so that a consistent on-state is achieved.

What might sabotage a dose of carbidopa/levodopa? The major culprit is what you eat. If you take carbidopa/levodopa immediately before or within a couple of hours after a meal, the benefit tends to be blocked. Obviously you could simply take your doses at other times. However, it may not be that simple for people with very brief levodopa responses who need to take their doses at short intervals. If you take doses every 3 hours or less, some of the doses will fall close to meals. In this situation, we may need to consider the content of our meals and strategies to prevent them from blocking the levodopa effect.

DIETARY PROTEIN AND LEVODOPA

Protein is the problem. Although dietary proteins are crucial to good nutrition, they can block the levodopa response. The basis for this relates to the similar chemical configuration of levodopa and the products of protein digestion.

When we digest protein, it is broken down into smaller elements, amino acids. Amino acids are the building blocks of protein; they are attached in long chains to constitute specific proteins. When we consume proteins, a variety of amino acids are liberated by the digestive process and circulate in our bloodstream.

Levodopa is also an amino acid and, when administered on an empty stomach, is the primary amino acid circulating in the bloodstream. However, when taken with a meal, levodopa is but one of several amino acids of similar configuration in the circulation. All of these amino acids compete for transport into the brain and into brain cells. Only a limited amount of amino acids can pass at any one time. Levodopa and similar amino acids all fight for the same seats on the train. This is a numbers game and the massive influx of other amino acids may overwhelm the levodopa from your pill. Unfortunately our digested food generates only small amounts of levodopa; most are other amino acids.

The important competition between administered levodopa and dietary amino acids is primarily at the blood-brain barrier. We previously learned how this natural barrier protects the brain from the biochemical fluxes that are constantly occurring in our bloodstreams. For amino acids to cross this barrier requires a specific transport mechanism. For each class of amino acids, there is a specific transporter that recognizes the appropriate amino acids and then carries them across the barrier. Otherwise, they would be excluded. These transporters do not have infinite capacity; rather, they can be filled up and then have no room to transport more. This is what can happen when we take levodopa with food. Dietary amino acids compete with levodopa for access to this transporter. These amino acids can knock levodopa off the train, so to speak. The other amino acids from our diet take up the space on the transporter and levodopa is prevented from getting into the brain.

MEALS AND SUSTAINED-RELEASE
CARBIDOPA/LEVODOPA (SINEMET CR)

The interaction between meals and levodopa is relatively straightforward. However, when levodopa is formulated in a controlled-release pill (Sinemet CR, sustained-release) this becomes much more complicated. On the one hand, levodopa from this sustained-release formulation competes with dietary amino acids just like regular (immediate-release) carbidopa/levodopa. However, this controlled-release pill doesn't release the levodopa very readily when the stomach is empty. In that case, the pill tends to sit in the stomach, undigested; eventually the release occurs, but slowly. With food in the stomach, levodopa is much more readily released from this CR tablet. Thus the blood levels of levodopa are greater when Sinemet CR is taken with food. However, the same food (protein) that helped liberate the levodopa from the CR pill, competes with it at the blood–brain barrier. Restated, food increases the amount of levodopa reaching the bloodstream, but blocks it from going to the next destination (the brain).

The best strategy for getting levodopa into the brain from Sinemet CR tablets has not been systematically investigated and we can only speculate about this. My suspicion is that the most consistent responses are obtained when the sustained-release dose is taken a couple of hours before a meal with a full glass of liquid, and perhaps with a small portion of some nonprotein food (such as crackers, dry bread).

If you are taking sustained-release carbidopa/levodopa and experiencing a good effect, don't worry about any of this. However, if the response is not optimal and you are having trouble coordinating this with meals, you might do better to switch to the immediate-release form of carbidopa/levodopa.

SPECIAL STRATEGIES TO OVERCOME
MEAL EFFECTS

If meals are still preventing consistent levodopa responses despite doing all of the above, special meal strategies may be necessary. The scheme we will discuss is designed for those taking the immediate-release form of carbidopa/levodopa. People who may be appropriate candidates for these strategies generally have the following attributes:

- Good but brief levodopa responses

- Carbidopa/levodopa dosing intervals of 3 hours or less (due to short-duration responses)

- Levodopa doses taken around mealtimes don't kick in

The phenomenon of doses failing to kick in (no on-response) has been termed skipped-dose effect or dose failure. This relationship to meals is often not recognized. People report to their physician that some of their carbidopa/levodopa doses don't work, yet fail to appreciate the correlation with mealtimes.

THE CRITICAL MEAL INTERVAL

The time frame surrounding meals when the levodopa effect may be compromised is approximately *20 minutes before a meal persisting to 2 hours after completion of the meal*. In other words, if you take carbidopa/levodopa within 20 minutes prior to a meal, during a meal, or within 2 hours after eating, you may experience a poor response. It is during this time that the meal-derived amino acids are in the bloodstream competing with levodopa. Note that this persists to 2 hours after the meal ends, not after it starts.

Is it really this precise? No; for some people the critical meal interval may be a little shorter or a little longer. Actually, the guidelines in chapter 12 recommended taking carbidopa/levodopa doses an hour before meals; this is because the meal effect may extend that far in occasional people. Thus the time frame given above (20 minutes before, to 2 hours after meals) is only an approximation. The meal contents and size as well as the function of your own gut will determine the exact margins of this critical meal interval.

MEAL STRATEGIES

If you find that carbidopa/levodopa doses taken within the critical meal interval don't kick in or kick in inconsistently, then we have methods to deal with this. We can't guarantee that these methods will work 100 percent of the time, but you should do considerably better. We will start with the simpler strategies first.

For some people, simply avoiding high-protein foods is sufficient. They may do fine on their regular diet but experience problems if they order a large steak at a restaurant. Or a hamburger and a milkshake may turn off their levodopa effect. After a while, you learn the foods with high protein content that cause trouble.

Foods high in protein are shown in table 17.1. You should not avoid these altogether; obviously you need some protein in your diet. However, you may choose to consume these in moderation. This is not an all-inclusive list and if you wish to address this in more detail, you could consult a dietitian.

Table 17.1.   Protein Foods

- Milk products (including ice cream, yogurt, butter, cheese, cottage cheese)
- Eggs and egg substitutes
- Meats of all types
- Poultry (including chicken, turkey)
- Fish of all types (including shellfish)
- Puddings, custards
- Dietary supplements, such as Ensure or Slim-Fast
- Nuts (including peanut butter)
- Beans, peas
- Soybeans (including tofu, which is soybean curd)
- Sunflower seeds

A second strategy is to shift the times of certain meals to match your social and occupational schedule. If you have an important engagement that may be sabotaged by a meal, avoid eating before or during that event. For example, if you have a golf tee-time at 1:00 P.M., defer lunch until after; alternatively, eat it much earlier (making it brunch). There is no law that stipulates that you must eat at the standard mealtimes. Change your mealtimes to match your day's activities. If the social engagement is a luncheon or dinner with friends and you are sensitive to proteins, order a salad. Remember, however, that some ingredients used to top off salads are high in protein, such as chunks of grilled meats, chicken, cheese, cottage cheese, and even nuts and seeds. Hence you might push some of these aside if they appear on your salad.

Bear in mind that protein snacks are often as problematic as regular meals. A big bowl of ice cream in the midafternoon may translate into a late afternoon off-state. Snack if you like, but recognize the potential relationship to your levodopa responses.

There are also more complex strategies for dealing with dietary protein. Another option focuses on meals, with redistribution of protein away from the first two meals of the day. The other focuses on levodopa, employing larger doses when taken around mealtimes. Let's consider these in more detail.

PROTEIN REDISTRIBUTION DIETS

We have a daily requirement for protein, but it is not necessary to consume protein with each meal. Consuming your daily protein requirement with just one of your meals should be sufficient. Thus, if you eat three meals a day, two can be low in protein. Most people choose to lower the protein content of breakfast and lunch, to optimize responses during the main part of the waking day. They accept the fact that their higher-protein supper will later tend to turn off their levodopa effect. This is a reasonable fit with our typical American diet, with the largest meal of the day being supper. However, you may choose to make lunch or even breakfast your high protein meal if that fits best with your needs.

To make certain that you will not become malnourished, it is wisest to seek advice from a dietitian/nutrition specialist before embarking on one of these protein redistribution diets. They can advise exactly which foods to avoid and which to substitute to make for palatable meals. This is a dietary strategy that has been employed for over a decade and dietitians are typically familiar with it. If not, show them this chapter and they should have no trouble devising an appropriate diet for you.

Theoretically, this should be a very effective approach to this difficult problem. However, in my experience, it works inconsistently but is worth trying.

MORE LEVODOPA WITH MEALS

Sometimes a simpler strategy is to simply take more levodopa when your carbidopa/levodopa dose falls around mealtimes. We already defined the times when your carbidopa/levodopa dose will potentially be compromised: *20 minutes before a meal persisting to 2 hours after completion of the meal.* Doses falling into this critical meal interval can be increased. In other words, employ two different doses throughout the day. One dose is for when your stomach is empty; the other, larger dose is for when your stomach is full (falls into this critical meal interval).

How does one establish these two different doses? Generally, we have already determined the carbidopa/levodopa dose that works when your stomach is empty. In fact, this was how we established the proper dose in the first place, taking it an hour before each meal. If you are unsure whether you know the optimal dose for times when your stomach is empty, make that determination first. Focus on this as the initial step in this process, using the principles we discussed in chapter 12. Once you have identified the ideal empty stomach dose, we use that as a reference point and make adjustments from there for the mealtime doses. Specifically, for the remaining doses falling into the critical meal interval, we simply increase that dose by small increments till we find a dose that also reliably kicks in during mealtimes. Thus we will have one dose taken when our stomach is empty and a larger dose for times of the critical meal interval.

So how much should you raise the dose during these critical meal intervals? Assuming that you are using the immediate-release carbidopa/levodopa 25-100 size, raise these mealtime doses by 1/2 tablet increments. In other words, start with the dose that works when your stomach is empty and add an extra 1/2 tablet during mealtimes. Try this for about a week. If you still don't experience a satisfactory response to these mealtime doses, raise them by another 1/2 tablet (i.e., a whole tablet more than your empty-stomach doses). Usually this will be sufficient. If still not sufficient, you could increase again by another 1/2 tablet. Typically, I do not find it necessary to raise these doses beyond 3–3 1/2 tablets, but there may be some rare exceptions.

With this scheme, you need to ask yourself a question each time you are due for another carbidopa/levodopa dose: Does this fall into the critical meal interval? If yes, take the larger dose; if not, take the smaller.

If you take your carbidopa/levodopa with meals and it still seems to work, don't worry about it. If your parkinsonism is well controlled, don't change anything.

SWEETS AND THE LEVODOPA RESPONSE

Sugary foods that are devoid of protein may enhance the levodopa response. For example, a large candy bar without nuts (nuts contain protein) may induce a more potent effect from your dose of carbidopa/levodopa. Presumably this is because the sugar (glucose) triggers your body to release insulin. Insulin is known to increase the exit of amino acids from the bloodstream into cells. Without the competition from other amino acids, administered levodopa can cross the blood–brain barrier more readily.

Taking your carbidopa/levodopa with candy bars, and so on, is not a good general strategy. Most of the time it is unnecessary, and if you do this frequently, the high sugar will suppress your appetite for other important components of your diet (and may cause tooth decay). Furthermore, if you have a tendency to obesity, all this candy will be detrimental.

FAVA BEANS AS A SOURCE OF LEVODOPA

Fava beans are a staple of some Mediterranean diets. They are high in levodopa. Limited studies have identified an antiparkinsonian effect from eating fava beans, and this has appeared on the Internet. However, if you are already taking carbidopa/levodopa, you don't need this other source of levodopa. If you are marooned on an island without your medications, then this might be important to you (provided fava beans are growing on your island).

When Levodopa Takes a Long Time to Kick In

If you lapse into a levodopa off-state, you want a quick response from your next dose of carbidopa/levodopa. With immediate-release carbidopa/levodopa, this should take about 30–60 minutes. However, certain factors will make it closer to 60 rather than 30 minutes.

Perhaps the major impediment to a quick start is when the carbidopa/levodopa pill sits undissolved in the stomach. To enter the bloodstream, it must dissolve and then get released into the small intestine. Absorption into the bloodstream takes place exclusively in the small intestine (see figure 17.5).

Perhaps the best way to jump-start the process is to drink adequate fluids each time you take your carbidopa/levodopa pills. This (1) helps dissolve the pill(s) and (2) stimulates the stomach to release the contents into the small intestine. (When the stomach is completely empty, the valve between the stomach and small intestine tends to stay closed.) On the other hand, if you take your carbidopa/levodopa without drinking something, the pills tend to sit in the stomach. I have been impressed with the number of people who tell me they swallow their pills dry.

The drug metoclopramide (Reglan) is sometimes used to facilitate stomach opening, allowing passage of contents into the intestine. Metoclopramide, however, is a bad choice for those with PD, since it blocks dopamine receptors; it may aggravate parkinsonism.

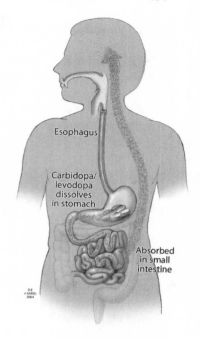

17.5 A carbidopa/levodopa pill has several hurdles before the levodopa reaches the blood stream. Once in the stomach it must be dissolved, and then the stomach must open to allow passage into the small intestine; absorption into the bloodstream takes place there.

Q: Does it make any difference what I drink with my carbidopa/levodopa?

A: Anything is okay as long as it is not a protein drink. In other words, you should *not* take your carbidopa/levodopa with milk, or with milk products such as Ensure or milkshakes.

Q: I take Sinemet CR. Will it also help this to kick in by drinking fluids?

A: Absolutely. However, if you are troubled by the slow response, you may well prefer immediate-release carbidopa/levodopa. It takes up to 2 hours for sustained-release carbidopa/levodopa to kick in, often twice as long as with the immediate-release formulation.

Q: What if I simply dissolve the carbidopa/levodopa in juice? Won't that help it kick in quicker?

A: Yes. In fact, this is a form of rescue therapy that may be used for a quick response when trapped in an off state. However, the benefit is also short-lived. If you dissolve your carbidopa/levodopa in 6–8 ounces of juice or soda pop, it will kick in within about 20 minutes, but the effect will only last 60–90 minutes. We consider this in more detail later in this chapter.

Q: If I chew my carbidopa/levodopa, won't it kick in more quickly?

A: This may help, but I don't recommend it. People whom I have watched do this end up with yellow carbidopa/levodopa between their teeth. Not only is this unsightly, but I suspect they leave behind some of the levodopa in their mouth, on their teeth.

The Effect of Exercise on Levodopa Fluctuations

Exercise is an important factor in managing PD. If we give in and become couch potatoes, the lack of exercise and consequent deconditioning adds to disability. However, those with fluctuations in their levodopa response need to be aware that physical exercise tends to use up the levodopa faster. In other words, the short-duration levodopa response often does not last quite as long during exercise. Think of this as burning the fuel faster. For example, if the effect from each carbidopa/levodopa dose normally lasts 4 hours, it may only last up to 3 1/2 hours if playing tennis, jogging, and so on. Sometimes even less rigorous exercise, such as walking or playing golf, may have the same effect. Thus, although vigorous exercise may contribute to control of your PD in the long term, be aware of the possible short-term effects.

So what should you do to deal with this? First, pay attention to what happens when you exercise. If your levodopa response tends to be consistently shortened, you can then change your dosing schedule. If your normal levodopa response is reduced from 4 to 3 hours while exercising, take your doses at 3-hour intervals during the time of the exercise. Once the exercise is over, you can revert to the 4-hour intervals. Don't worry about how many doses you take per day. If you burn the fuel faster, you simply need to fill the tank a little more often.

May I Take Any Dose Early If the Levodopa Effect Wears Off?

Yes. This option of taking a dose early is not only for times of exercise. If you recognize that your carbidopa/levodopa has kicked in and later is starting to wear off, you have essentially started to empty your fuel tank; your gauge is reading "low fuel." Sometimes this is signaled by recurrence of tremor or the dystonic curling of toes mentioned earlier. You will learn the signals, which differ from person to person. If it is getting close to the time for your next dose and these signals are going off, don't worry if you are a little early. You may take the dose when your body tells you it is time.

If you take a dose a little early, should you take as much? Answer: You should take your full dose, rather than a partial dose. When the tank is empty, you want to fill it full, not half full.

Here are a couple of case studies that illustrate how to deal with this.

Mr. Thompson normally takes his carbidopa/levodopa every 3 hours. This afternoon at the shopping mall, he noticed that his leg was cramping and his tremor returned a half hour before he was due for his next dose. Thus, rather than waiting until 5:00 P.M., he took his full dose at 4:30 P.M., a half hour early. What about his next dose, which would have been due at 8:00 P.M.? If he took it then, that would have been 3 1/2 hours after that 4:30 P.M. dose; this would have been a half hour too long. Hence, he took that next dose at 7:30 P.M. to maintain the 3-hour dosing schedule.

Mrs. Mulligan was putting on the golf course at 8:00 A.M. when she recognized that her levodopa effect was starting to wear off. This was an hour before she was due to take her next dose. She took that dose an hour early and found it necessary to do that again, later in the day. Moving those doses earlier required her to take 2 extra doses that day, which is not of concern.

These examples illustrate two key points:

- If you take a dose a little early, subsequent doses will need to be moved up in your schedule to avoid a big gap later in the day.

- Don't worry about the number of carbidopa/levodopa doses per day, with more doses necessary if you take doses earlier than scheduled.

Bear in mind that we are talking about taking a dose a little early. This implies that the levodopa effect has occurred and is starting to wear off prematurely. This is different from a dose failing to work, which requires a different strategy (see below).

Q: Why do most of my doses wear off early?

A: If this is your problem, the interval between doses is too long. Shorten the interval to match the duration of the typical response. Take as many doses each day as necessary to maintain an on-response.

Q: Should I be compulsive about treating these wearing-off problems?

A: You do not need to do this if the wearing-off effect is not a problem for you. Some experience a mild decline in their levodopa effect each dose cycle but without any compromise in their functioning. If this does not get in the way, and is not troublesome, stick with your current dosing schedule, rather that trying to compulsively adjust your medication doses. You are better off living with mild wearing-off effects as opposed to becoming obsessed with tightly regulating your dosing schedule.

Q: I often forget to take my pills and then I go off.

A: Buy a pill box timer. Most medical supply stores and many pharmacies carry these timers, which are made exactly for this purpose. The standard models allow you to set the dosing interval. Once you have set this interval, you don't need to set the timer again until the battery dies. You run the timer off a single button, which will recycle the timer to go off again according to your setting. If you can't hear high-pitched sounds, similar devices are made which signal by vibrating.

What Can I Do When My Levodopa Doesn't Work?

People with PD are especially prone to bad days: you are going out for the afternoon and your carbidopa/levodopa doesn't kick in. Or guests are coming over and the carbidopa/levodopa dose that you took 90 minutes ago has done nothing. Now what? If this is recurring frequently, you may be underdosed and need a slightly higher dose (see above). Or meals may be the culprit, as we just discussed. However, the primary concern is now. How can you get your levodopa effect to turn on? Obviously, there are a variety of things you could try, such as the following.

- Take another full dose of carbidopa/levodopa now (i.e., 60–90 minutes after the dose that failed). Result: This probably will kick in, but you may experience an excessive effect with dyskinesias.

- Take a fraction of your usual dose now (i.e., 60–90 minutes after the dose that failed). This partial dose might be half of a 25-100 immediate-release carbidopa/levodopa tablet, or even 1 tablet if your usual dose is much higher. Result: This may allow you to lapse into an on-state in 30–60 minutes; however, sometimes partial doses fail to kick in.

- Wait until it's time for your next dose and then take your full carbidopa/levodopa dose. Result: this will likely kick in, but the wait may be frustrating.

- Wait until about an hour before your next dose is due and then take another full carbidopa/levodopa dose. Result: You still will have to wait, but not as long.

These are all reasonable but imperfect options that you may consider.

RESCUE THERAPY WITH LIQUID SINEMET

You are playing golf on the 13th hole and suddenly your levodopa effect wears off. It's hard to walk, much less hit a golf ball. How can you reverse this off-state and finish the round of golf? Liquefying your full dose carbidopa/levodopa is the simplest solution. You do this by crushing your tablets (the full dose) and dissolving this in soda pop or some other liquid. Thus if you usually take 2 of the 25-100 carbidopa/levodopa tablets four times daily, crush 2 of these tablets, dissolve and drink; this will be in addition to what you would have taken that day. It will start to work in about 20 minutes. Is there a downside? Yes, the effect only lasts about an hour. However, this buys you time. Soda pop or carbonated water works best for this purpose, probably because the carbonation stimulates the stomach to contract, facilitating digestion. Juice or water is also okay, but water may not be very palatable. Obviously, do not mix it in milk or other protein drinks. In general, about 4–6 ounces of fluid is appropriate. However, remember that the entire contents of your mixture must be drank; otherwise you will only be receiving part of your levodopa dose.

Before you use this strategy, exercise appropriate patience with your conventional carbidopa/levodopa pills. If you just took your pills 20 minutes ago, and they still haven't kicked in, you should wait a little longer. If you now also took the liquid rescue dose, this would kick in about the same time as the pills and you would then experience a double effect; the consequence would probably be dyskinesias.

The exception to these dosing guidelines relates to those who are very prone to dyskinesias and who took their pills within the last couple of hours. Even if that dose failed, there still may be enough levodopa in the brain to summate with your rescue dose of carbidopa/levodopa. If dyskinesias are a major concern, you may need to use a lesser amount of carbidopa/levodopa as rescue. In that case, you could experiment on several occasions to find out what works for you. It's okay to try different doses. If you take too much, dyskinesias will result, but these will be over in perhaps 60–90 minutes. If you take too little, then the rescue dose won't work.

Anticipate that this effect won't last long, only about an hour. You will need to take your carbidopa/levodopa pills shortly after the liquid Sinemet kicks in. Since it takes up to an hour for your carbidopa/levodopa tablets to kick in, you probably need to take them right after you recognize that the liquid rescue dose is starting to work. Don't forget to do this or you will lapse into another off-state.

There is no limit to how often you add extra doses of liquid Sinemet. However, if you need to do this often, this means that your responses are fluctuating a lot. In that case, be sure that you have adjusted your regular carbidopa/levodopa dosage as best you can. You may then be a good candidate for one of the dopamine agonist drugs that we will discuss in chapter 18.

This extra dose of levodopa, in the form of liquid Sinemet, may cause dyskinesias. This will happen if this effect is superimposed on the effect from your regularly scheduled carbidopa/levodopa doses. However, this is not dangerous and most would prefer dyskinesias to an immobile state. Moreover, since the liquid Sinemet response is brief (60–90 minutes), any dyskinesias that develop from this extra dose should be short-lived.

An injectable drug (apomorphine) for rescue therapy was recently introduced for prescription use. This dopamine agonist is discussed in chapter 18.

Liquid Sinemet As Ongoing Therapy

You just learned about dissolving your carbidopa/levodopa dose to use as rescue therapy from an off-state. Actually, this strategy has also been used as ongoing treatment of PD, specifically, using "liquid Sinemet" for every dose. Instead of taking pills throughout the day, you drink your carbidopa/levodopa dose mixture. I've saved the discussion of liquid Sinemet for last because it tends to be the least practical approach to these problems of wearing-off. You can't buy liquid Sinemet in stores; you need to mix this yourself. This strategy was in vogue about a dozen years ago, but few people stuck with it because of the hassle factor.

You can fine-tune your levodopa dosage with great precision using liquid Sinemet. The standard recipe allows you to vary the amount of levodopa in your dose by as little as a few milligrams. Contrast this to the pills; suppose that a dose of two 25-100 carbidopa/levodopa tablets is too much (causing dyskinesias) but 1 1/2 tablets is too little (too much parkinsonism). With pills, the best you could do is to split the difference and quarter the tablets. With liquid Sinemet you can take any milligram amount.

With the standard liquid Sinemet recipe, the levodopa dose in milligrams (mg) corresponds to the volume you drink in milliliters (mL). In other words, you mix it up so that 1 mg is equal to 1 mL. If you decide you want 175 mg (the equivalent of 1 3/4 pills), you simply drink 175 mL of your solution. Moreover, the response is quick; it will kick in within 20 minutes. Some people also find that this is a little more reliable than pills; that is, it is more likely to kick in.

So why not do this? The practicalities dissuade most people. First, you need to mix it each morning and then carry the container of medicine around all day. If you currently take about ten 25-100 tablets during the day, you will need to carry around a liter container (the recipe calls for one liter of fluid for every ten 25-100 pills). Moreover, you will need some type of milliliter measuring cup so that you take the right amount; this also needs to be carried with you. Perhaps the most dissuasive factor, however, is the brevity of the response. The effect typically lasts about an hour, occasionally slightly longer, but no more than 90 minutes. The advantages and disadvantages to liquid Sinemet are summarized in table 17.2.

A trial of liquid Sinemet is never dangerous. However, it is impractical if you now can get by with taking your carbidopa/levodopa pills at intervals of 3 hours or more. With the switch to liquid Sinemet, you will probably need to take it hourly. It becomes a reasonable option only if your carbidopa/levodopa tablet dosing interval is already close to 60–90 minutes.

Table 17.2.   Advantages and Disadvantages of Using "Liquid Sinemet" as Your Primary Therapy

Advantages	Disadvantages
• Quick responses (about 20 minutes)	• Must be mixed daily (or every 2–3 days if preservative Vitamin C added)
• Precise titrations of the dose are possible	• Inconvenient to carry around
• It may be a little more reliable than pill form (fewer doses that fail to kick-in)	• Need a measuring cup to get correct dose
	• Effect only lasts 60-90 minutes

HOW TO MIX AND USE LIQUID SINEMET

If you decide to try liquid Sinemet, you don't need to ease into this like you do when you start a dopamine agonist. You just start the new day with the liquid form rather than your usual pills. If you don't like it after a day, week, or month, just switch back to pills.

The standard recipe for liquid Sinemet calls for 2000 mg of vitamin C (ascorbic acid) as a preservative. Vitamin C comes in a variety of pill forms; buy whatever size you like and just use enough of these pills to total approximately 2000 mg. Liquid Sinemet is prepared as follows.

1. Grind up ten 25-100 carbidopa/levodopa tablets (immediate-release formulation) plus 2000 mg vitamin C.

2. Mix this in 1000 milliliters (mL) of tap water, juice, or soda pop; dissolve well.

3. If the tablets are mixed in water, you will probably want to add some flavoring such as Kool Aid or Tang. Sugar-free flavorings are better for your waistline and your teeth. Theoretically, the artificial sweetener NutraSweet (aspartame) may work against levodopa, but in practice, this has not appeared to be a problem.

Each mL of this mixture contains one mg of levodopa. This makes it easy to determine the dose. For example, 100 mL contains 100 mg of levodopa, which is equivalent to one 25-100 pill. Thus, if you have been taking two 25-100 tablets of carbidopa/levodopa at a time, the same amount of levodopa would be found in 200 mL of your solution. You just need a measuring cup.

When you use liquid Sinemet, it goes through your system quicker. Consequently, the amount of levodopa you take per day will likely increase. Don't worry about that. There are two principles that apply to the switch to liquid Sinemet:

1. For each dose of liquid Sinemet, take the same amount as you took in pill form. If you previously took one 25-100 carbidopa/levodopa pill every 2 1/2 hours, take 100 mL of your liquid Sinemet each dose.

2. Take this dose at intervals that match the duration of the effect. Start out taking it at intervals of a little longer than an hour (perhaps at 90 minute intervals so that you can get a good feel for the duration of the response as it kicks in and later wears off). You can reduce this interval depending upon how long the effect lasts. Anticipate that it will be about an hour.

Don't worry about the number of doses per day or about how much levodopa you are taking daily. Both the number of doses and the mg of levodopa per day will increase substantially with this transition to liquid Sinemet.

Buy a pill-box timer to stay on schedule. These are sold at most pharmacies and medical supply stores. Buy one that allows you to set the dosing interval once without the need to reset it every time. These cost about $20.

Once you have made this transition, you are then in a position to fine-tune your levodopa response. For example, if you are taking 200 mL of liquid Sinemet (i.e., 200 mg levodopa) and experience frequent dyskinesias, you can lower the doses by small decrements, for example, 10–20 mL reductions. As you continue to reduce the dose by small amounts, you should eventually arrive at a dose that is less likely to cause dyskinesias. However, if you go too low and parkinsonism is poorly controlled, you could then do the opposite, and raise it by 10–20 mL increments. Find the dose providing the best balance between over- and underdosage effects.

Q: How long can I keep the liquid Sinemet?

A: If you use the standard recipe, it should be good for two days and may even be good for a third day, especially if you keep it refrigerated. Keep it out of the heat.

Q: How do I know if my liquid Sinemet isn't any good?

A: There will be one of two clues: (1) it doesn't work or (2) the color turns dark. If you're trying to stretch this out over three days and one of these clues surfaces, then discard and mix another batch.

Q: Must I mix vitamin C (ascorbic acid) in my liquid Sinemet?

A: Although the standard recipe calls for this as a preservative, it may not be necessary if you prepare a new batch every day. My recommendation is to include the vitamin C for at least a couple of weeks. Then, if things are going well, you could try cutting corners and leave this out. At least one study suggests that if you use your liquid Sinemet within a day and don't allow it to get hot, it should be stable even without the vitamin C.

WHAT ABOUT MY OTHER PD MEDICATIONS IF I SWITCH TO LIQUID SINEMET?

When switching to liquid Sinemet, don't change your other medications. The liquid Sinemet only replaces the levodopa in pill form. You will still need to take your other medications in pill form, as you have been doing, generally at the same times and in the same doses. For the dopamine agonist drugs, this is straightforward. However, if you have also been taking entacapone (Comtan) with each of your carbidopa/levodopa doses, you may need to rethink this slightly. Since entacapone enhances the levodopa effect for about 4 hours, you should take the entacapone at 4-hour intervals. If you end up taking liquid Sinemet every hour, you could then take your 200 mg entacapone dose with every fourth dose of liquid Sinemet.

CAN I EXPERIENCE A QUICKER RESPONSE FROM THE NEW ORALLY DISINTEGRATING CARBIDOPA/LEVODOPA TABLET (PARCOPA)?

Data available from the pharmaceutical company suggests that this formulation kicks in about the same as conventional immediate-release carbidopa/levodopa. Hence, it does not produce a quicker response. It may be advantageous, however, when water or other liquid isn't available (e.g., on the golf course), or when socially conspicuous (e.g., at a party).

Special Cases and Rare Problems

The vast majority of people with PD can optimize their carbidopa/levodopa treatment using the above guidelines. If these fit your needs, you might skip the rest of this chapter, which deals with some very unique and complex problems.

DYSKINESIAS WITH SMALL DOSES OF CARBIDOPA/LEVODOPA

A small minority of people develop dyskinesias from very low carbidopa/levodopa doses. For these people, the only doses that don't provoke dyskinesias are those too low to control their parkinsonism. Fortunately, this is rare, but it can be disabling. Consider the person who tolerates no more than one 25-100 tablet three times daily; with 1 1/2 tablet doses, dyskinesias develop and worsen further when the dose is raised to 2 tablets three times daily. In this example, 1 carbidopa/levodopa tablet three times a day barely improves this person's parkinsonism. What to do? There are two options: (1) employ a special carbidopa/levodopa dosing schedule to avoid dyskinesias or (2) switch to a dopamine agonist drug in place of carbidopa/levodopa.

In the long run, the dopamine agonist medications ultimately fail to control parkinsonism; levodopa therapy is almost always necessary after a few years or less. Also, starting a dopamine agonist drug is fairly complex. Hence I favor the first option, the special carbidopa/levodopa-dosing scheme. The alternative strategy, switching to a dopamine agonist medication, is discussed in the next chapter.

So what is this special carbidopa/levodopa dosing scheme? This strategy for avoiding dyskinesias provoked by even low levodopa doses capitalizes on two principles. First, dyskinesias are short-duration responses. When dyskinesias occur, they are tied to each individual carbidopa/levodopa dose, but are not directly related to the total daily dose. The potential for dyskinesias lasts for no more than a few hours after each dose, tending to follow the blood levels of levodopa (peaking shortly after a dose and then declining within a few hours or less). There is no build-up, unless doses are too close together.

Second, the *beneficial* (antiparkinsonian) responses to levodopa are both short-duration and long-duration. The long-duration antiparkinsonian response to levodopa builds up over about a week or so with continued treatment. This is the exclusive response in early PD. However, the potential for a long-duration response persists, even when overshadowed later in PD by the short-duration response. With advancing PD we become oblivious to this long-duration response unless levodopa is discontinued, which we almost never do.

If dyskinesias are provoked by even low doses of carbidopa/levodopa, we can capitalize on the fact that this is a short-duration response. We can focus on capturing a long-duration levodopa response as the primary source of benefit. Furthermore, if you have early PD, the long-duration response may be all that you need.

Recognizing these levodopa dynamics, let us design a treatment scheme that emphasizes the long-duration aspect of levodopa therapy. There are two steps in constructing this scheme.

First, progressively lower carbidopa/levodopa until you find a dose that does not provoke dyskinesias. If the starting dose causes dyskinesias, then reduce by 1/4 tablet decrements until you come up with a dose that can be taken without dyskinesias. If one 25-100 tablet provokes dyskinesias, try 3/4 tablet; if necessary, reduce to 1/2 tablet doses. You will not need to go any lower than that. We want to identify the largest dose that comes up short of the dyskinesia threshold.

Once this dose has been determined, take it as often as you can, short of overlapping the effects. Obviously, if the doses are too closely spaced, they will summate and dyskinesias will occur. However, if spaced far enough apart the short-duration dyskinesia potential from one dose will have dissipated before the next dose kicks in. This allows you to take multiple doses per day and build-up a long-duration antiparkinsonian response. What should be the interval between doses? You can experiment and see how close together you can space the doses without overlapping the effects, and causing dyskinesias. You might start out by spacing the doses about 4 hours apart. With this scheme, work in doses at bedtime and during the night (e.g., take a dose if you wake up to go to the bathroom). We want as many doses as we can work in, per 24 hours. Also, bear in mind that if you are asleep, dyskinesias will not occur; hence, if you can sleep through the night, you might get by with taking higher nighttime doses.

How much levodopa is necessary to capture the full long-duration response? This has not been systematically investigated; however, my own experience suggests this to be about 600–800 mg daily. In other words, if your total daily dose of levodopa is in this range, you probably have achieved the full long-duration levodopa effect. Lower doses may capture only part of this effect.

A RARE, PARADOXICAL DYSKINESIA PATTERN

There is an unusual pattern of involuntary movements termed biphasic dyskinesias. I see this in perhaps less than 1 percent of the people with PD in my clinic. Biphasic dyskinesias begin just as the levodopa dose is *starting* to kick in; they then subside and recur later as the levodopa effect is wearing off. The term biphasic implies that there are two phases of dyskinesias, one at the beginning and one at the end of the levodopa response cycle. It is usually the dyskinesias at the end of the cycle that are problematic.

If your toes curl or your foot turns in as your levodopa effect is wearing off, this is not a biphasic dyskinetic pattern. Rather this is the more common *dystonia* that occurs when the levodopa effect is starting to wear off. This is sometimes called end-of-dose dystonia. Cramp-like sensations among those with PD are typically dystonia and are a symptom of PD, rather than a medication effect. These occur in untreated people with PD and also may be experienced as your levodopa effect is wearing off. The dyskinesias experienced by those with the biphasic dyskinetic response include prominent chorea.

TREATMENT OF BIPHASIC DYSKINESIAS

There are two alternative strategies for controlling this rare pattern of dyskinesias.

1. Overlap the carbidopa/levodopa doses so that the end-of-dose dyskinesias are avoided until after the last dose of the day. Thus you adjust the timing of the levodopa doses just as you would to treat wearing-off problems.

2. Switch to a dopamine agonist drug in place of carbidopa/levodopa. This is less desirable and reserved for only the most difficult to control cases of biphasic dyskinesias. Dopamine agonist therapy is not nearly as effective in controlling PD symptoms as carbidopa/levodopa. This strategy is detailed in the next chapter.

BRIEF TREMOR JUST BEFORE SINEMET KICKS IN

This is an occasional observation and should not be confused with biphasic dyskinesias. Specifically, an occasional person with PD may experience a typical parkinsonian tremor about 20–30 minutes after a dose of carbidopa/levodopa, which lasts minutes and then goes away. It seems to be triggered by levodopa and may occur in someone who otherwise has no tremor or only mild tremor. The rhythmic movements characteristic of tremor should be easy to distinguish from the chaotic, dancing movements of dyskinesia. Typically, no specific treatment is directed at this levodopa kick-in tremor since it is so brief.

18

◆ ◆ ◆

Supplemental Drugs for Motor Fluctuations and Dyskinesias

Levodopa is a very effective drug for treating the symptoms of PD. However, after several years, the response often becomes uneven. The effect may no longer last around the clock (the long-duration effect); rather, the primary benefit lasts a few hours or less after each levodopa dose (the short-duration effect). This results in response fluctuations. In this chapter, we consider adding another medication to smooth the response and control the symptoms. Note that these drugs are supplemental and do not substitute for carbidopa/levodopa. Levodopa is the most potent medication and remains the foundation of treatment.

When to add another drug is sometimes an arbitrary decision. Simply adjusting the carbidopa/levodopa dosing scheme may fix the problem and would obviously be a cheaper solution. You often can fine-tune the levodopa dose quite precisely. In fact, my usual strategy is to do this first. If substantial fluctuations in the response persist, then I add a second drug.

One factor that may persuade me to add the second drug earlier is the age of parkinsonism onset. Young-onset PD is associated with early development of levodopa dyskinesias and fluctuations. These problems are especially likely if PD started before age forty. When troublesome levodopa complications are anticipated, combination therapy using carbidopa/levodopa plus a dopamine agonist often works best.

The drugs we consider in this chapter may also exacerbate dyskinesias, since they enhance the levodopa effect. Anticipate this happening so that you will know what to do if it occurs. The appropriate strategy is to reduce the carbidopa/levodopa doses. This is done in small decrements, such as by 1/4 or 1/2 of the 25-100 tablets (immediate-release), as discussed in the previous chapter. The idea is to strike an optimum balance between the supplemental drug and levodopa, which often requires a lower levodopa dose. Note that if you lower the levodopa doses too much, parkinsonism increases.

The Medication Options

There are several medications that may be added to your carbidopa/levodopa regimen if you are experiencing fluctuations in the response. First, we will focus on treating short-duration responses and wearing-off; supplemental drugs targeting dyskinesias are discussed later. Drugs for motor fluctuations include the following.

Dopamine agonists are the *most effective*. They have a longer duration of action than the levodopa short-duration response; because their effects last longer, they can reduce wearing-off symptoms. They include:

- Pramipexole (Mirapex)

- Ropinirole (Requip)

- Pergolide (Permax)

- Bromocriptine (Parlodel)

The catechol-O-methyltransferase (COMT) inhibitors are *moderately effective*. They block one route of levodopa metabolism, allowing levodopa to remain longer in the bloodstream. Examples of COMT inhibitors include:

- Entacapone (Comtan)

- Tolcapone (Tasmar)

Monoamine oxidase-B (MAO-B) inhibitors are the *least effective*. They block one route of dopamine breakdown. An example is selegiline (Eldepryl).

My first choice is typically a dopamine agonist drug because of its efficacy. My second choice is the COMT inhibitor, entacapone, which is much easier to dose than the dopamine agonist drugs. The MAO-B inhibitor selegiline is not very effective but is simple to use.

EXPENSE

These supplemental drugs are expensive and, unfortunately, cost occasionally plays a role in choice of medications. Table 18.1 lists the typical retail cost for a monthly supply of these medications when taken in sufficient doses to be helpful.

Table 18.1. Expense of Supplementary Medications for Motor Fluctuations*

Drug	Typical Therapeutic Dose	Cost per Tablet	Cost per Month
Dopamine agonists			
Pramipexole (Mirapex)	1.5 mg tablet 3 times daily	$2.60	$234
Ropinirole (Requip)	5 mg tablet 3 times daily	2.62	236
Pergolide (Permax)	1 mg tablet 3 times daily	4.63	417
Bromocriptine generic	Two 5 mg capsules 3 times daily	3.41	614
Bromocriptine, brand name Parlodel	Two 5 mg capsules 3 times daily	5.29	952
COMT inhibitors			
Entacapone (Comtan)	200 mg tablet 4 times daily	2.22	266
Entacapone plus carbidopa/levodopa (Stalevo)	One tablet of Stalevo-150 four times daily**	2.36	283
Tolcapone (Tasmar)	100 mg tablet 3 times daily	2.83	255
MAO-B inhibitor			
Selegiline generic	5 mg tablet daily	2.58	77
Selegiline, brand name Eldepryl	5 mg tablet daily	2.98	89
Comparison: Generic carbidopa/levodopa 25-100 immediate-release	Two tablets 5 times daily**	0.26	78

*Retail cost, based upon large community pharmacy prices, 2004.

**One of many possible dosages used by those with fluctuations.

My Usual First Choice: Dopamine Agonist Drugs for Treatment of Short-Duration Levodopa Responses

The dopamine agonists' long-lasting effect can bolster the response when the levodopa effect is wearing off. The agonists are similar in potency, but what sets them apart are expense, side effects, and dosing complexity, as explained in chapter 13. These considerations clearly favor pramipexole and ropinirole over bromocriptine and pergolide. Personally, I prefer pramipexole because the dosing scheme is a little easier to employ than the ropinirole schedule. Otherwise, these two medications are quite similar and either is a good first choice as a supplemental drug.

ADDING A DOPAMINE AGONIST TO LEVODOPA THERAPY

To start an agonist, refer to the dosing schedules in chapter 13. Dopamine agonist drugs are always started low and slowly raised. How high to go? Continue to raise it until you have smoothed out the fluctuations in your levodopa response. Focus on your off-states. These should become less pronounced. This is because these agonist drugs have a longer-lasting effect, which spans into the levodopa off-states.

Improvement of parkinsonism will be minimal with the initial doses, and you will probably require several weeks of dosage escalation to appreciate any benefit. Be patient! Once you start to experience the good effects, you may stick with a given dose if you are satisfied with the response.

TAKING CARBIDOPA/LEVODOPA LESS OFTEN

People with short-duration levodopa responses often must take their carbidopa/levodopa doses frequently and at short intervals to maintain their good effect. This can be quite inconvenient and make life very complicated. Adding a dopamine agonist may allow fewer carbidopa/levodopa doses and longer intervals between those doses.

Once the dose of the agonist is sufficiently high (i.e., close to the target dose), try increasing the interval between your carbidopa/levodopa doses. You may experiment with this by delaying your next carbidopa/levodopa dose by thirty to sixty minutes; if the effect doesn't wear off, try this a few more times. If this continues to work, then lock in this new dosing schedule. The idea is to arrive at the longest duration between carbidopa/levodopa doses that still allows continuous control of parkinsonism.

LEVODOPA ADJUSTMENTS AFTER STARTING A DOPAMINE AGONIST

Don't reduce your carbidopa/levodopa doses just because you are starting one of these drugs. Remember, these initial doses are too low to have much of an effect. If you reduce your carbidopa/levodopa dose too early, your parkin-sonism will suffer. Wait until there are side effects that tell you it's time; usu-ally, dyskinesias are the signal to lower your carbidopa/levodopa dose. Once those develop, then reduce your carbidopa/levodopa dose (or increase the interval between doses).

Sometimes it is easier to grasp these concepts by discussing typical cases where these medication strategies are being employed. Let's go over a few of these.

> Mrs. Jackson was taking carbidopa/levodopa at three-hour intervals and was still experiencing 20 minutes of off-time at the end of each dose. She started ropinirole and by the seventh week, these off-periods were essentially abolished (7.5 mg ropinirole daily). She decided to raise the dose even higher to allow her to increase the intervals between her carbidopa/levodopa doses. Several weeks later on twice the dose of ropinirole, she was able to lengthen the interval between carbidopa/levodopa doses to four hours. Since she didn't experience dyskinesias, the individual carbidopa/levodopa doses were kept the same.

> Mr. Grant started pramipexole to reduce his levodopa off-time. However, he also experienced mild levodopa-induced dyskinesias despite carbidopa/levodopa adjustments. By the fourth week of his pramipexole dosing sched-ule, he began to experience increased dyskinesias. To manage these, he re-duced his carbidopa/levodopa (25-100) doses from 2 to 1 3/4 tablets. He then raised pramipexole further. By the sixth week, the dyskinesias increased again and he controlled those by lowering his carbidopa/levodopa doses to 1 1/2 tablets. By the seventh week he realized that he could increase the interval between his carbidopa/levodopa doses to every three hours instead of every 2 hours; he did this without increasing his off-time.

To summarize, the carbidopa/levodopa dose can be manipulated in two ways. Lower each dose if dyskinesias become a problem. Do this by 1/4 to 1/2 tablet decrements. Second, once the dopamine agonist dose is high enough to do some good, you can try increasing the interval between your doses of carbidopa/levodopa. Don't concern yourself with how much carbidopa/levodopa you are taking per day, since this is not very important in this scheme. Note that you may take your dopamine agonist medication at the same time as your carbidopa/levodopa doses if you are not nauseated (for increased convenience).

I TRIED PRAMIPEXOLE (OR ROPINIROLE, PERGOLIDE, BROMOCRIPTINE); IT DIDN'T DO ANY GOOD

This comment should elicit this question: How much did you take? The most common reason people experience inadequate responses to dopamine ago-nist drugs is failure to raise the dose into the therapeutic range. Recall that they are started in very low doses, too low to do any good. This is to avoid side effects. With all the dosing schemes for these drugs, it takes several weeks of increments to achieve a dose that is even mildly beneficial.

I TRIED ROPINIROLE (OR PRAMIPEXOLE, PERGOLIDE OR BROMOCRIPTINE); IT MADE MY PARKINSONISM WORSE

I've heard this comment more than once. However, these drugs do not worsen parkinsonism. The usual explanation is premature levodopa reduction. Specifically, when the agonist was started, the carbidopa/levodopa dose was simultaneously lowered. Don't do that. The starting doses of these agonist drugs are too low to benefit. If the levodopa dose is reduced when the agonist is started, parkinsonism will predictably worsen. Don't lower your carbidopa/levodopa dose until dyskinesias or other side effects develop. In some cases, you may not need to lower the carbidopa/levodopa dose at all.

FREQUENT OVERSIGHT WHEN STARTING A DOPAMINE AGONIST MEDICATION

Don't forget to have your standing blood pressure checked as you start one of these drugs. These medications, like levodopa, can lower the blood pressure, especially the blood pressure when you stand up. If it gets too low, you will feel lightheaded when you stand up; activities may be compromised by fatigue. If even lower yet, you might faint. If your standing blood pressure is around 90/60, this could be a problem. It is better to recognize the problem and treat it rather than confronting it only after you have fainted. This issue is discussed in detail in chapter 21.

WOULD TAKING TWO DOPAMINE AGONIST DRUGS BE HELPFUL?

There is no obvious benefit to adding a second agonist drug if you are already taking another. Taking two of these agonist drugs at the same time makes dosing more confusing and may increase the side effect spectrum. If the effects from one of these are insufficient, there are two options: (1) raise the dose or (2) switch to another drug. The dose can be raised if side effects are not a problem. The usual maximum doses were provided in chapter 13. On the other hand, if you are considering switching to another drug, read on.

SWITCHING DOPAMINE AGONIST MEDICATIONS DUE TO SIDE EFFECTS

What if side effects develop while you are starting one of the dopamine agonist drugs? Would it be worthwhile to try another of these medications or would the same problem be just as likely with another agonist? There have been few clinical trials comparing these drugs head to head. My own sense is that all four dopamine agonist drugs have approximately equal propensity to provoke the same side effects except for the following.

- Sleepiness: Pramipexole seems a little more likely to induce daytime sleepiness than ropinirole, in my view. Pergolide and bromocriptine seem to be the least likely.

- Leg swelling: This may be more common with pramipexole and ropinirole than with pergolide or bromocriptine.

- Dyskinesias: The potential for dyskinesias seems similar among these drugs but may be a little greater with pergolide.

- Ergot side effects: These are unique to pergolide and bromocriptine and include the potential heart and lung problems discussed in chapter 13; these do not occur with pramipexole or ropinirole.

Nausea, hallucinations, delusions, and low blood pressure (orthostatic hypotension) may be provoked by any of the dopamine agonist drugs with equal propensity; switching to another agonist probably won't help with these side effects.

THIS AGONIST INITIALLY WORKED BUT DOESN'T NOW; COULD I TRY ANOTHER?

After many months, the benefits of a dopamine agonist medication may become less pronounced. Why? Perhaps the brain has habituated to the drug. Or perhaps this reflects the normal progression of PD; it may still be helping but no longer is sufficient. What can you do in this circumstance? Again, the options are to (1) raise the dose or (2) switch to another drug. Increasing the dose makes the most sense as the initial strategy. If you are not very close to the maximum dose specified in chapter 13, you could try further increments.

But what if your dose is maxed out? How helpful would it be to switch to one of the other dopamine agonist medications? The answer depends upon what you are currently taking.

- Switching from pramipexole to ropinirole, or vice versa, may not prove very helpful (assuming that side effects are not the reason for switching). These drugs are very similar in potency (recognizing that there is no milligram-to-milligram correspondence). It's okay to try the switch, but I wouldn't expect the response to the second drug will be much different from the first.

- Switching between pergolide and one of these drugs may be helpful on occasion, given that pramipexole and ropinirole have a slightly different spectrum of effects at dopamine receptors.

- A switch from any of these drugs to bromocriptine is unlikely to prove beneficial, so we won't consider that.

Such switches are complicated and may cause some upheaval during the transition. Since they are not likely to provide dramatic benefits, I generally don't do this. However, if you recognize the limitations, it's okay to try.

There are two ways to do this. One is to taper off the first agonist drug over a few weeks and then start the second with the same dosage escalation schedules outlined in chapter 13. However, this takes a long time. A simpler strategy is to do this overnight. This requires estimating equivalent doses between the two drugs. In other words, one has to guess the dose of the new drug that would approximately match the first drug. The approximate equivalent doses of the four drugs are:

- Pramipexole 4.5 mg per day (1.5 mg three times daily)

- Ropinirole 12–15 mg per day (4–5 mg three times daily)

- Pergolide 3 mg per day (1 mg three times daily)

- Bromocriptine 30 mg daily (10 mg three times daily)

Thus, if you are taking 1 mg of pergolide three times per day and wish to switch to pramipexole, a similarly potent dose is 1.5 mg three times daily. To make the transition, stop pergolide after your last dose of the day and the next day, start pramipexole in its place in a dose of 1.5 mg three times daily. Bear in mind, however, that the doses may not be exactly equivalent and you may be under- or overdosed after the transition. Thus there could be some upheaval in your parkinsonism control and further adjustment of the new drug may be necessary. In our example, if the switch to pramipexole proved to be more potent, dyskinesias might develop. To counter this, small reductions of your carbidopa/levodopa doses or reduced pramipexole would be appropriate. Conversely, if it seems that the switch to pramipexole was even less effective than pergolide, you could try raising the pramipexole doses by 0.25 mg increments.

What if the pergolide dose was 4 mg a day and you want to convert to pramipexole? You can still use the conversion values shown above. A pergolide dose of 4 mg is a third larger than the 3 mg dose shown above. Simply make the pramipexole dose a third larger to come up with the equivalent dose. In other words, 3 mg of pergolide is equivalent to 4.5 mg of pramipexole; correspondingly, 4 mg of pergolide is approximately equivalent to 6 mg of pramipexole.

These overnight switches of dopamine agonist drugs may not always go smoothly, especially at higher doses. Hence you should work closely with your physician if you choose to do this.

SPECIAL CASE: WHEN DYSKINESIAS FORCE A SWITCH FROM CARBIDOPA/LEVODOPA TO A DOPAMINE AGONIST

There are two rare but troublesome situations where a switch from carbidopa/levodopa to a dopamine agonist medication may be appropriate: (1) When levodopa in even low doses provokes prominent dyskinesias and (2) when biphasic dyskinesias from levodopa treatment cannot otherwise be controlled. Both of these problems relating to dyskinesias were discussed in the last chapter. If these are not your problem, you may skip this section and move on to the section below on COMT inhibitors.

The dopamine agonists (pramipexole, ropinirole or pergolide) only rarely cause dyskinesias if used alone, in the absence of carbidopa/levodopa. The downside is that they are not as potent as carbidopa/levodopa and parkinsonism may not be satisfactorily controlled. If your parkinsonism is relatively mild, this might be an acceptable strategy to counter these dyskinesias. Read on.

How to Phase in the Dopamine Agonist If Replacing Carbidopa/Levodopa

Substituting a dopamine agonist drug for carbidopa/levodopa can't be done overnight. That's because the dopamine agonists are not started in high doses; the starting doses are too low to be helpful. They are phased in over a number of weeks. If we abruptly stop carbidopa/levodopa and begin one of these, using the typical starting dosage, your parkinsonism will worsen due to lack of a medication effect (assuming you were taking enough levodopa to do some good).

Make the transition from carbidopa/levodopa to the dopamine agonist drug in three steps.

1. Lower the dose of carbidopa/levodopa to levels that fall short of causing troublesome dyskinesias.

2. Begin to phase in the dopamine agonist. The guidelines for starting a dopamine agonist are found in chapter 13. Choose one of the three: pramipexole, ropinirole, or pergolide. Their potencies are not dramatically different but the side effects and expense place pergolide last. Hence the favored choices are pramipexole or ropinirole. Continue the carbidopa/levodopa while the dopamine agonist drug is initiated and the dose raised.

3. After several weeks of agonist dose escalation, dyskinesias may recur. Then lower each dose of carbidopa/levodopa by 1/4 tablet decrements until the dyskinesias resolve. After that, you may continue to raise the agonist drug. Likely you will need to taper off carbidopa/levodopa altogether to avoid dyskinesias; thus you will manage your parkinsonism with the dopamine agonist alone. To capture enough of a therapeutic effect, you will probably need to raise the dopamine agonist dose to the maximum levels, as outlined in chapter 13 (if tolerated).

Catechol-O-methyltransferase (COMT) Inhibitors

Recall that COMT is an enzyme that breaks down levodopa (and dopamine). Inhibitors of COMT prevent this from happening. COMT inhibitor drugs

Table 18.2. COMT Inhibitor Drugs

Drug	Tablet Size	Dose	Notable Side Effects
Entacapone (Comtan)	200 mg	One tablet with each dose of carbidopa/levodopa (but no more frequently than every 3 to 4 hours)	• Enhances levodopa side effects, especially dyskinesias • Occasional diarrhea
Entacapone plus carbidopa/ levodopa (Stalevo) Stalevo - 50 Stalevo - 100 Stalevo - 150	200 mg entacapone in each tablet plus: 50 mg levodopa* 100 mg levodopa* 150 mg levodopa*	Dosage varies depending upon the levodopa requirements	• Same as above
Tolcapone (Tasmar)	100 mg, 200 mg	One 100 mg tablet three times daily**	• Same as above, plus rare serious liver disease

*And proportionate amounts of carbidopa.

**The 200 mg tablet is usually not employed since this dose appears to have at least a slightly greater risk of liver problems and does not add much to the benefit.

produce no benefit when used alone, but enhance the levodopa effect. Their sole role is to supplement carbidopa/levodopa when there are fluctuations in the levodopa response. In other words, they help counter the levodopa short-duration response, which results in wearing off.

Two COMT inhibitor drugs are available, entacapone (Comtan) and tolcapone (Tasmar); their characteristics are outlined in table 18.2. The more potent of the two, tolcapone (Tasmar), is a last choice among all the supplemental drugs due to side effects. It has potential for serious and life-threatening liver toxicity. The other drug, entacapone, appears to have no significant potential for liver damage.

Entacapone is less effective than the dopamine agonist drugs but is much easier to use. There are no dose adjustments necessary; you start the same dose that you intend to maintain. Side effects also tend to be less with entacapone, with the most common being increased dyskinesias.

Recently a tablet that combines entacapone with carbidopa/levodopa was introduced and marketed under the brand name Stalevo. Its primary utility is convenience, supplying all three drugs (carbidopa, levodopa, and entacapone) in a single pill.

WHO IS A BAD CANDIDATE FOR A COMT INHIBITOR DRUG?

These drugs are notorious for enhancing levodopa-induced dyskinesias. If dyskinesias are a troublesome problem for you, they are probably not a good choice. Obviously you can always lower your carbidopa/levodopa doses to reduce dyskinesias; however, if they are a major problem in the first place, you won't accomplish much by adding a COMT inhibitor.

ENTACAPONE (COMTAN)

Entacapone prolongs the duration of levodopa in the bloodstream by virtue of COMT inhibition. It does this for about four hours after each dose. Usually, it is taken with each dose of carbidopa/levodopa, since the intent is to enhance the levodopa effect. However, if your carbidopa/levodopa doses are taken at very short intervals, you may not need to take entacapone with each carbidopa/levodopa dose. For example, those taking carbidopa/levodopa every two hours could take a dose of entacapone with every other carbidopa/levodopa dose.

Entacapone comes in only one size tablet, 200 mg. It is typically started in a dose of 1 tablet with each dose of carbidopa/levodopa, up to 8 tablets a day. Once started, you do not need to make any further adjustments of the entacapone dose.

The carbidopa/levodopa dose may need to be reduced since entacapone increases levodopa potency and dyskinesias may develop or exacerbate. If this happens, reduce each dose of carbidopa/levodopa (25-100) by 1/4 to 1/2 tablet decrements until the dyskinesias are controlled.

ENTACAPONE PLUS CARBIDOPA/LEVODOPA: STALEVO

Stalevo combines all three ingredients into one pill: carbidopa, levodopa, and entacapone. If entacapone therapy is chosen, my recommendation is to start with plain entacapone using the strategy described above. In other words, I would not start Stalevo in place of carbidopa/levodopa, even though Stalevo combines carbidopa/levodopa with entacapone. Why? Because levodopa adjustments may be necessary once entacapone is initiated. It's a lot simpler in the beginning to use separate pills. Thus simply add plain entacapone (Comtan) to your regimen; adjust the levodopa dosage as necessary and only then consider conversion to Stalevo.

Stalevo comes in three sizes, each containing 200 mg of entacapone:

- Stalevo 50 contains 12.5 mg carbidopa and 50 mg of levodopa

- Stalevo 100 contains 25 mg of carbidopa and 100 mg of levodopa

- Stalevo 150 contains 37.5 mg carbidopa and 150 mg levodopa

The cost per tablet is the same for each of these, despite different doses of carbidopa and levodopa.

Some combinations of entacapone and carbidopa/levodopa can easily be converted to Stalevo. For example, if you initially settled on 1 1/2 carbidopa/levodopa 25-100 tablets plus one 200 mg entacapone tablet four times daily, you could simply substitute one Stalevo 150 tablet for each of the four doses. Or, 200 mg entacapone plus two 25-100 carbidopa/levodopa tablets three times daily could be switched to two Stalevo 100 tablets three times daily.

ENTACAPONE SIDE EFFECTS

Entacapone's primary side effects occur by making carbidopa/levodopa more potent. Hence levodopa side effects may be provoked or enhanced (e.g., hallucinations, low blood pressure, nausea, as well as dyskinesias). Entacapone has two unique side effects, however. First, it may cause diarrhea in a small minority. Second, it discolors the urine, which is not of any concern.

HOW MUCH WILL ENTACAPONE HELP?

In my experience, this is a mildly effective drug. If there are major problems with off-states, the benefits may come up short. Adding entacapone to your carbidopa/levodopa regimen may allow you to extend the interval between your carbidopa/levodopa doses, but typically by no longer than 30–60 minutes.

The major advantage of entacapone over the dopamine agonists is ease of use and the immediate effect. No dosage escalation is necessary.

ENTACAPONE DIDN'T HELP; MAY I STOP IT?

Yes, you may. Tapering off is not necessary. If you stop it and deteriorate, you can always restart it.

TOLCAPONE (TASMAR)

Head-to-head trials comparing tolcapone to entacapone are lacking, but my experience suggests that tolcapone is a slightly more effective drug. Unfortunately, shortly after tolcapone was released for prescription use, three cases of fatal liver toxicity surfaced. Subsequently no additional fatal cases have been reported, perhaps due to stringent blood monitoring guidelines. However, this potential side effect has rendered tolcapone a third-line drug. Entacapone does not appear to share this liver toxicity.

Tolcapone comes in two sizes: 100 mg and 200 mg tablets. It is taken three times per day (it has a longer duration of action than entacapone). Because the 200 mg size may be more likely to cause liver problems, the 100 mg size is recommended. Thus the dose should be one 100 mg tablet three times daily.

HOW LONG SHOULD I TRY TOLCAPONE?

Give tolcapone about three weeks. If adding this to your carbidopa/levodopa seems to provide little benefit, then stop this drug.

BLOOD TEST MONITORING WHEN TAKING TOLCAPONE

Before starting tolcapone, your physician will need to perform two blood tests to assess your liver function: measurement of SGPT/ALT and SGOT/AST. If these are abnormal, then you should not be started on tolcapone (anyone with preexisting liver disease may be more likely to experience a serious liver problem with tolcapone). Once tolcapone is started, this blood testing should be repeated at the following intervals:

- Every two weeks for the first year
- Monthly for the next six months
- Every two months for the remainder of time you continue to take tolcapone

If these blood tests (SGPT/ALT and SGOT/AST) turn abnormal, then tolcapone should be stopped immediately. As with entacapone, it may be stopped abruptly.

OTHER TOLCAPONE SIDE EFFECTS

Apart from liver toxicity, it has the same side effect spectrum that we described above for entacapone. It is a little more likely to cause diarrhea, however. As with entacapone, if you have prominent problems with dyskinesias, don't start tolcapone.

WHAT SHOULD I EXPECT FROM TOLCAPONE?

This may improve wearing-off of the levodopa response to a moderate degree. Hence you may be able to increase the interval between your carbidopa/levodopa doses. However, this effect is not highly dramatic and you shouldn't anticipate being able to increase this interval by much more than an hour or two.

Treating Wearing-off with Selegiline (Eldepryl, Deprenyl)

Selegiline is the least effective of the drugs discussed in this chapter for treating short-duration levodopa responses (wearing-off). A number of years ago, there was a general belief that it slows the progression of PD, based upon indirect evidence. Studies failed to confirm this, however, as explained in chapter 9. Currently the primary indication for selegiline is to enhance the effect of carbidopa/levodopa. In addition, some physicians prescribe it as the first drug for PD, especially if the symptoms are mild and don't demand aggressive treatment. When taken in the absence of levodopa, it has very mild effects on the symptoms of PD. When added to levodopa therapy, it enhances the levodopa effect.

Selegiline inhibits one of the enzymes that break down dopamine, monoamine oxidase (MAO). There are two major forms of this enzyme and selegiline blocks one of these, the B form of MAO. This tends to raise brain dopamine levels. We considered this in more detail in chapter 10.

Selegiline is conventionally administered twice daily, with one 5 mg tablet taken in the morning and the second at midday (lunchtime). However, the blockade of MAO-B can be achieved with a single 5 mg dose. Hence many physicians prescribe one 5 mg tablet taken either at breakfast time or with the first morning dose of carbidopa/levodopa. In my own experience, the clinical effect is the same whether 1 or 2 tablets a day are prescribed.

The timing of the selegiline dose is not important except from the standpoint of side effects. It can cause insomnia since one of its byproducts is a weak form of amphetamine (a distant cousin of "speed"). This insomnia effect is typically brief, spanning just a few hours after a dose. Hence the reason for giving the single dose in the morning.

Selegiline has a long-lasting effect on brain MAO-B, persisting for weeks after it is stopped. This has several implications:

- If you decide to discontinue selegiline, you may stop it abruptly.
- If you stop it, there may be a decline in control of your PD symptoms that may not be appreciated for many days to weeks.

- You can be late with your dose or even occasionally skip a dose and you won't miss a beat.

To summarize, selegiline is easy to use and requires no dose adjustments. I prescribe it as a single 5 mg tablet taken in the morning. Either it helps or it doesn't. Any improvement should be apparent within a few weeks. No further adjustments need to be made.

SELEGILINE SIDE EFFECTS

Insomnia has already been noted, although this is usually not a problem if the single dose is taken in the morning. The other side effects relate to enhancing the levodopa effect. Hence such side effects as hallucinations, dyskinesias, nausea, or low blood pressure (orthostatic hypotension) could be provoked or increased by adding selegiline.

Hallucinations deserve special comment. I have seen occasional people who experienced hallucinations when they combined selegiline with carbidopa/levodopa but could tolerate carbidopa/levodopa alone. This can be a source of confusion if these two drugs are started around the same time; the blame may be inappropriately placed on carbidopa/levodopa. If you are experiencing hallucinations, don't start selegiline or if you are taking it, discontinue it.

Occasionally, people taking selegiline are told that they need a special diet. However, this is not necessary if they are taking selegiline as directed: 1–2 tablets daily. Special diets are necessary for the more potent MAO blocking drugs that inhibit both the A and B forms.

SELEGILINE CAVEATS

- Taking high doses of selegiline may not be safe, such as 4 tablets daily or more. In higher doses, it blocks MAO completely (i.e., both the A and B forms). This can result in serious elevations of blood pressure. If MAO is completely blocked, then the aforementioned special diet is critical to minimize risk.

- If taking selegiline, you should not be administered the narcotic drug, meperidine (Demerol). Rarely this combination can result in a serious reaction. This narcotic is sometimes used for severe pain, such as pain after surgery. If you are taking selegiline and surgery is being contemplated, advise your surgeon to avoid Demerol. Other narcotics are acceptable.

Many of the medications used to treat depression are also said to adversely interact with selegiline, including the commonly prescribed SSRI drugs (see chapter 22). However, these serious interactions are very rare, and, in practice, these drugs are often used concurrently without any problems.

Anticholinergic Drugs for Uncontrolled Tremor or Dystonia

Medications that block the brain chemical, acetylcholine, were used well before levodopa became available as treatment for PD. These are called anticholinergic drugs (anti = block; cholinergic = acetylcholine). These are only infrequently used today since they are not very effective and have a variety of side effects. Personally, I almost never prescribe these because the side effects usually offset the benefits. However, in rare patients they might have unique utility. They may be useful in two specific cases where other drugs prove insufficient: tremor and dystonia.

Parkinsonian tremor typically improves, and may even be abolished by, carbidopa/levodopa, dopamine agonists, and other medications that work through dopamine systems. Where they fail to control this sufficiently, an anticholinergic drug might be added.

Similarly, troublesome dystonia may be treated with this class of drug. Dystonia represents a muscle contraction state sometimes experienced as a cramp-like sensation or extreme muscle tightness. Often it affects the feet (in-turning of the foot), toes (curling or pointing up), calf or thigh (cramp-like sensation), or occasionally neck. Dystonia can usually be controlled with proper adjustment of carbidopa/levodopa and perhaps with addition of the other drugs we discussed earlier in this chapter. Where these fail, however, you could try an anticholinergic agent.

There are numerous drugs with anticholinergic properties. The two most frequently used in the treatment of PD are trihexyphenidyl (Artane) and benztropine (Cogentin). Other anticholinergic drugs include procyclidine (Kemadrin) and biperiden (Akineton); however, we will examine only trihexyphenidyl and benztropine.

These are the only medications considered in this chapter that are inexpensive. Trihexyphenidyl and benztropine each costs approximately $0.25 a tablet, and a month's supply will be a little over $20.

ANTICHOLINERGIC SIDE EFFECTS

The side effects from these drugs are not particularly dangerous; however, they may be aggravating. If you push the dosage high enough, most people will experience at least one, if not more, of these:

- Mild memory impairment or worsening of preexisting dementia
- Dry mouth
- Dry eyes
- Visual blurring
- Constipation

Table 18.3. Anticholinergic Drugs

Medication	Tablet Size	Starting Dose*	Typical Maintenance Dose*	Usual Maximum Dose*
Trihexyphenidyl (Artane)	2 mg, 5 mg	Half of the 2 mg tablet once daily, then 3 times daily	One 2 mg tablet three times daily	One 5 mg tablet three times daily
Benztropine (Cogentin)	0.5 mg, 1 mg, 2 mg	0.5 mg tablet once daily, then twice daily, then 3 times daily	One 1 mg tablet 3 times daily	One 2 mg tablet three times daily

*How high and how rapidly you raise the dose depends on side effects. Doses less than the typical maintenance amounts are sometimes employed with benefit.

- Reduced ability to urinate
- Reduced sweating (important if you work in the extreme heat; in that case reduced sweating may predispose to heat stroke)

If you have a propensity to hallucinations or delusions, these drugs may exacerbate that. They may also worsen glaucoma, primarily narrow angle glaucoma.

ANTICHOLINERGIC DRUG DOSING

Trihexyphenidyl and benztropine pill sizes and dosing strategies are shown in table 18.3. One usually starts with a low dose and observes for a few days. If that is tolerated, it can then be slowly raised every few days thereafter. With each of these drugs, a three times daily dosing scheme is usually employed, although twice daily dosing is also appropriate. The strategy is to slowly raise the dose until either the tremor or dystonia is improved, or side effects develop. The usual maximum doses are shown in table 18.3.

If you have been taking one of these drugs for more than a couple of weeks and decide to discontinue it, do this slowly; even if it hasn't been very beneficial, it should be tapered off, rather than stopped abruptly. If you have been taking one of these for no more than a few months, you should taper off over approximately two weeks. If you have been taking one of these for years, you should taper off even more slowly, perhaps reducing the dose gradually over several weeks.

HOW MANY OF THESE DRUGS MAY BE USED AT THE SAME TIME?

Often the supplemental drugs discussed in this chapter are used in combination. Hence it is not uncommon to see someone who is taking carbidopa/levodopa, a dopamine agonist, a COMT inhibitor, and perhaps even selegiline. This is acceptable, provided you tolerate such a combination. Two rules should generally be followed, however:

- Make only one medication change at a time and then let the dust settle.
- Optimize the dosage of your current medications before adding another. In other words, if you are taking carbidopa/levodopa and a dopamine agonist, adjust the doses of these two drugs as best you can before adding a third drug.

Adding a third or fourth drug may improve control of parkinsonism sufficiently to justify the expense and complexity. However, certain side effects may limit this in some cases. As we add more drugs, the likelihood of hallucinations or paranoia increases, especially among seniors. This is not a high likelihood if your mind is clear to begin with. However, if such problems develop, this is a signal to reduce your supplemental drugs, one by one. Adding medications may also increase dyskinesias. However, that often can be countered by simply reducing your doses of carbidopa/levodopa by 1/4 to 1/2 tablet decrements until these are better controlled.

Summary: My Approach When Fluctuations in the Levodopa Response Become Problematic

There are a variety of means to arrive at satisfactory control of parkinsonism. The approach that I take is based on what has seemed to work in the clinic. For those with short-duration levodopa responses and wearing-off problems, I address medication adjustments in the following order.

1. I initially optimize the dosage of levodopa, adjusting each dose so that the peak response is neither excessive (resulting in dyskinesias), nor insufficient (resulting in poor parkinsonism control). I then adjust the interval between doses to match the response duration; this may entail adding extra doses to provide continuous coverage.

2. Although one could switch to the sustained-release formulation of carbidopa/levodopa, I rarely do that in this circumstance. It only adds about an hour to the response and is less predictable. However, some physicians may consider this strategy. I often use a single dose of Sinemet CR at bedtime, however, when coverage is needed into the night (see chapter 20).

3. If optimizing levodopa is insufficient, I then add a dopamine agonist. My usual first choice is pramipexole, since it is a little simpler to use than ropinirole and with fewer troublesome side effects than pergolide (or bromocriptine). If someone is already on a dopamine agonist, I make sure the dosage is adequate. I usually don't add a dopamine agonist if someone is experiencing prominent thinking and memory problems, orthostatic hypotension, or prominent daytime sleepiness; I never start it in people with hallucinations or paranoia. Once the dopamine agonist dose has been raised to the therapeutic range, I then reduce the levodopa dose if dyskinesias become a problem.

4. If fluctuations are still a problem, I consider adding entacapone next. However, I don't do this if levodopa dyskinesias are a prominent problem. Occasionally I will add entacapone before starting a dopamine agonist if the wearing-off problems are mild and a quick fix seems most appropriate. Recall that no adjustment of entacapone is necessary (although you may need to reduce your carbidopa/levodopa dose if dyskinesias become a problem).

5. I could add selegiline at some point in the above sequence. Usually I don't do this, since the added benefit is rather modest. However, it

could be considered if the wearing-off problems are relatively mild. Certainly, an advantage of selegiline is simplicity. A single 5 mg tablet each morning is the starting and finishing dose; either it works or it doesn't. When people come to see me who are taking the conventional dosage of one 5 mg tablet twice daily, I usually lower the dose to a single tablet each morning, since 2 tablets does not seem to add any substantial benefit.

6. I rarely start an anticholinergic drug and if I do, it is in desperation to treat tremor or dystonia that has been hard to control.

In this setting I could add tolcapone, although I rarely do. I believe this drug is more effective than entacapone, but the potential for serious liver problems and the need to frequently check blood tests dissuades me from prescribing this drug. Or I could switch from one dopamine agonist to another. If high doses of one agonist are ineffective, trying another will not likely prove much more successful. Typically I try a second dopamine agonist only if the first was not tolerated due to side effects. Even then, I may not try a second if the side effect was common to all these drugs, such as hallucinations, paranoia, severe nausea or low blood pressure. However, if the side effect seemed unique to a particular agonist drug, I may then try another. For example, sleepiness is most common with pramipexole, perhaps less with ropinirole (although debatable) and least with pergolide or bromocriptine.

This sequence of medication adjustments is my approach to chronic treatment of fluctuations in the levodopa response—wearing-off. Bear in mind that other aspects of parkinsonism may respond to other medication strategies, as we discuss in subsequent chapters.

Apomorphine Rescue Therapy

The U.S. Food and Drug Administration recently approved injectable apomorphine for use as rescue therapy in PD. This is employed in the same type of situation we discussed in the previous chapter for liquid Sinemet. Specifically it is intended for people with rapidly occurring and severe levodopa off-states. It is for the person who suddenly experiences an off-state at the shopping mall, or on the golf course. Injected apomorphine can quickly recapture an on-state (in 10 minutes or less).

Apomorphine is a dopamine agonist and, therefore, mimics the effect of dopamine. It is a very potent agonist, more potent than any of the four dopamine agonists that are currently available. It is not a new drug and has been used outside the United States for treatment of PD for many years; thus there is widespread experience with apomorphine.

In initial PD treatment trials thirty years ago, apomorphine was administered in pill form. Although efficacious, kidney toxicity precluded developing this drug further as oral therapy. It was soon recognized, however, that administration by other routes, such as injection, carries no risk of kidney damage. Investigators outside the United States subsequently developed injectable forms of apomorphine with demonstrable safety and efficacy.

Apomorphine is an ideal drug for rescue therapy from levodopa off-states. It is rapidly effective when administered by injection under the skin (subcutaneous); it typically reaches full potency in less than ten minutes, allowing quick reversal of a levodopa off-state. Although the response is brief, lasting 60–90 minutes, the antiparkinsonian effect is pronounced, similar to levodopa.

Apomorphine side effects are much the same as the other dopamine agonist medications, including potential for nausea, dyskinesias, hallucinations, paranoia, and delusions. It can cause orthostatic hypotension (low standing blood pressure), and if this is a preexisting problem, apomorphine is best avoided. Irritation around the injection site can occur, but usually is not severe. The apomorphine solution contains sodium metabisulfite and should not be used by people with know sulfite sensitivity. Sudden sleepiness may occur with apomorphine administration; avoid driving when using apomorphine until you have taken it sufficiently often to be sure sedation will not occur.

INITIATING APOMORPHINE

For apomorphine to reverse your levodopa off-state, it must be administered in an appropriate dose. This varies from person to person. Determination of the correct dose is initially done in the clinic where your doctor or nurse can observe the responses. This includes not only monitoring your parkinsonism, but also assessing for side effects such as low blood pressure. During this evaluation in the clinic, the doctor or nurse also must instruct you in the administration of apomorphine.

Apomorphine is packaged in two types of containers: a 3.0 milliliter (mL) cartridge, and a 2.0 mL ampule. Your physician's prescription will indicate one or the other. The cartridge fits into an injector pen that is relatively easy to self-administer, provided you understand the dosing scheme. The injector pen may be reused but the needle must be changed after each injection. The 2.0 mL glass ampule is administered with an injection syringe that must be manually filled; for people unfamiliar with injections, this may be the less preferable choice.

Each milliliter contains 10 milligrams (mg) of apomorphine; hence the cartridge contains 30 mg of apomorphine and the ampule contains 20 mg. However, be aware that the dose you will be administering is conventionally given in milliliters (mL), not milligrams (mg); there is a tenfold difference in these numbering schemes, so do not mix this up. The injector pen has a dial that allows you to determine the dose.

Dose determinations in your physician's office start with you in an off-state. Then, if the administered apomorphine dose is sufficient, an on-state will be triggered in ten minutes or less. Your doctor or nurse will likely start with a 0.2 mL (2 mg) apomorphine dose. If you develop a good on-state, this is probably the correct dose. They will also observe the duration of the response, so that you will know how long this effect lasts (usually 60–90 minutes). If the initial 0.2 mL (2 mg) dose fails to produce a satisfactory on-state, a higher dose is tried, usually 0.3 mL or 0.4 mL (3–4 mg). You will need to allow a minimum of two hours to elapse before injecting again, however. If still an inadequate response, further trials are conducted up to a dose of 0.6 mL (6 mg). Thus the typical dosing range for apomorphine is 0.2 to 0.6 mL (2–6 mg). During each of the dosing assessments, the sitting and standing blood pressure should be checked.

Where do you inject the apomorphine? It is injected subcutaneously, which means under the skin. You can pick up a fold of skin and insert the needle into that fold. Usually it is injected into the thigh, upper arm, or stomach area. You should shift the injection sites each time; if you inject into the same region, it may become irritated. You must wipe clean the injection site with an alcohol swab before each injection, and use a new, sterile needle each time. Don't inject through your clothes since they are not sterile. Also, do not inject it by some other route, such as into a vein.

What if you're out in public wearing a suit or dress, and don't want to be conspicuous with the injection? The easiest strategy is to unbutton a couple of the lower buttons on your shirt or blouse, exposing a limited area of your abdomen for the injection. (Don't wear an undershirt.) If the weather is nice and you're wearing shorts, then injection into the thigh is an easy strategy.

Apomorphine may induce nausea. Consequently an antinausea drug is conventionally started as many as three days before the first apomorphine injection. Trimethobenzamide (Tigan) in a dose of 250 mg three times daily is recommended (outside the United States, the more potent antinausea drug domperidone is available). As we discussed in chapter 6, the other antinausea drugs worsen parkinsonism and should not be used (i.e., don't use metoclopramide/Reglan or prochlorperazine/Compazine). This begs the question, Do you need to stay on trimethobenzamide indefinitely? What if you plan to use apomorphine only occasionally? If you have tolerated apomorphine on numerous occasions without nausea, you might try omitting trimethobenzamide to see if you can get by without it. Do not use ondansetron as the antinausea drug since this combination may cause a severe drop in blood pressure; also avoid other drugs in the ondansetron class: dolasetron, granisetron, palonosetron, and alosetron.

Once you determine the ideal dose in your doctor's office, you can use this medication on your own. Use your regular pills (carbidopa/levodopa, etc.) to keep you in an on-state throughout the day as best you can. However, if you get stuck in an off-state, anticipate that within 10 minutes after the injection, you should be mobile again. Plan ahead, recognizing that the effect will wear off in 60–90 minutes. However, this gives you time for your pills to start working.

How often can you safely administer apomorphine injections? There are no recognized limits; however, there are some practical constraints. The brief response, skin irritation from too many injections, hassle factor, and the cost will limit how often you choose to use this medication.

OTHER ROUTES OF APOMORPHINE ADMINISTRATION

Apomorphine is also very effective as rescue therapy when administered by intranasal inhalation. However, it may cause nasal irritation and even ulcers of the lining of the nose in some people. Sublingual (under the tongue) and rectal administration of apomorphine are also feasible, although these routes are not as quick to kick in. Apomorphine by these other routes, including intranasal, is not approved by the United States Food and Drug Administration but may be available in the future.

Supplemental Drugs for Dyskinesias

Although we have already considered dyskinesias, let's be certain we understand this term. Dyskinesias are the involuntary movements that reflect an excessive response to levodopa. People affected by them look fidgety; they are always moving. They may look like they are dancing in place. These dyskinetic movements have no pattern or rhythm. They may affect only one part of the body, such as the head and neck or one arm. They may affect the entire body or only one side. Occasionally they only affect muscles of the face.

Dyskinesias are not tremor, which is a rhythmic, to-and fro-movement. Tremor may affect not only the hands but also the legs, giving the appearance of someone tapping out a beat or nervously moving a knee up and down while seated. PD tremor may also cause the chin or jaw to move up and down. These to-and-fro tremulous movements are signs of PD, not a side effect of levodopa.

Dyskinesias are not feelings of restlessness. A restless, nervous, or very anxious feeling that comes and goes typically represents parkinsonism, rather than a levodopa medication effect. People tend to feel restless during their levodopa off-states and this resolves during the on-state. Since dyskinesias occur during the on-state, people typically do not feel restless at that time.

The dyskinesias we are discussing also need to be distinguished from the simple dystonia that is a primary symptom of PD. Dystonia is a muscle contraction state—sustained tension in a leg or foot. It is an abnormal posture of some part of the body. This frequently occurs in untreated or undertreated PD. It often feels like a cramp. Common dystonias include toes curling or turning up, calf cramps, turning in of a foot; eye closure (blepharospasm). These are all primary symptoms of PD, rather than due to levodopa.

TREATMENT OF DYSKINESIAS

If adjustments of carbidopa/levodopa have failed to satisfactorily control dyskinesias, then we can consider supplemental medications. Bear in mind, however, that it is not imperative that we control these dyskinesias. If they don't bother you and don't get in the way, it is acceptable to do nothing further.

What additional drugs might we consider? There are several options:

- Dopamine agonists (which allow levodopa reduction)
- Amantadine (Symmetrel)
- Mirtazepine (Remeron)
- Propranolol (Inderal)

These medications may be helpful but rarely abolish dyskinesias. For those occasional people with extremely troublesome and uncontrollable dyskinesias, surgery, as discussed in chapter 33, may be a consideration.

DOPAMINE AGONISTS FOR DYSKINESIAS

We just discussed how a dopamine agonist may be added to help control fluctuations in the levodopa response (i.e., wearing-off; short-duration levodopa responses). When this is done, typically the carbidopa/levodopa dose ultimately is lowered. This combination of dopamine agonist plus lower doses of carbidopa/levodopa may also reduce dyskinesias. Hence you could employ the same dosing strategies described above. Although this makes good sense, in my experience, this often fails to optimally control dyskinesias. It may indeed reduce these, especially among those where the dyskinesias are not too troublesome. However, when dyskinesias are a major problem, this strategy typically comes up short.

Should a dopamine agonist be the first choice for dyskinesias that can't be controlled by levodopa adjustments?

- Yes, if fluctuations in the levodopa response are also a problem. You then are treating two problems by adding one new drug.

- No, if levodopa fluctuations don't demand treatment. In that case, I would try something simpler first—amantadine—as we will consider next.

- Possibly, if you are one of those rare people who find that even low doses of carbidopa/levodopa cause troublesome dyskinesias or dyskinesias develop during the time your levodopa is wearing off (i.e., biphasic dyskinesias). These unusual problems were examined above and in chapter 17.

AMANTADINE REDUCES DYSKINESIAS

Amantadine has been around for several decades, first introduced around the time levodopa initially became available. It was recognized to have a mildly beneficial effect on parkinsonian symptoms. Interestingly, it took about twenty years for physicians to recognize that it also tends to reduce levodopa dyskinesias. Currently that is its primary role in PD treatment.

Amantadine does many things in terms of brain chemistry, none very prominently. There has been much debate about which of these is responsible for the beneficial effect. Likely, this relates to blocking a brain neurotransmitter, glutamate. There has been emerging research indicating that drugs blocking glutamate neurotransmission tend to reduce levodopa dyskinesias. Unfortunately the most potent drugs in this category have too many side effects to allow these to be used. Amantadine has a mild glutamate blocking effect, which is enough to reduce dyskinesias but not so potent as to provoke troublesome side effects.

Amantadine Dosing

Amantadine comes in only one size: 100 mg tablets. You may take this with food or on an empty stomach. Amantadine is taken in addition to carbidopa/levodopa and other medications.

Start with one amantadine tablet in the morning and then after a week, raise the dose to 1 tablet twice daily. See how things go for a couple of weeks. If dyskinesias are still troublesome, raise the dose to 1 tablet three times daily. This is the typical dose. Give this a few weeks to work before raising the dosage any higher. Then, if dyskinesias are still problematic, increase the dose to 2 tablets twice daily. Ultimately you may go as high as 5 tablets a day. If you go that high, distribute these in three doses, two of which are 2 tablets and last dose, 1 tablet. Unless dyskinesias are a problem at night, take the last dose well before bedtime.

Amantadine Side Effects

In low doses, amantadine is typically well tolerated. A common side effect is redness or reddish purple discoloration of the legs, often with swelling. This is not worrisome and if it doesn't bother you, the dose does not need to be lowered.

Among those who are disposed, amantadine may provoke hallucinations, paranoia, or confusion. This is more likely to occur with the higher doses, beyond three tablets daily. This happens in only a small minority of people, but when it occurs, it usually signals the need to taper off the amantadine altogether.

OTHER DRUGS FOR DYSKINESIAS

Mirtazapine (Remeron) is a medication used to treat depression. Several years ago, one published report indicated that it had potential for reducing levodopa-induced dyskinesias. In my own experience, it reduces dyskinesias in only occasional patients and not dramatically. It may be worth trying but do not expect a dramatic benefit.

An appropriate starting dose of mirtazapine is 1/2 of a 30 mg tablet at bedtime. It may make you sleepy, even persisting into the next morning but your body may get used to this if not too troublesome. If you tolerate the 1/2 tablet dose, stick with this for a week or two and then raise the dose to a full 30 mg tablet at bedtime. Any reduction in dyskinesias should be apparent in a few weeks on that dose. It may be tapered off if not helpful.

Besides sedation, mirtazapine may also increase your appetite and result in weight gain. It may also lower your standing blood pressure (orthostatic hypotension). This may be a problem if you are already experiencing symptoms from orthostatic hypotension, as is common in PD.

Propranolol (Inderal) has been used for years as treatment for rapid heart beating, angina (heart pain) or high blood pressure. It has a variety of other uses, as well, including treatment of tremor, migraine headaches and stage fright. Several years ago, a single medical report indicated that it might be useful in treating levodopa dyskinesias. It has not gained wide acceptance for this purpose, probably because it is not very effective in that capacity. Propranolol is from a class of drugs called beta-blockers. These drugs block one of the two main effects of adrenalin-like substances (the "beta" but not the "alpha" effect). There are several medical conditions that preclude using beta-blockers:

1. Low blood pressure (orthostatic hypotension)

2. Asthma (works opposite to many asthma drugs)

3. Diabetes mellitus when low blood sugar reactions to insulin are common

4. Severe congestive heart failure

5. A very slow heart rate

Propranolol may also cause fatigue and exercise intolerance, or it may worsen depression.

Propranolol comes in both an immediate-release form and a sustained-release (LA or long-acting) form. For dyskinesias, the immediate-release form is used, with a typical dose from one to two of the 10 mg tablets three times daily. Start with one 10 mg tablet once a day and check your standing blood pressure; if the pressure remains consistently above 90, then you may increase to one 10 mg tablet three times daily. You may take this with food or on an empty stomach. See how this goes for a couple of weeks. If dyskinesias are still a problem, raise one of your three doses to two 10 mg tablets and again check the standing-up blood pressure. If it is still okay, then make all three doses two 10 mg tablets. Give this a couple of weeks to determine if propranolol is worth continuing. If not, taper off by dropping to one tablet three times daily for a week and then stopping it altogether.

We considered propranolol for treatment of refractory tremor in chapter 14. We used a different dosing strategy since tremor is typically treated with higher propranolol doses.

COST OF THESE SUPPLEMENTARY DRUGS FOR DYSKINESIAS

In contrast to other supplementary PD drugs, amantadine and propranolol are cheap, primarily because they have been around for years and are available as generics. At community pharmacy prices, amantadine costs about $0.70 a tablet or $63 monthly, if you take a tablet three times daily. A 10 mg propranolol tablet costs about $0.30 and a 20 mg tablet, $0.35. Mirtazepine (Remeron) is more expensive but is a little cheaper in generic form. A generic 30 mg tablet costs about $3.12 (month's supply, $94); brand-name Remeron runs $3.46 per tablet ($104 monthly).

◆ ◆ ◆

PART NINE

Other Treatment Problems: Not Just a Movement Disorder

19

♦ ♦ ♦

Subjective Symptoms That May Respond to Levodopa or Dopamine Agonists

We usually think of Parkinson's disease (PD) as a disorder of movement. The signs are apparent to family and friends, who see variable degrees of slowness, tremor, and gait difficulties. These movement problems primarily reflect brain dopamine deficiency, and they respond to medications that restore the effect of dopamine. However, the problems of PD are not confined to these *objective* movement manifestations. Many *subjective* symptoms are also a part of the PD experience, which are only apparent to the person with PD. Because these symptoms cannot be seen, they often go unrecognized as components of PD. They may be attributed to other conditions, and treatment may get

Table 19.1. Subjective Symptoms That May Respond to Levodopa or Dopamine Agonists*

• Anxiety	• Cramps
• Panic attacks	• Sciatica and other pain
• Restlessness (akathisia)	• Tingling (paresthesia)
• Inner tremor	• Increased urinary urgency
• Fatigue	• Hot flashes, sweating (diaphoresis)
• Shortness of breath (dyspnea)	• Poor concentration; slowed thinking (bradyphrenia)

*Sleep disorders, restless legs syndrome, and depression may also benefit from these PD drugs, but are discussed in subsequent chapters.

sidetracked. Like tremor, slowness, or walking problems, these subjective symptoms may also respond to levodopa or dopamine agonist medications. Pain, anxiety, and shortness of breath are examples, with the most common listed in table 19.1 (not an exhaustive list). These sometimes take center stage, with PD medications adjusted to treat these subjective symptoms. Levodopa or dopamine agonists do not adequately treat these problems in every case but may be very effective, suggesting that brain dopamine deficiency is responsible. In this chapter we focus on these symptoms, plus consider alternative causes that also need to be entertained.

How Can You Tell If These Subjective Symptoms Are Due to PD?

We shouldn't simply jump to the conclusion that each and every symptom listed in table 19.1 is always due to PD. For example, if you are short of breath, heart and lung problems should be excluded before considering PD as the cause. Similarly, sciatica is a common problem and may have nothing to do with PD. Thus clinical acumen is often necessary to sort this out. When PD is the cause, the response to levodopa (or a dopamine agonist) may be a clue, such as the following. (1) PD symptoms resolve with carbidopa/levodopa or dopamine agonist drug therapy, if the dosage is sufficient. (2) After PD has been present for a few years, the PD symptoms often come and go, time-locked to the levodopa response. PD symptoms resolve at the time of the peak levodopa effect (assuming the dose is adequate); this peak effect begins about one hour after a dose of immediate-release carbidopa/levodopa (or two hours after sustained-release carbidopa/levodopa). PD symptoms recur later, two to six hours after a dose of levodopa, when the levodopa effect has worn off.

Because carbidopa/levodopa is the most potent of the antiparkinsonian drugs, administration of this drug may be necessary to determine if the symptoms will be medication-responsive. The other antiparkinsonian medications may fail to completely alleviate symptoms, which ultimately respond to levodopa therapy.

On the other hand, what clues suggest these symptoms are not due to PD?

1. The symptoms have been lifelong, predating parkinsonism by years.

2. The symptoms fail to respond to aggressive carbidopa/levodopa therapy (as outlined in chapter 12).

3. There is some other obvious cause, such as low thyroid or anemia in the case of fatigue.

Sometimes it is initially unclear whether PD, and hence a brain dopamine deficiency state, is responsible for certain of the symptoms listed in table 19.1. In that case, your physician may then perform tests to exclude other treatable or worrisome causes and subsequently proceed with carbidopa/levodopa or dopamine agonist therapy. Let's now consider each of these symptoms, since these are fairly common and may affect you either now or later.

Anxiety, Panic Attacks, and Akathisia

ANXIETY IS A COMMON SYMPTOM OF PD

Anxiety implies nervousness, apprehension, or worry. In the mildest form, it may simply represent an uneasy feeling that something will go wrong. In its most severe form, it is experienced as a panic state without insight or objectivity. Sometimes anxiety is appropriate, such as the nervousness that precedes a college examination or starting work in a new job. However, it becomes problematic when it is out of proportion to life's events or develops in the absence of any inciting factors.

Among those with PD, the origin may go unrecognized, with bewilderment why this nervousness should have developed without good reason. It later may become apparent when these symptoms resolve with levodopa or dopamine agonist therapy.

Anxiety may be one of the first symptoms of PD, preceding the tremor, gait, and movement problems by many years. Among people of Olmsted County, Minnesota, those with PD were significantly more likely to have experienced anxiety states early in life, compared to the general population. These anxiety problems were documented well before the onset of parkinsonism, suggesting that these may have been among the earliest PD symptoms. Obviously anxiousness is common in general, and most people who are anxious worriers will not ultimately develop PD.

AKATHISIA

Akathisia implies an inner restlessness or an inability to sit still or get comfortable. It is experienced as an antsy feeling, causing you to feel like you might jump out of your skin. Occasionally it is confused with anxiety and sometimes they occur together. Akathisia is among the more common subjective symptoms of PD and responds to levodopa and often dopamine agonist therapy.

Some people with PD also experience an inner tremor that cannot be seen. It is debatable whether this is a variant of akathisia or actually a low-grade, imperceptible tremor.

PANIC

Panic is anxiety taken to its highest level. Panic states are uncommon among those with PD, but in rare cases may be the most troublesome symptom. When it occurs, it typically is experienced in discreet episodes. Most often, panic will occur as a manifestation of a levodopa off-state. In other words, it represents loss of the levodopa effect, when the response has worn off. When this occurs, the relationship to levodopa often goes unrecognized. For those with PD and panic, the physician's antianxiety drugs may not be nearly as effective as carbidopa/levodopa.

Panic attacks also occur in those who do not have PD. In that setting, the drugs for PD are ineffective. Thus not all panic attacks are due to PD.

TREATMENT OF ANXIETY AND PANIC ATTACKS

Minor anxiety due to PD, as well as akathisia, typically resolve as the movement symptoms are effectively treated with levodopa, a dopamine agonist, or both. Hence they usually need no additional treatment. For most people with PD, these symptoms never become substantial issues as long as they maintain their antiparkinsonian medications.

Severe anxiety and frank panic attacks from PD are uncommon. When these occur, they typically develop later in the course of PD, rather than as an early symptom; most often, these develop in one of two situations: (1) in a generally underdosed parkinsonian state (too little or no levodopa) and (2) as a manifestation of a levodopa off-state. Frequently the relationship to PD and levodopa is unrecognized.

Let's address the strategies for treating this problem, recognizing that PD drugs are often the crucial therapy. I don't jump to the conclusion that PD is responsible in every case; appropriate questions need to be asked.

Have You Been Anxious All Your Life?

Is this a lifelong problem? If the answer is yes, treatment will likely need to include psychiatric medications. Although optimal doses of PD drugs may prove helpful, these alone will be inadequate in these cases. In these situations, a psychiatrist should advise. Chronic, long-standing anxiety is often a complex problem with depression sometimes contributing (depression tends to make people worry and ruminate). A psychiatrist should be able to sort this out and choose the appropriate medications.

Even in the case of lifelong anxiety that predates PD, I find that optimal adjustment of the PD medications facilitates the response to the psychiatric drugs. It is hard to treat anxiety effectively if parkinsonism is poorly controlled.

Is Your Parkinsonism Controlled?

Symptoms and signs tell us if we are adequately controlling parkinsonism. I inquire and look for the following:

- Tremor (tremor at rest)
- Shuffling gait or other major walking problems

- Prominent slowness (bradykinesia)

- Markedly reduced facial animation (limited facial expression)

These are markers of brain dopamine status in PD. If these and related signs are present, we may not have adequately replenished brain dopamine. Thus, this brain dopamine deficiency could also underlie the anxiety state.

I also consider the medications and doses, and especially whether carbidopa/levodopa is maxed out. Is there room to escalate? Recall from chapter 12 that when starting immediate-release carbidopa/levodopa, we allowed for dosage escalation up to two-and-a-half 25-100 tablets, three times daily on an empty stomach. Doses that are substantially less than 2 1/2 tablets, or if taken with meals, leave us room to treat more aggressively. This focus on the motor signs of PD are relevant because *PD-related anxiety responds to PD medications in parallel to tremor, gait, and slowness.* If parkinsonism is poorly controlled, we can simply treat as we would otherwise and anticipate that the anxiety may fall into place. If the parkinsonism is well-controlled and the medications maxed out, we turn to the psychiatrists, who have different medication options.

Do Your Parkinsonism and Anxiety Fluctuate?

Is there a short-duration pattern, as described in chapter 17? Clues suggesting that anxiety is part of this pattern include the following:

- The anxiety states come and go. (This should lead the physician to inquire whether they have a relationship to the times of the levodopa doses.)

- A dose of carbidopa/levodopa is followed by resolution of the anxiety state.

- Anxiety is minimal when the levodopa effect is most prominent (i.e., during the on-state).

- The anxiety state tends to occur during times when no levodopa doses have been administered, such as in the middle of the night.

- Anxiety tends to occur around the time that the next dose of carbidopa/levodopa is due (i.e., at the time of wearing-off).

This fluctuating pattern suggests that the anxiety is occurring when the levodopa effect has worn off. Just as tremor and stiffness may recur several hours after a dose of carbidopa/levodopa, so may anxiety. Fluctuating anxiety can be treated the same as fluctuating movement problems.

DOPAMINE AGONISTS AND PD-RELATED ANXIETY

Dopamine agonists (pramipexole, ropinirole, pergolide, and bromocriptine) improve parkinsonism and may therefore treat PD-related anxiety. However, these drugs are not as potent or as fast working as carbidopa/levodopa. The dosage adjustments take many weeks to accomplish (see chapter 13). Hence, if anxiety is a major issue, optimization of the carbidopa/levodopa doses is the appropriate first step. The dopamine agonists, however, are good choices for smoothing out fluctuations in the levodopa response. Thus as supplemental therapy, they may effectively reduce fluctuating anxiety, just as they help control fluctuating parkinsonism in general (see chapter 18).

OTHER DRUGS FOR ANXIETY

Levodopa and related drugs may not adequately treat all anxiety states encountered in PD. Brain dopamine deficiency may not be responsible for each and every case of anxiety. Antianxiety drugs may then have a role and the more commonly prescribed medications from this class are listed in the table 19.2. Although they do have a calming effect, they also have a downside, especially as it relates to long-term treatment.

- These drugs work best when initially prescribed, but are not as effective in reducing anxiety after weeks to months of treatment.

- They cause sleepiness, clumsiness, and dulled thinking (a little like drinking a couple of martinis).

- They may be habit forming.

On the other hand, these drugs tend to relax people who are driving themselves crazy with worrying and nervousness.

For people with PD, I tend to avoid these drugs, although I do prescribe them when acute anxiety needs more immediate treatment. If I start one of these medications, it is with anticipation that they may be tapered off in the future. When long term use seems necessary, I ask one of my psychiatry colleagues to advise.

Almost all of the conventional antianxiety drugs are compatible with PD treatment. However, most of the major tranquilizers (neuroleptics) should not be prescribed since they may worsen parkinsonism (listed in chapter 6).

Buspirone (Buspar) is a unique antianxiety drug that differs in its mechanism of action from the other medications listed in table 19.2. Buspirone interacts with brain dopamine receptors and, for that reason, I have generally avoided it, to make certain that the effects of levodopa and dopamine agonists are not inhibited. It probably does not have any major potential to block dopamine receptors, but when there is even the small chance, I prefer to avoid this.

Table 19.2. Some Commonly Prescribed Antianxiety Medications

Generic Name	Brand Name
Diazepam	Valium
Chlordiazepoxide	Librium
Alprazolam	Xanax
Clorazepate	Tranxene
Lorazepam	Ativan
Clonazepam	Klonopin

ANTIDEPRESSANT MEDICATIONS FOR ANXIETY STATES

Depression is a distinctly different symptom than anxiety. People who are depressed feel sad, blue, unsatisfied, or unable to see the bright side of their lives. However, the same medications used to treat depression sometimes have a role in treatment of anxiety. There are two reasons. First, anxiety often accompanies depression. Second, depression makes people worriers; they tend to see the dark side of things and focus on that. They tend to ruminate about little things and this makes them anxious. What if I fail? What if the stock market goes down? What if I can't make any friends in this new community? Antidepressant medications may have a place in the treatment of people who are anxious or depressed worriers. The SSRI drugs for depression (discussed in chapter 22) are often used in this setting and are effective.

DON'T MISTAKE DYSKINESIAS FOR A SIGN OF ANXIETY

You will recall that dyskinesias are involuntary movements sometimes provoked by levodopa treatment. These are the dancing, fidgety movements that occur when the levodopa effect is too prominent. These may convey the appearance of nervousness, but just the opposite is true. People with PD and anxiety will be the least nervous when their PD medications are working; obviously, their PD drugs are working maximally when dyskinesias are present. Don't confuse dyskinesias with anxiety or your treatment could make these worse.

Fatigue and Shortness of Breath

FATIGUE

Fatigue is a common experience among those with PD. Fatigue implies poor energy and tiredness; however, it must be distinguished from sleepiness, which is not the same as fatigue. It may be a direct consequence of PD and therefore improve with levodopa and related medications. However, fatigue is a common symptom that may be provoked by a variety of factors. Thus other treatable conditions should also be considered if fatigue is a prominent complaint.

1. Other medical problems. A general medical examination and routine blood tests may be appropriate to exclude other disorders. Appropriate blood tests include a complete blood count, thyroid and chemistry panel, plus whatever other studies seem warranted by the medical history.

2. Medications. Some drugs cause fatigue, such as:

   Sleep medications, primarily those that are long-acting like clonazepam

   Certain antihypertensive drugs, such as the beta-blockers (e.g., propranolol)

   Some allergy medications, most notably diphenhydramine (Benadryl)

Many of the medications for psychiatric symptoms, especially medications for "nerves" (anxiety), as well as some of the older antidepressant medications (e.g., amitriptyline)

Seizure medications

Muscle relaxants or drugs for spasms (such as cyclobenzaprine, baclofen, or tizanidine)

3. Low blood pressure (orthostatic hypotension). People with PD are predisposed to orthostatic hypotension and this is exacerbated by the medications used to treat PD, as already noted. Although lightheadedness and faintness are typical symptoms of orthostatic hypotension, general fatigue may also be a consequence. This is diagnosed by blood pressure readings taken during times of fatigue. If the systolic blood pressure is less than 90, this could be your problem. Remember to check it when standing, since it may be normal when seated. See chapter 21 for more details.

4. Poor sleep at night. Poor energy during the day may be a consequence of inadequate sleep at night. There are various reasons the person with PD may experience poor nighttime sleep. Contributing factors include inadequately controlled parkinsonism at night, periodic leg movements of sleep (which partially arouse, preventing deep sleep), or sleep apnea (impaired breathing during sleep, often with the clinical clue of loud snoring). These conditions and their treatment are discussed in chapter 20.

5. Depression. Lack of energy and interest are common depressive symptoms. Depression is common in PD and often requires medical treatment, which is addressed in chapter 22.

6. Deconditioning. Lack of exercise may also contribute to fatigue, although it is unlikely to be the primary cause. It may initially seem that your fatigue makes it too difficult to be physically active. However, if you can get over the hump, you may find that with a good exercise program, your energy level increases.

When these causes have been treated or excluded, we are left with PD as the probable cause of fatigue. PD-related fatigue typically improves, but rarely resolves with PD medications. Those who were energetic prior to PD may find that their high energy levels never return, despite otherwise optimum treatment. They may no longer be able to burn the candle at both ends. However, this is not to say that they cannot continue to have productive careers and hobbies; they simply must pace themselves appropriately.

SHORTNESS OF BREATH

The medical term for shortness of breath is "dyspnea." It is occasionally experienced as a symptom of PD and may dramatically respond to levodopa and related medications. Obviously lung conditions (such as pneumonia or asthma) or heart failure may cause dyspnea. Additionally, a variety of advanced medical conditions, such as liver or kidney failure, may cause shortness of breath. When physicians hear the complaint of dyspnea, they appropriately think first about lung, heart, or other serious medical conditions. The physician should consider such serious causes before jumping to the conclusion that PD is responsible for the shortness of breath. However, if these have been excluded, then PD should be considered.

Q: Does PD affect the lungs?

A: Lung damage does not occur in PD. On microscopic examination of the lungs, the appearance is normal for age. The same is true for the heart; PD results in no damage to heart muscle and does not cause the heart to fail.

Q: If my lungs and heart are okay, why should PD cause dyspnea?

A: Consider what happens when we breathe. We repetitively contract and then relax our breathing muscles. Back and forth, the muscles of the diaphragm and rib cage contract to expel air and then relax to expand the lung cavity. (The diaphragm is the large breathing muscle underneath the lungs.) These repetitive movements by the breathing muscles move air in and out of the lungs, and PD occasionally affects these unconscious repetitive breathing movements.

Let's digress for a minute to think about what happens to any repetitive movement when you have PD. You have probably already noticed that repetitive movements of your hands don't flow normally. The back-and-forth movements of handwriting or brushing teeth are slowed and the excursions are reduced. This is typical of PD; repetitive movements of any part of the body may be similarly slowed and dampened in amplitude. Doctors test for this as part of the routine PD exam, termed "alternate motion rate" or "repetitive alternating movement"; your doctor observes as you rapidly and repetitively tap your thumb and index finger. How does PD affect these movements? Typically the amplitude of these finger-thumb excursions dampens and the speed diminishes.

Now apply what I just explained to the repetitive movements of your breathing muscles. Just like handwriting, the repetitive breathing movements may have a tendency to diminish—the amplitude of the excursions dampens. The reduced contractions of the breathing muscles result in less airflow into and out of the lungs; dyspnea is consequently experienced. Is this common among those with PD? No, but when it develops, it is important to keep this in mind so that it can be appropriately diagnosed and treated.

Q: Is PD dyspnea dangerous?

A: No. There is no threat to life or any risk to your heart or lungs. However, it is uncomfortable and may compromise your activities. For that reason, it is important to recognize and treat.

Q: How can I tell if my dyspnea is from PD?

A: Sometimes it is difficult to be certain whether shortness of breath is linked to PD or has some other cause. Generally, it is wise to err on the side of caution and investigate heart and lung function, even if clues suggest that PD is the cause. Having stated that, let's go ahead and consider the clues that point toward PD as the cause of dyspnea.

CLUES THAT DYSPNEA MAY BE DUE TO PD

Shortness of breath could have a variety of other causes, some serious. The serious causes should always be considered and an appropriate workup performed. If this evaluation is negative, then we focus on PD as possibly responsible. The first question to ask is: Does the dyspnea come and go? If the answer is yes, dyspnea may be occurring as a levodopa off-state symptom. Thinking about this in more detail, consider the following.

- Is the dyspnea primarily experienced when tremor, gait freezing, slowness, and stiffness are prominent (levodopa off-state)?

- Is the dyspnea absent when tremor and slowness are gone (levodopa-on-state)?

- Is the dyspnea gone during times of levodopa dyskinesias? Dyskinesias are a marker of levodopa on-states.

- Does the dyspnea tend to occur during times of uncomfortable dystonia, such as accompanying foot, calf, or toe cramps? Painful dystonias are generally signs of a levodopa off-state.

If the dyspnea is linked to levodopa off-states, then the treatment is obvious. We simply employ the strategies described in previous chapters for treating levodopa wearing-off problems. If the dyspnea resolves as we treat the off-states, this confirms that we are on the right track.

Not everyone with PD-related dyspnea experiences this as a levodopa off-state phenomenon. If your parkinsonism is inadequately treated in general (underdosed), you may not experience response variability (fluctuations); you may simply be slow and stiff all the time. Correspondingly, just as you are continuously slow and tremulous, you will also be persistently short of breath. With a more aggressive treatment strategy to improve control of your parkinsonism, not only should tremor and slowness improve but also dyspnea (if it is due to PD). If the dyspnea improves in parallel with your parkinsonian symptoms, this confirms parkinsonism was likely the cause.

ASIDE: DOPAMINE AGONIST DRUGS AS A CAUSE OF DYSPNEA

Two of the available dopamine agonist medications, bromocriptine (Parlodel) and pergolide (Permax), may cause an inflammatory reaction of the lungs or heart. Anyone taking either of these medications should have this suspected first and foremost if dyspnea develops. These are serious reactions and, if confirmed, require discontinuation of these drugs. We considered this in chapter 13. A drug available in Europe, cabergoline, is from the same ergot drug class and may also cause these same heart and lung reactions. The other two available dopamine agonist medications, pramipexole (Mirapex) and ropinirole (Requip), appear to have no risk for these problems.

ASSESSMENT OF DYSPNEA

Identifying a cause for shortness of breath is bread-and-butter medicine and your physician will know the appropriate tests to order. The evaluation typically starts with a general medical history and examination, including listening to your heart and lungs. Tests may include a chest X ray, electrocardiogram, breathing tests (pulmonary function tests), and routine blood tests (complete blood counts and a chemistry profile). An echocardiogram may also be performed (which evaluates the function of the heart muscle and valves). When someone is short of breath, this evaluation is typically appropriate. If all is negative, then the focus can be on parkinsonism.

Cramps, Sciatica, Pain, and Tingling

Pain and a variety of abnormal sensations may be due to PD. Sometimes this is associated with tense muscles or cramps. Obviously pain is a universal human experience and most pain is not caused by PD. As we already saw, if the pain abates when your levodopa kicks in, then PD may well be the cause. If your pain comes and goes, pay close attention to whether it cycles with your levodopa effect.

CRAMPS

Almost everyone has experienced cramps. These are severe muscle spasm states, often provoked in tired muscles after extreme exercise. Cramps are common in PD relating to the brain dopamine deficiency state. Most commonly, it affects toes and calves; often the toes curl under or turn up. The calf may go into a spasm. Unlike common cramps, these are not linked to exercise but occur spontaneously. Like typical cramps, they are often painful.

Cramps occurring among those with PD may represent a form of dystonia. Dystonia is an abnormal muscle contraction state triggered in the brain.

TREATMENT OF CRAMPS

In the general population, quinine is typically prescribed for cramps. Similarly, cramps after exercise are often treated with fluid intake and sodium/potassium/glucose supplements, contained in some sport drinks. However, these may not be effective if your cramps are due to PD. Among people with PD, cramps are typically due to a deficiency of brain dopamine and usually respond best to levodopa and related medications. Cramps may signal a levodopa off-state occurring (1) in the middle of the night or the early morning, when no

PD medications have been taken for many hours, and (2) close to the time for the next levodopa dose, at the time it is wearing off. Some people recognize cramps as a signal to take their next dose of levodopa (especially toe or foot cramps). Cramps in the middle of the night that awaken you from sleep may respond to a dose of controlled-release carbidopa/levodopa at bedtime, as explained in more detail in chapter 20.

SCIATICA

Sciatica, experienced as pain down a leg, may be due to a lumbar disc irritating a nerve in your back. However, a similar pain may also be caused by the brain dopamine deficiency state of PD. If this is the cause, it should resolve with adequate dopamine replacement therapy.

UNDERTREATED PD AND NON-PD PAIN

Non-PD pain is worse when PD is undertreated. People with PD experience the same pains as everyone else. Injuries, arthritis, inflammations are all sources of pain that may be superimposed on PD. People with PD have provided me with interesting and important insight into their pain experiences. *Pain from any source is worse during levodopa off-states or when PD is inadequately treated.* Thus, if someone with PD fractures a leg, the resulting pain will be magnified if PD drugs are withheld. If his general levodopa response fluctuates, his pain will cycle with the levodopa effect. Hence controlling parkinsonism may also help control pain due to other causes.

Surgery is associated with incision pain. Hence potent pain medications are typically administered after any surgery. This is not the time to stop your PD medications; carbidopa/levodopa and related drugs that maintain your on-state will help you tolerate the surgical pain.

TINGLING (PARESTHESIA)

A pins-and-needles sensation, numbness, or tingling is sometimes a symptom of PD, most often in an arm or a leg. This could also be a symptom of one of a variety of other neurologic conditions. However, if it began around the time that parkinsonism first developed, or if this fluctuates with the levodopa response, it may well be a parkinsonian symptom. Usually it resolves or improves with medical treatment of parkinsonism.

Other Symptoms That May Relate to PD

EXACERBATION OF URINARY URGENCY

Urinary symptoms are common among those with PD and relate to problems with nervous system control of the bladder (so-called neurogenic bladder); this is discussed in chapter 27. These symptoms of a neurogenic bladder do not respond to levodopa therapy. However, an occasional person with PD will experience troublesome increases in urinary frequency and urgency during levodopa off-states. These exacerbations of urinary symptoms can be controlled with improved levodopa coverage.

HOT FLASHES, SWEATING (DIAPHORESIS)

Hot flashes or hot flushes are common among women, in general, who experience these symptoms after menopause. In that setting, estrogen therapy is very effective. Men and women with PD may experience a similar phenomenon, but which has nothing to do with estrogen, and does not respond to estrogen supplementation.

Occasionally in PD, a sense of heat or flushing may signal wearing-off of the levodopa response. In other words, those with short-duration levodopa responses may experience this several hours after the last dose, as control of parkinsonism is starting to decline. Sometimes this is associated with profuse sweating (diaphoresis). Occasionally pronounced sweating may occur during nighttime sleep, sufficient to soak the bedclothes, as a consequence of sleeping beyond the time of the next scheduled levodopa dose. Typically these flushing or sweating episodes do not persist with the off-states, but develop during the transition.

Minimizing levodopa off-states effectively treats episodes of profuse sweating. Nighttime diaphoresis is usually the most troublesome, and strategies for improving nighttime levodopa coverage may be effective; these are explained in the next chapter. Nighttime diaphoresis has also been treated with medications already mentioned. This includes propranolol (20–40 mg at bedtime) or anticholinergic drugs such as trihexyphenidyl (2 mg at bedtime). These may not prove highly effective but in some cases may be worth trying.

SLUGGISH THINKING

Impaired concentration and slowed thinking are common experiences in PD. Physicians call this bradyphrenia. The slowed thinking of PD improves with optimum medical treatment of PD. More profound cognitive problems may also develop that do not respond to levodopa or other PD medications and this is addressed in chapter 23.

A variety of other subjective symptoms may also occur as part of the parkinsonian process. If the symptoms abate when the levodopa effect kicks in, parkinsonism is likely responsible.

20

◆ ◆ ◆

Sleep Problems: Insomnia, Daytime Sleepiness, and Disruptions During the Night

How we sleep affects our waking hours. Poor sleep translates into poor day-time performance. For those with PD, sleep is frequently disordered and this affects the waking day, including control of parkinsonism.

Insomnia

Insomnia is a common problem in the general population and increases with aging. When we are young, we typically have no trouble getting adequate sleep. Teenagers left undisturbed on a Saturday morning will sleep till noon. As we age, getting to sleep or staying asleep often becomes increasingly diffi-cult. Sometimes this relates to life stressors; lying in bed ruminating about the day's events is a frequent cause of insomnia. Depression is a common human affliction and insomnia may be one symptom. Finally, some people simply have insomnia as part of their constitutional makeup.

Insomnia, however, is especially frequent and troublesome among people with PD. They have trouble getting to sleep and, once they do, may awaken after a few hours and experience another cycle of sleeplessness. Consequently many with PD are chronically sleep deprived and, hence, sleepy during the daytime.

A variety of factors may contribute to insomnia among those with PD and these are summarized in table 20.1. By far, the most common and significant reason for insomnia, however, is the parkinsonism itself. Since this is highly treatable with our PD medications, we will focus first on this.

Table 20.1. Common Causes of Insomnia in PD

Cause	Comments
Primary insomnia	Predates onset of parkinsonism and is an unrelated problem
Insomnia due to PD	Typically relates to insufficient treatment of parkinsonian symptoms at bedtime and during the night
Urge to urinate	Common among seniors, who awaken to urinate and have trouble returning to sleep
Depression	Improves with treatment of the depression
Medications	Selegiline (Deprenyl, Eldepryl) and certain antidepressants may cause insomnia if taken in the evening

Insomnia Due to PD

People with PD often have problems getting a good night's sleep because the dopamine-deficient state of PD makes it impossible to get comfortable and relax. The stiffness and muscle tension (rigidity) of parkinsonism are not compatible with a sleep-inducing state. For those with rest tremor, the repetitive shaking may prevent sleep, just as noisy neighbors in the next apartment might keep you awake. Parkinsonism may also limit your movement in bed. We normally toss and turn throughout the night to optimally position our body for comfort. The reduced mobility of parkinsonism may inhibit these normal nocturnal movements, leaving you stuck in the bedcovers. Perhaps the most important factor, however, is the akathisia of PD. Akathisia is experienced as an inner restlessness, an inability to feel relaxed, a sense of nondescript discomfort when sitting or lying still. Very few with PD volunteer such a complaint to their physician, but they recognize akathisia if asked.

Akathisia, rigidity, tremor, and immobility in bed are all treatable symptoms. Hence insomnia linked to PD is treated with the same general strategies used for daytime movement problems. The most effective drug remains carbidopa/levodopa, the same medication used for slowness, gait problems, and tremor experienced during the waking day. Does insomnia experienced by those with PD always respond to levodopa therapy? It will if parkinsonism is the cause of your insomnia. Obviously a variety of other factors may also contribute, as listed in table 20.1.

Ideally, the medication chosen to treat nighttime akathisia, rigidity, and tremor would be long lasting, with an effective single dose taken before bedtime. However, many with PD experience only a shorter response to levodopa therapy and more than a single bedtime dose is often required. Although the dopamine agonist drugs (pramipexole, ropinirole, pergolide, and bromocriptine) have longer durations, they often are not sufficiently potent by themselves to cover the nighttime needs. This does not mean they cannot be tried. However, the drug of choice for this problem is typically carbidopa/levodopa.

How you take carbidopa/levodopa to treat insomnia depends on whether you are having trouble getting to sleep, staying asleep, or both. A useful treatment strategy is to consider sleep in three stages:

- *Falling asleep*. Do you fall asleep within about 30 minutes of going to bed?

- *Early part of the night*. Do you awaken after 1–3 hours, unable to return to sleep?

- *Last part of the night*. Are you awake at 4:00 or 5:00 A.M., unable to sleep?

We will address each part of the sleep cycle and how to treat.

WHY CAN'T I GET TO SLEEP?

You go to bed at your usual time and can't fall asleep. Even when you do, you sleep lightly. This never happened before you developed PD. What is going on? For those with PD, this is typically due to the brain dopamine deficiency state. When did you take your last dose of carbidopa/levodopa (or dopamine agonist)? Often the last dose was around suppertime; now, five or six hours later, you can't get to sleep. A long interval since your last medication dose may be the problem. If you have a short-duration levodopa response, your medication effect probably wore off before bedtime.

The solution should be obvious. You need another medication dose a little before bedtime. Will adding a bedtime dose be too much? Should I reduce one of my daytime medication doses? In this situation, there is no concern about overdosing. Exactly how you reorganize your medication schedule is a bit arbitrary, but this is how I would do it.

- If you are taking only a dopamine agonist drug with each meal and your daytime parkinsonism is well controlled, you have two options. First, you can simply take your third agonist dose a little before bedtime instead of at suppertime. The alternative is to add a fourth dose before bedtime. If you still can't get to sleep, you may need to either raise the agonist dose (chapter 13) or add carbidopa/levodopa, including a bedtime dose (chapter 12).

- If a dopamine agonist is your only medication and is not controlling your daytime parkinsonism, you may need to add carbidopa/levodopa, including a bedtime dose (assuming that the dopamine agonist drug has been raised to the target doses, as described in chapter 13).

- If you are taking carbidopa/levodopa one hour before each of three meals, you could add a fourth dose at bedtime, using the same amount you take during the daytime. Alternatively, you could simply move your third carbidopa/levodopa dose to bedtime, instead of before supper; however, if you have a short-duration levodopa response, this will cause an evening off-state because of the long duration since the noontime dose.

- If you have had PD for a number of years and have a short-duration carbidopa/levodopa response, add another dose about an hour before bedtime.

One common mistake is to take a lower dose of carbidopa/levodopa (or dopamine agonist) at bedtime. People sometimes assume that since they are asleep, they don't need as much medication. Although this makes sense, it doesn't work that way. Whatever dose you take during the day to control your parkinsonism is the same dose you should take at bedtime or during the night.

I WAKE UP AFTER A COUPLE OF HOURS AND CAN'T GET BACK TO SLEEP.

For those with a short-duration levodopa response, the last evening dose may wear off *after* going to sleep. This is common in PD, with awaking at 1:00 or 2:00 A.M., unable to return to sleep.

For this problem, the sustained-release formulation of levodopa is helpful. The sustained-release drug, Sinemet CR (CR = controlled-release), is slow to kick in, often requiring two hours. During the daytime, this slow release is less than ideal; a quick response is preferable during an active day. This slow kick-in, however, is helpful if you awaken after one to three hours, unable to return to sleep. If properly timed, the delayed effect from sustained-release levodopa will just start to kick in as the benefit from the last evening dose is declining.

In this situation, Sinemet CR, or its generic equivalent, should be taken just as your head is hitting the pillow. Remember that this is not being used to get you to sleep; you will need to have taken an evening carbidopa/levodopa dose for that purpose. That evening carbidopa/levodopa dose (taken an hour or more before bedtime) is to induce a comfortable state so that you can initially fall asleep. Then take the sustained-release carbidopa/levodopa right at bedtime for its delayed effect, which will help you stay asleep; it will kick in while you are sleeping. As long as you separate these doses by at least an hour, the overlapping effects shouldn't be a problem. Let's consider a couple of typical situations.

Mrs. Smith was having no problems during the day taking 2 immediate-release carbidopa/levodopa tablets four times daily. However, she couldn't get to sleep. Following our guidelines, she added 2 immediate-release carbidopa/levodopa tablets at 9:00 P.M., an hour before her 10:00 P.M. bedtime. With that, she easily fell asleep but couldn't sleep past 2:00 A.M. Again, following our guidelines, she then added a controlled-release carbidopa/levodopa dose right at bedtime, 10:00 P.M. This probably kicked in around midnight when she was asleep and allowed her to sleep well beyond 2:00 A.M.

Mr. Jones has a 3-hour levodopa effect and takes 2 immediate-release tablets every 3 hours during the day and through the evening. He falls asleep when he goes to bed at 11:00 P.M. but awakens feeling stiff and uncomfortable at 1:00 A.M. His last evening carbidopa/levodopa dose is at 10:00 P.M. Obviously his 10:00 P.M. levodopa dose wore off while he was asleep, awakening him. The appropriate strategy is to add a dose of controlled-release carbidopa/levodopa at his 11:00 P.M. bedtime. With its delayed effect it will kick in at around 1:00 A.M., just when his prior dose of regular carbidopa/levodopa is wearing off.

How close to the last evening dose of carbidopa/levodopa may the Sinemet CR be taken?

In most cases, at least an hour should elapse between these doses to avoid too much overlap. For example, if the last evening dose of immediate-release carbidopa/levodopa is taken at 9:30 P.M. and Sinemet CR at 10:00 P.M., the effects will combine. This is not dangerous, but the combination might provoke dyskinesias.

What dose of Sinemet CR should be used at bedtime?

This depends on your optimal daytime dose of immediate-release carbidopa/levodopa. It should be approximately as potent (assuming the daytime doses are adequate). If Sinemet CR is also used during the daytime, then this is simple; just use the same dose at bedtime. However, if immediate-release carbidopa is the daytime medication, then we need to make a dosage conversion. Recall that there is no milligram-to-milligram correspondence between the levodopa content of these two formulations. Less levodopa is absorbed from the sustained-release (CR) than the immediate-release carbidopa/levodopa. To provide similar potency, a higher levodopa dose is necessary when using Sinemet CR.

The general rule of thumb is that the levodopa dose must be about 30–50 percent greater with the sustained-release (CR) drug, compared to immediate-release carbidopa/levodopa, as noted in chapters 12 and 17. Recall that the sustained-release tablets come in two sizes: 25-100 and 50-200. Thus, if the daytime dose of immediate-release carbidopa/levodopa is 200 mg of levodopa (e.g., two 25-100 tablets), the corresponding dose of Sinemet CR is around 300 mg (i.e., one 50-200 plus one 25-100 Sinemet CR tablet). Remember that we are focusing on the second number (e.g., "200" with a 50-200 tablet), since this is the levodopa content of these pills. If the daytime 25-100 immediate-release doses are 1 1/2 tablets, then the bedtime dose of sustained-release carbidopa/levodopa should be either one 50-200 tablet or perhaps even slightly higher, such as one 50-200 tablet plus one-half 25-100 sustained-release tablet.

What if the bedtime dose of Sinemet CR is not high enough?

The answer is that it won't work. In that case, you will still awaken shortly after you have fallen asleep (when your last evening dose of carbidopa/levodopa wore off). This reflects the fact that there is a dose threshold for this effect; if the Sinemet CR dose does not reach a certain level, no sleep benefit will occur. If the Sinemet CR is adequate (comparable dose to your daytime carbidopa/levodopa), it will sustain sleep; if not high enough, you awaken. I stated that the Sinemet CR dose must be 30–50 percent higher than the daytime immediate-release dose to be comparable. For this purpose, it often requires doses closer to 50 percent. You can experiment with the Sinemet CR doses, perhaps raising them by small increments until you capture the effect. If 400 mg of Sinemet CR (two 50-200 tablets or four 25-100 tablets) is not effective, there may be other problems and this should specifically be addressed with your physician.

Will a bedtime snack interfere with this medication strategy?

It may, especially if it contains protein (e.g., milk, cheese, meat, etc.). If the bedtime Sinemet CR strategy is not working, try eliminating the bedtime snack or at least eliminating bedtime protein.

AWAKENING AT 3:00 OR 4:00 A.M.

For many, that bedtime dose of Sinemet CR does not last throughout the night. You can anticipate that the sustained-release carbidopa/levodopa will take an hour or two to kick in and last about an hour longer than immediate-release carbidopa/levodopa. Thus, in many cases, the effect wears off in the wee hours of the morning, perhaps around 4:00 A.M. The strategy in this situation switches back to immediate-release carbidopa/levodopa; this is taken upon awakening. There are also occasional individuals who don't require bedtime Sinemet CR and sleep well during the first two-thirds of the night, but awaken at around 4:00 A.M., unable to return to sleep. For these people the strategy is the same: immediate-release carbidopa/levodopa upon awakening.

Q: Why should I choose immediate-release carbidopa/levodopa for these early morning problems?

A: Obviously the slow (often 2-hour) kick-in time of Sinemet CR is a disadvantage in the middle of the night when a quick response is desirable. The immediate-release carbidopa/levodopa works in half the time or less. Put your dose of immediate-release carbidopa/levodopa and a glass of water on your nightstand, ready to take when you awaken.

Q: What dose is best to take at this time?

A: The immediate-release carbidopa/levodopa dose should be the same as used for the daytime doses. Don't take less or it won't work.

Q: What if Sinemet CR is the daytime drug?

A: In that case, a dose conversion is necessary, as explained in chapter 12. To be similarly potent to the Sinemet CR dose, the immediate-release dose should be about 2/3 the amount of levodopa. For example, if one 50-200 Sinemet CR tablet several times daily is the daytime dose (200 mg levodopa), this corresponds to about 1 1/2 of the 25-100 immediate-release tablets (150 mg levodopa). Thus 1 1/2 of these tablets should be sufficient for the 4:00 A.M. dose.

Q: How soon after the bedtime dose of Sinemet CR can the dose of immediate-release carbidopa/levodopa be taken?

A: Ideally, these doses should not overlap too much or the responses will summate. This won't cause any serious problems but could result in dyskinesias. Usually allow at least 4 hours after the bedtime Sinemet CR dose before taking the immediate-release carbidopa/levodopa to get back to sleep. For those with very brief levodopa responses, however, a shorter interval may be necessary.

Q: What about the new, orally disintegrating carbidopa/levodopa tablet (Parcopa)?

A: This is a reasonable alternative to the immediate-release tablets in the middle of the night. Although more expensive, the convenience of not having to wash your pills down with water may offset the expense. You simply need to place this on your tongue; when it dissolves in your mouth, swallowing this with your saliva will get it into your system.

Summary: Carbidopa/Levodopa Treatment of Insomnia

Based on the above principles, patients with Parkinson's disease who have trouble both getting to sleep and staying asleep may find that they need three separate carbidopa/levodopa adjustments. First, they will need an evening dose of carbidopa, so that they are feeling relaxed and comfortable as they are getting into bed. Second, they may take a dose of Sinemet CR (sustained-release carbidopa/levodopa) just as they are getting ready to fall asleep. This drug's delayed effect will kick in perhaps two hours later carrying them into the wee morning hours. Third, if they awaken in the middle of the night, after the effects from the Sinemet CR have worn off, they could then take a dose of immediate-release carbidopa/levodopa (or the orally disintegrating tablet). Supplement 20.1 at the end of this chapter summarizes this strategy; photocopy this and have your physician fill in the blanks.

Other Treatable Contributors to Insomnia

Although inadequate levodopa coverage during the night is the most common cause of insomnia among those with PD, other factors or conditions may also play a role. This includes restless legs syndrome, urinary symptoms, and depression, as well as other medications. Let's think about these as well.

RESTLESS LEGS SYNDROME

Restless legs syndrome is a ubiquitous disorder, estimated to occur in 3 percent to 8 percent of all people. This may be even more frequent in those with PD. Other conditions have also been associated with restless legs syndrome, including iron deficiency, kidney failure, and peripheral neuropathy. Peripheral neuropathies are disorders affecting the nerves to the limbs, such as might occur in diabetes mellitus.

Those with restless legs syndrome describe an uncomfortable sensation in their legs when trying to sleep at night or when relaxing. These leg sensations are described in a variety of ways: crawling, itching, pulling, tension. People with this disorder cannot lie still and need to move their legs or get up and walk to relieve this. Obviously this can severely interfere with sleep.

Most with restless legs syndrome also have periodic limb movements of sleep. These are jerks of the legs occurring during sleep. They are "periodic" in that they typically recur about every 20–30 seconds throughout the night. People with these periodic movements will be unaware, since they are asleep; however, the sleep partner may be keenly aware! This periodic kicking of the legs may force a spouse into another bed.

Periodic limb movements affect the quality of sleep, since they may prevent deep sleep. We all cycle through stages of sleep, going from light sleep to deeper sleep and back. The periodic movements tend to inhibit deep sleep stages. Just as the person is cycling into deeper sleep, they are slightly aroused by the jerk and remain in the lighter sleep stage, so-called mini-arousals. As a consequence, they will not experience restful sleep and will be tired the next day.

Iron deficiency occasionally causes restless legs syndrome and blood iron studies are an appropriate part of the evaluation. Iron supplementation reverses the symptoms in these people. Most people with restless legs are not iron deficient, however, and therefore do not respond to iron therapy.

The subjective symptoms of restless legs syndrome resemble akathisia, described in chapter 19. It may be difficult to distinguish these two conditions among those with PD. However, those with restless legs syndrome primarily focus on their legs, whereas akathisia is typically not confined to legs or one part of the body.

The medications that effectively treat restless legs syndrome in the general population are the same drugs used to treat PD. Relatively low doses of levodopa therapy or the dopamine agonist medications are often dramatically beneficial. The dopamine agonist drugs (pramipexole, ropinirole, pergolide) are usually the most effective in the long term. The same medications that treat the restless sensations are also effective in treating periodic limb movements of sleep.

For restless legs syndrome in the general population, the dopamine agonist drugs are preferred over levodopa for several reasons:

- They appear to be at least slightly more effective and more consistent in their benefits.

- Often lower doses of these medications are sufficient.

- They are much less likely to result in "augmentation." Augmentation implies that with treatment, the restless legs sensation spills over from the evening to earlier in the day. This then requires medication doses during the daytime, as well. This is more likely with carbidopa/levodopa than dopamine agonist drugs. It is not a substantial issue among those with PD since they take these same medications anyway during the day-time for parkinsonism.

Among those with both PD and restless legs syndrome, adding a dose of antiparkinsonian medication at bedtime is an appropriate treatment. A bed-time dose of carbidopa/levodopa for parkinsonian symptoms during the night should also treat the restless legs. However, if restless legs is your only night-time problem, a bedtime dose of a dopamine agonist drug is appropriate. The dosing strategy for these dopamine agonist medications is shown in table 20.2. Whichever of the three drugs you choose, start with the single tablet listed in the table. Take it an hour or so before retiring so that it will have a chance to work once you go to bed. This starting dose may be too low to help and, if so, take 2 tablets two to three nights later. Then, every two to three nights, you may increase the dose by adding another tablet until it takes away the restless legs sensation. The maximum doses are shown in table 20.2. Once you have arrived at an effective dose, you may simplify by switching to a larger tablet size. For example, rather than taking eight 0.25 mg ropinirole tablets, switch to a single 2.0 mg tablet. You can refer back to chapter 13 for the different dopamine agonist tablet sizes that are available.

Other medications besides those used for PD are also helpful for restless legs. This includes gabapentin (Neurontin) and certain narcotic drugs. How-ever, among people with PD and restless legs, one drug treats both, and a dopamine agonist or levodopa therapy is preferred.

Table 20.2. Dopamine Agonist Drugs for Restless Legs
(Increase every 2–3 days by adding a tablet to the
bedtime dose until symptoms controlled)*

Medication	Starting Dose (1 Tablet at Bedtime)	Dosing Range, Bedtime Dose (mg)**
Pramipexole (Mirapex)	0.125 mg tablet	0.125–1.5
Ropinirole (Requip)	0.25 mg tablet	0.25–6.0
Pergolide (Permax)***	0.05 mg tablet	0.05–0.75

*For example, if one 0.125 mg pramipexole tablet was insufficient after two to three nights, increase to 2 tablets; two to three nights later, it could be increased to three 0.125 mg tablets at bedtime, and so on.

** Add another dose if breakthrough symptoms appear during the waking day.

***Last choice because of ergot side effects discussed in chapter 13.

FREQUENT URINATION

Those with PD often experience an urge to urinate during the night and this may affect sleep. The need to urinate, however, is often inappropriately blamed for awakenings during the night. Light sleepers may periodically cycle into near wakefulness and then begin to appreciate urinary symptoms. The urinary system gets blamed, but in fact it is the light sleep that allows the urinary symptoms to come into awareness. Improving sleep with adequate levodopa dosing, as described above, may be adequate to override most of the nighttime urinary urges.

Other medical options are available for urinary urgency causing sleep disruption despite adequate nocturnal levodopa coverage. Typically, however, urinary laboratory studies and review by a urologist are advisable to rule out any other cause.

Certain medications may be taken at bedtime to dampen the urge to urinate. These drugs share a common mechanism: They block the neurotransmitter acetylcholine, which makes them "anticholinergic" drugs. Commonly prescribed anticholinergic medications include oxybutynin (Ditropan) and tolterodine (Detrol). Sometimes low doses of the antidepressant medication amitriptyline are also used for this purpose (it has anticholinergic properties). We consider this in more detail in chapter 27.

Finally, avoid diuretics (water pills) in the evening since these make you urinate; common diuretics are listed in the next chapter. Similarly, don't drink caffeinated or alcoholic beverages before bedtime, which have a mild diuretic effect.

DEPRESSION AND SLEEP

Psychological depression is frequent in PD and insomnia is a common manifestation of this disorder. The person who frequently feels blue, has no appetite, has lost interest in life, and can't sleep may have an underlying depression that requires specific treatment.

Antidepressant medications may reverse insomnia due to depression, but some may also inhibit sleep if taken at bedtime. This includes SSRI drugs (selective serotonin reuptake inhibitors), such as fluoxetine (Prozac), sertraline (Zoloft), and paroxetine (Paxil). Also, antidepressants that block the neurotransmitter, norepinephrine, such as venlafaxine (Effexor), may cause insomnia. These are very effective medications, but if taken at bedtime, they may cause insomnia; hence, they are often administered in the morning. If insomnia remains a problem despite morning administration, another antidepressant that induces sleep is often added at bedtime. Typically trazodone (Desyrel) is used for this purpose, administered in a low dose of 50–100 mg. Trazodone is not a potent antidepressant, especially in this dosage, but is effective as a sleep aid. More is offered about depression and these drugs in chapter 22.

DRUGS THAT CAUSE INSOMNIA

Selegiline (Eldepryl, Deprenyl) is used in the treatment of PD and is notorious for inducing insomnia. The beneficial effects from this drug are very long lasting, whereas the insomnia-inducing effects are shorter-lived, lasting perhaps several hours. Hence this drug should not be administered much beyond noontime to avoid insomnia.

Selegiline is conventionally prescribed as a 5 mg tablet, twice daily, with doses at breakfast and lunchtime. If insomnia is a problem despite no doses in the afternoon or beyond, the dosage could be reduced to a single early morning tablet. The medical literature suggests that the main effect of selegiline on brain chemistry (blocking the enzyme monoamine oxidase-B) is essentially the same, whether the dose is 1 or 2 tablets daily.

Certain asthma drugs (such as dyphylline/Lufyllin, or theophylline/Theo-Dur) and medications for attention deficit (such as methylphenidate/Ritalin) may prevent sleep; avoid these later in the day, if possible. Don't forget that caffeinated beverages (e.g., colas, tea, coffee) also tend to cause insomnia and are best not consumed later in the evening.

Primary Insomnia

Insomnia may develop independent from PD, urinary symptoms, or depression. In other words, it may have its own origins and we will refer to this as primary insomnia ("primary" implying that it is not "secondary" to some other obvious cause).

Primary insomnia is common among all adults, and entire books and careers have been devoted to treatment. A detailed and comprehensive discussion of treatment is beyond the scope of this book, but some simple measures deserve discussion. Two basic strategies for treating primary insomnia include use of sleep-inducing medications and modification of behavior.

MEDICATIONS TO AID SLEEP

When simpler strategies fail, a medication for sleep taken at bedtime may be appropriate. Bear in mind, however, that these are not as effective as levodopa therapy for those who experience insomnia secondary to parkinsonism. Three basic categories of medications are used for sleep.

- Antihistamines
- Antidepressants
- Drugs designed specifically to induce sleep

Not all the drugs in the first two categories are appropriate as sleep aids, as we will see.

Table 20.3. Antidepressant Medications Used As Sleep Aids

Medication	Common Brand Names	Dose Range for Sleep (Administered at Bedtime)	Typical Dose Range for Depression
Amitriptyline	Elavil	10 mg–75 mg	50 mg–150 mg
Nortriptyline	Pamelor, Aventyl	10 mg–75 mg	50 mg–150 mg
Trazodone	Desyrel	50 mg–150 mg	150 mg–400 mg
Mirtazapine	Remeron	15 mg–30 mg	15 mg–45 mg

The antihistamine typically used for sleep is diphenhydramine. It is an over-the-counter drug that goes under a variety of names, such as Benadryl. It is an ingredient in Tylenol PM (Tylenol is the brand-name for acetaminophen). The usual dose of diphenhydramine for sleep is 50 mg. This is the amount contained in two Tylenol PM caplets. Some who take this medication feel drugged and don't like the effect. Diphenhydramine administration is compatible with PD and it may have a slightly beneficial effect on PD symptoms as well. Note that the newer antihistamines now commonly prescribed for allergies are not sedating and have no role as sleep aids; this includes such drugs as fexofenadine (Allegra), cetirizine (Zyrtec), and loratadine (Claritin).

Certain antidepressant medications have been used for years to treat insomnia. For this purpose, they are prescribed in low doses, too low to treat depression. They induce sleep regardless of whether the person is depressed or not. These medications include amitriptyline (Elavil), nortriptyline (Pamelor, Aventyl), and trazodone (Desyrel). More recently, mirtazapine (Remeron) has been added to this list. Doses commonly employed are shown in table 20.3. It is usually wise to start with the lowest amount shown in the table and then increase if necessary. As with other drugs for sleep, they may cause a hangover or grogginess the following day. Also, they have anticholinergic effects (greatest for amitriptyline; least for trazodone), which can result in dry mouth, constipation, and reduced urine flow from the bladder. For some, the reduction in urination may be beneficial during the night. Note that these drugs are from different classes than the SSRI antidepressant drugs mentioned above. The SSRI drugs, such as fluoxetine (Prozac), sertraline (Zoloft), and paroxetine (Paxil), often are mentally activating and are not used as sleep aids. Rather, they may induce insomnia and are best taken in the morning.

There have been a variety of medications specifically designed as sleep aids. Some of the older medications in this category, such as flurazepam (Dalmane), have longer durations of action and may cause daytime grogginess or clumsiness. Shorter-acting drugs, such as zolpidem (Ambien; doses 5 mg to 20 mg), have been better tolerated. It is generally recommended that they not be used for long-term treatment of insomnia, since they might cause dependency. However, this advice is not always followed.

MODIFYING SLEEP BEHAVIOR

Primary insomnia, or insomnia due to any cause, may improve with measures directed at lifestyle, stressors, and behavior. Experts in sleep disorders typically counsel their insomniac patients about sleep hygiene. Sleep hygiene tips include the following.

- Avoid caffeine beyond the early afternoon.

- Avoid alcoholic beverages; these may induce sleep, but they increase the likelihood of awakening in the middle of the night.

- Avoid evening activities that increase stress. This includes good stress, such as late-night sporting events.

- Sleep in a quiet, dark room. Clock watchers should move their alarms out of sight. Slightly cooler room temperatures are often the most conducive for sleep (but with adequate bed covers).

- Avoid doing other activities in bed such as homework from the office, balancing the checkbook, and so on. Reserving the bed for sleep allows the bedroom environment to trigger sleep-related thoughts.

- Avoid daytime naps. A single, relatively brief nap after lunch is usually not a problem, but specifically avoid naps after supper. If tempted, leave the easy chair and engage in some stimulating activity, such as walking or working on a hobby.

- Establish fairly regimented sleep patterns. Avoid having to reset your biological clock repeatedly.

- Get adequate exercise. Avoid exercise right before bedtime when it can produce a stimulating effect.

- Figure out ways to manage your stress. Don't be a ruminator; avoid carrying unpleasant thoughts.

One common reason for nighttime insomnia among seniors with PD is *reversal of the day-night cycle*, and this deserves further emphasis. Retirees have the luxury of sleeping during the day if they don't get a good night's sleep; sometimes this habit evolves, and most of one's sleep occurs during the daytime. If this is becoming a problem, specific measures to revert to a more normal sleep pattern are necessary.

If your day-night cycle is reversed, transition to a more conventional sleep pattern will be aided by the following measures:

- Avoid naps beyond the early afternoon.

- Limit the afternoon nap to 60–90 minutes.

- Avoid sedentary activities after supper (don't sit in the easy chair to read the paper or watch TV, where sleep is inevitable).

- Stay active during the daytime. If you are feeling sleepy when engaged in some sedentary activity, force yourself to get up and go for a walk, or do something active.

It may also be necessary to use a sleep medication at bedtime to help the body retime the sleep cycle. If forcing yourself to stay up during the day does not result in sleepiness at bedtime, you can use one of the medications from the section above to elicit sleep and get the body back on track. It may not be necessary to use this for long, once the normal sleep cycles are restored and the body gets used to this new schedule.

I'm Sleepy All the Time

A variety of factors may contribute to daytime sleepiness among those with PD and most of these are treatable. A poor night's sleep from insufficient control of parkinsonism or other causes will cause drowsiness during the day, as we just discussed. Sleepiness may also be a side effect from certain medications. Finally, some with PD sleep through the night but obtain insufficient deep sleep. This may be due to recurrent arousals caused by a breathing disorder (sleep apnea) or involuntary movements (periodic leg movements of sleep). These causes are summarized in table 20.4.

If you are troubled by daytime sleepiness, ask yourself the following questions:

- How is your nighttime sleep?

Table 20.4. Treatable Causes of Daytime Sleepiness

Causes	Comments
Insomnia	
Insomnia due to parkinsonism	Inadequate control of parkinsonian symptoms during the night is a common cause of insomnia.
Primary insomnia	If insomnia predated the onset of PD, it may be a separate condition.
Disruptions during sleep	
Sleep apnea	Breathing interruptions prevent deep sleep.
Periodic leg movements of sleep	Often associated with restless legs syndrome, but may occur separately.
Medications	
Drugs that cause daytime sleepiness	Includes drugs for PD and others.
Drugs that cause insomnia	Drugs preventing nighttime sleep secondarily may cause insomnia.

- Do you feel rested after a night's sleep?
- Do you take any medications that make you sleepy (or cause insomnia)?

The answers to these questions help focus on the cause, which could be night-time insomnia, medications, or disruptions of deep sleep.

INSOMNIA RESULTING IN DAYTIME SLEEPINESS

A poor night's sleep because of parkinsonian symptoms is a very common contributor to daytime sleepiness. People with PD often sleep poorly due to stiffness, akathisia, and trouble turning over in bed. Consequently they are sleep deprived and sleepy during the daytime. Treat the insomnia from parkinsonism (as discussed above) and the daytime sleepiness should also respond.

Insomnia is common among people in general and for some is a lifelong problem. If difficulty sleeping began before the earliest signs of PD, this may be a separate disorder. In that case, it may not respond to PD medications at bedtime and during the night. You then need to focus on sleep hygiene and perhaps a sleep medication, as we discussed above.

MEDICATIONS THAT CAUSE SLEEPINESS

A wide variety of drugs may induce drowsiness, both those used in the treatment of PD and others. It may be helpful to think back to when the sleepiness first started and consider whether any new medications were initiated around that time. Although any drug that passes into the brain could potentially be a cause of daytime sleepiness, some drugs are much more likely to do this than others.

Certain general categories of drugs are notorious for causing daytime drowsiness, listed in table 20.5. If daytime drowsiness is a problem, then drugs from these classes should be minimized if possible. This is not an exhaustive list and other drugs may also be offenders. The physician prescribing the medication should be a party to the decision to discontinue the drug. Often drugs need to be slowly reduced before stopping and your physician can advise you how best to do that.

It is also helpful to know which medications are unlikely to cause daytime drowsiness. General classes of drugs unlikely to induce sleepiness are shown in table 20.6. If you are taking one of these, there should be no reason to worry that it is making you sleepy.

DRUGS FOR PD THAT MAY INDUCE SLEEPINESS

Almost all of the medications used in the treatment of PD movement symptoms may cause sleepiness; however, this is not a frequent problem with any of these. Some do this rarely, whereas others induce drowsiness occasionally. If sleepiness has been only a recent problem, consider whether this began after starting one of these medications for PD.

Table 20.5. General Classes of Medications That May Cause Daytime Sleepiness

Medication Classes	Examples of Drugs from Each Class
Antianxiety drugs	Alprazolam (Xanax), diazepam (Valium), clorazepate (Tranxene), lorazepam (Ativan)
Muscle relaxants, drugs for spasticity	Cyclobenzaprine (Flexeril), orphenadrine (Norflex), tizanidine (Zanaflex), baclofen (Lioresal)
Narcotics	Codeine (in Tylenol #3), hydrocodone (in Vicodin), oxycodone (in Percodan, Oxycontin)
Nonnarcotic prescription pain relievers	Tramadol (Ultram)
Seizure drugs	Phenytoin (Dilantin), carbamazepine (Tegretol), phenobarbital
Nonprescription antihistamines	Diphenhydramine (Benadryl)*
Longer-acting drugs for insomnia (may carry over to next day)	Clonazepam (Klonopin), flurazepam (Dalmane)
Drugs for hallucinations/ psychosis	Quetiapine (Seroquel), clozapine (Clozaril), olanzapine (Zyprexa)
Certain drugs for depression	Amitriptyline, nortriptyline, mirtazapine (Remeron)

*The newer prescription antihistamines such as fexofenadine (Allegra) are unlikely to cause drowsiness.

The two dopamine agonist drugs, pramipexole (Mirapex) and ropinirole (Requip), received recent notoriety for occasionally causing sleepiness, including while driving an automobile. The other two dopamine agonist drugs, pergolide (Permax) and bromocriptine (Parlodel), are much less likely to do this. If drowsiness from an agonist drug is troublesome, it might be best to taper off and focus on carbidopa/levodopa. This is especially appropriate if you need to drive, and your driving safety is threatened by drowsiness.

Carbidopa/levodopa may cause drowsiness, but infrequently. It does this in one of two ways. (1) It may directly cause drowsiness, but this is uncommon. (2) It may indirectly cause drowsiness by reversing parkinsonism in those sleep-deprived from lack of nighttime levodopa coverage. After a night of sleeplessness because of untreated nighttime parkinsonism, the first morning dose of carbidopa/levodopa reverses the pent up akathisia and rigid, tense muscles. Relief of these symptoms may translate into a relaxed state, where someone who has been awake most of the night can now fall asleep. Thus the

Table 20.6. Commonly Prescribed Medications Unlikely to Be the Cause of Daytime Sleepiness

Medication Classes	Examples of Drugs from Each Class
Drugs for lowering cholesterol	Atorvastatin (Lipitor), pravastatin (Pravachol), simvastatin (Zocor)
Most drugs for lowering blood pressure	Amlodipine (Norvasc), enalapril (Vasotec), losartan (Cozaar)
Diabetic agents	Insulin, metformin (Glucophage), glipizide (Glucotrol)
Most antibiotics	Penicillins (Amoxacillin), sulfa/trimethoprim (Bactrim, Septra)
Diuretics (water pills)	Furosemide (Lasix), hydrochlorothiazide (Hydrodiuril)
Prescription anti-inflammatory drugs	Celecoxib (Celebrex), diclofenac (Cataflam), etodolac (Lodine), fenoprofen (Nalfon), ketoprofen (Orudis), ketorolac (Toradol), nabumetone (Relafen), oxaprozin (Daypro), rofecoxib (Vioxx), sulindac (Clinoril), tolmetin (Tolectin)
Nonprescription anti-inflammatory drugs	Aspirin, ibuprofen (Motrin, Advil), naproxen (Aleve)
Non-prescription pain relievers	Acetaminophen (Tylenol)
Estrogen, progesterone or thyroid hormones	Premarin, oral contraceptives, levothyroxine (Synthroid)
Bronchodilators for asthma (but may cause insomnia)	Dyphylline (Lufyllin), Theophylline (Theo-Dur)
Steroids (but may cause insomnia)	Prednisone
Anti-coagulants	Warfarin (Coumadin)
Drugs for gastritis, ulcers, acid reflux	Cimetidine (Tagamet), famotidine (Pepcid), nizatidine (Axid), omeprazole (Prilosec), pantoprazole (Protonix), ranitidine (Zantac), sucralfate (Carafate),
Drugs for osteoporosis	Alendronate (Fosamax), risedronate (Actonel), calcitonin (Miacalcin)

initial morning levodopa dose facilitates a belated sleepy state. A typical case illustrates the second scenario:

> Mrs. Good complained to her husband's doctor that every morning at 7:00 A.M. her husband takes his first dose of carbidopa/levodopa and then promptly falls asleep on the couch. He wakes up around 10:00 A.M., takes a second dose a little later, and then falls asleep again. He sleeps away much of the morning and his wife thinks the levodopa dose must be excessive. His physician appropriately inquired about his nighttime sleep habits. It turns out that he has trouble getting to sleep, and when he does, he often awakens during the night, unable to return to sleep. He takes no medications for PD after suppertime.

How to treat? You have probably already figured this out. Mr. Good should follow our previous directives for levodopa coverage at night. If this restores his nighttime sleep, his morning doses of carbidopa/levodopa may no longer make him sleepy.

What about the first, less common scenario where levodopa directly induces drowsiness in someone who is not sleep deprived? We can't blame it on poor sleep at night; rather, this is a direct side effect of levodopa. Since levodopa is crucial in the management of PD, substituting another drug is usually not practical, except early in the course when symptoms are mild. Hence strategies are necessary for working around this problem. There are three alternatives.

1. The simplest approach is to briefly nap after each carbidopa/levodopa dose. This can be scheduled into the day, using an alarm that awakens after 20–30 minutes of sleep.

2. The times of the carbidopa/levodopa doses can be shifted to evening and night. This works if the primary levodopa response is of the long-duration type; that is, you don't require precisely timed carbidopa/levodopa doses because of a short-duration levodopa effect. If varying the times of your carbidopa/levodopa doses doesn't cause deterioration in your parkinsonism, simply take them all in the evening and at night. If they make you drowsy, that's okay since they are being taken at times you want to sleep. Thus the total daily levodopa requirement can be administered in two to three doses, with the first dose in the evening and additional doses during the night when you awaken to go to the bathroom.

3. Stimulating medications can be administered to offset the sleepiness from carbidopa/levodopa. Starting with the simplest, a cup of strong coffee could be consumed around the time of each levodopa dose. If this is insufficient, prescription medications such as modafinil (Provigil) or methylphenidate (Ritalin) may be considered. This is discussed in more detail later in this chapter.

IS YOUR MEDICATION RESPONSIBLE FOR YOUR SLEEPINESS?

Occasionally it is unclear whether one of the drugs for PD is causing sleepiness or if you're always sleepy at a particular time every day for some other reason. For example:

Mrs. Schwartz is sleepy every morning after breakfast. She takes carbidopa/
levodopa an hour before eating and pramipexole with breakfast. Are one of
these drugs the cause?

To sort this out Mrs. Schwartz may wish to omit her morning dose of one of
these two drugs for a few days and observe whether the sleepiness persists.
She may omit one and then the other. If she is still sleepy despite omitting
each of the drugs, one at a time, then they are probably not responsible.
There is no danger in doing this, although her parkinsonism may not be
adequately treated those mornings.

SLEEP APNEA

In the general population, disrupted breathing patterns during sleep are a frequent cause of daytime sleepiness. The term for this is "sleep apnea"; apnea
implies cessation of breathing. Those with PD are even more likely to experience this problem. Periodically during the night, breathing ceases briefly. Typically this is unrecognized since the person with sleep apnea remains asleep and
only appreciates lack of restful sleep after awakening in the morning. The spouse
or bed partner usually does not appreciate the apnea in the darkened bedroom
and only hears the loud snoring, which is often a red flag for sleep apnea.

People with sleep apnea breathe normally until they fall into deeper stages
of sleep. As they cycle into deep sleep, breathing stops. The consequent drop
in blood oxygen triggers the body's internal alarm. Two things then occur:
(1) breathing resumes, often with snorts and snoring, (2) deep sleep is aborted,
with a return to light sleep stages. The snoring represents the sounds made
when the airway is partially obstructed. This process recurs throughout the
night; each apneic episode partially arouses the sleeper, who returns to a lighter
stage of sleep. Hence people with sleep apnea do not experience adequate
deep sleep, which leaves them tired and sleepy the next day. With prominent
and persistent sleep apnea, other medical problems may also develop, including headaches and elevated blood pressure.

How can you detect sleep apnea? Clues to this condition include loud
snoring and daytime sleepiness. Those with more severe forms of sleep apnea
may become so tired that they fall asleep at very inappropriate times such as
driving a car or eating. Obesity predisposes to sleep apnea and is an additional clue to this disorder, although it also occurs in the nonobese.

If sleep apnea is suspected, a special overnight sleep study, termed
polysomnography, is typically performed to make this diagnosis. During this
study, your brain waves, breathing, and blood oxygen are recorded to document the presence and extent of the problem. Sleep laboratories that perform
polysomnography are located at most larger medical centers. Your physician
likely knows the closest sleep centers and can refer you. Sometimes physicians
will do a screening test to see if polysomnography is necessary. This employs

a simple device you use at home to measure your blood oxygen while asleep in your own bed (oximeter). If the blood oxygen periodically plummets during sleep, then sleep apnea is suspected.

If sleep apnea is documented during polysomnography, treatment is usually initiated the night of this study. This typically consists of a trial of continuous positive airway pressure (CPAP). CPAP is administered via a mask that fits over your mouth and nose. It is connected via a tube to a bedside compressor that generates higher air pressure, which keeps the airway open. This is effective in most people with sleep apnea. People generally feel so much better after treating their sleep apnea that they gladly put up with the minor aggravation of the CPAP device.

PERIODIC LIMB MOVEMENTS OF SLEEP

Periodic limb movements of sleep are jerks that occur during sleep, mainly of the legs, but also in arms or trunk. The typical movement is a sudden drawing up of one leg, which then quickly relaxes after no more than a few seconds. This is termed periodic because they recur periodically throughout the night at fairly constant intervals, often 20–40 seconds apart. If these are frequent and prominent, they may prevent deep sleep. In other words, as you are drifting off into a deeper stage of sleep, the periodic limb movements cause a partial arousal; this returns you to a lighter sleep stage and may even awaken you. The loss of deep sleep with these mini-arousals can result in sleep deprivation and consequent daytime sleepiness.

Most people with restless legs syndrome (discussed above) also have periodic leg movements of sleep (about 80–85 percent). However, periodic leg movements of sleep frequently occur in the absence of restless legs syndrome, and, in fact, most with this condition do not have restless legs.

Periodic limb movements are fairly common among those with PD and may be a cause of daytime sleepiness. Exactly how frequently this occurs in PD is not known. At least some of the observed frequency in PD is due to the fact that periodic limb movements of sleep are a more common condition among seniors, in general.

How to recognize and diagnose periodic limb movements of sleep as a cause of daytime sleepiness? This usually requires study in a sleep laboratory. Although the sleep partner may note movements during sleep, it is very hard to correctly diagnose this without these special studies.

Treatment involves the same medications and strategies used to treat the restless legs syndrome, specifically carbidopa/levodopa and the dopamine agonist medications. These are very effective in most cases, as previously noted. Thus, if periodic leg movements are suspected of disrupting sleep, a trial of bedtime carbidopa/levodopa or a dopamine agonist might be tried even without confirmation by polysomnography.

DRUGS TO COMBAT SLEEPINESS

Stimulant drugs may counter drowsiness. However, these should be employed only after other causes have been considered and addressed, such as medications producing drowsiness or conditions compromising nighttime sleep. In fact, the stimulant drugs are not consistently effective for the drowsiness that occurs in PD.

Starting with simple strategies, a cup or two of strong coffee might be used at times during the day when sleepiness is anticipated. This is compatible with the medications used in the treatment of PD.

Modafinil (Provigil) is a prescription medication that is used for treatment of daytime drowsiness. It is a long-acting drug that may take two or three days to become fully effective. It is administered in a dose of one 200 mg tablet once daily, in the morning. Side effects include headache, nausea, and anxiety; not surprisingly, it can also cause insomnia.

Methylphenidate (Ritalin) has been used for years in the treatment of daytime drowsiness. This is the same drug used to treat attention deficit hyperactivity disorder in children. Among those with PD, this medication is usually tried only when all other measures have failed and daytime drowsiness is a substantial problem.

PSEUDO-SLEEPINESS: LOW BLOOD PRESSURE

If your blood pressure drops too low, you may faint. People with PD are prone to low blood pressure due to a combination of their underlying condition plus medications, as we will address in detail in the next chapter. Sometimes, fainting from low blood pressure can be confused with sleep. Here is an illustrative case from the clinic.

> Mrs. Hill reports that her husband falls asleep after breakfast most mornings. "He just slumps over and sleeps with his head on the table." His blood pressure during that afternoon clinic appointment was normal in the lying position (130/70), a little low when sitting (85/60), but very low when standing (70/50).

How do these blood pressure readings relate to the morning sleepiness? Mr. Hill is an actual case (not his real name), and it was subsequently learned that his blood pressure would drop to around 50/30 following breakfast, sufficient to cause fainting. Thus he wasn't falling asleep after breakfast, he was losing consciousness. His afternoon sitting blood pressure (85/60) in the clinic was not sufficiently low to cause fainting but it raised suspicions; if this low in the afternoon, it might be even lower in the morning. Three factors converge after breakfast that can bring this problem to a head.

1. Levodopa may markedly drop the blood pressure in susceptible individuals for a few hours after each dose. The levodopa effect is fully present after breakfast since this medication is typically taken before.

Also, dopamine agonist drugs may contribute and they are typically administered with meals, including breakfast.

2. In those prone to this problem, meals cause a drop in blood pressure.

3. A night's sleep exacerbates these low blood pressures in susceptible individuals.

From my experience with Mr. Hill, I learned to become suspicious of people who fall asleep right after breakfast. This is uncommon, but important to recognize. These problems of low blood pressure are discussed further in the next chapter.

Disruptions During the Night

A variety of happenings may occur while you are asleep. Some of these may be disruptive and prevent you or your sleep partner from getting a good night's sleep.

VIVID DREAMS AND NIGHTMARES

All of us have occasional nightmares or vivid dreams and the medications used to treat PD occasionally increase this tendency. This is not a serious problem, unless you find it disturbing. However, the development of vivid dreams needs to be distinguished from acting out your dreams, which we discuss in the next section. Acting out your dreams is due to PD, not your medications.

Bear in mind that any medication that passes into the brain could trigger nightmares. This includes our PD drugs, as well as medications for psychiatric conditions (e.g., anxiety), insomnia, nighttime urinary symptoms (e.g., oxybutynin), prescription pain medications, and muscle relaxants. As discussed in the sections below, these same medications may also contribute to nighttime confusion in susceptible individuals.

ACTING-OUT DREAMS (REM SLEEP BEHAVIOR DISORDER)

When humans dream, they typically are quiet and unmoving in bed. This is because the normal brain turns off the connection between the dreaming circuits and the movement control centers. Often in PD, however, the connection is not turned off, and people act out their dreams while asleep. Not only is this common in PD, it may precede parkinsonism by many years. The dream behavior may be dramatic, with thrashing, hitting, or yelling during sleep. Some people may actually jump out of bed to chase a character in a dream.

This phenomenon of acting out dreams is termed rapid eye movement sleep behavior disorder, or REM sleep behavior disorder for short. The term "rapid eye movement sleep" relates to a specific sleep state. We normally cycle through various stages of sleep over the course of the night, going from lighter to deeper stages and then back. Most dreaming occurs during the rapid eye movement (REM) stage of sleep. In this stage, our bodies are paralyzed except for our eye movements. Thus, in normal individuals, dreams are acted out only with eye movements (hence the term "rapid eye movements") but not with our bodies. This obviously has practical consequences, preventing us from injuring ourselves or our bed partners while fighting bad guys in our dreams.

People who act out their dreams are said to have REM sleep behavior disorder. PD predisposes to this dream enactment behavior; although the PD drugs may get blamed, they are not responsible. As mentioned, REM sleep behavior disorder may be an early sign of PD, predating any other manifestations by many years.

Those with REM sleep behavior disorder do not necessarily have a serious problem. It only becomes significant if the dream enactment behavior endangers the sleeper or sleep mate. Falling out of bed while mentally running from a dream state pursuer may result in injury. Hitting your spouse while dreaming is equally serious.

Treatment is considered if there is potential for injury. Otherwise, it requires no specific therapy. Practical strategies for the bedroom may be appropriate. This includes a separate bed for your sleep partner. For those who are at risk for falling out of bed, surround the bed with padding and remove furniture with sharp corners (such as a nightstand). Bedrails may also be devised to prevent falls to the floor.

If acting-out dreams are sufficiently troublesome, a medication may be appropriate, usually clonazepam (Klonopin). This drug is from the benzodiazepine class of medications, which includes diazepam (Valium). Clonazepam is typically administered as a single dose, a little before bedtime. It induces sleep, so may be additionally helpful for that reason. However, it does have side effects, which include potential for morning sleepiness as well as clumsiness. People with memory difficulties may experience increased nighttime confusion with clonazeapam.

Clonazepam is prescribed in low doses to avoid side effects, starting with one-half to one 0.5 mg tablet at bedtime. It may be raised to 1 mg if necessary and tolerated. When used for more than a few days, it may be difficult to sleep without it; however, this will resolve with continued abstinence.

Melatonin has also been advocated for this condition. This is available over the counter and doses from 3 to 10 mg at bedtime have been employed.

The medications we use to treat PD, carbidopa/levodopa and the dopamine agonists, do not improve REM sleep behavior disorder symptoms in most cases. However, occasional patients in my practice have reported benefit from these drugs, although they are the exception rather than the rule.

REM SLEEP BEHAVIOR VERSUS HALLUCINATIONS

REM sleep behavior disorder symptoms may sometimes be mistaken for hallucinations. Hallucinations are visual illusions—seeing things that aren't there. Hallucinations occur in a minority of people with PD and there are ways to control them (see chapter 24). However, the measures can be quite drastic and you don't want to do this inappropriately. If you were acting out a dream, your spouse might mistakenly perceive that your bizarre behavior represents hallucinations and you were psychotic during the night.

How can you be sure that what is occurring at night is really dream enactment and not hallucinations or delusional behavior? The primary distinction is based on whether you are asleep or awake. Hallucinations occur when you are awake, but REM sleep behavior occurs during sleep. The following are clues to help you sort this out.

- You can have a conversation with someone who is hallucinating. They respond to questions from their sleep partner and will engage in a conversation. Those acting out their dreams tend not to respond to questions and commands, or simply mumble, half asleep.

- Those acting out their dreams will do this for only the length of the dream, which may be a few minutes or less. Those hallucinating tend to persist in this state for longer periods of time.

- Those acting out their dreams can be awakened. If the dream has been very vivid, they may be mentally caught up in this for a few minutes after awakening, however.

- Those acting out their dreams may remember the dream the next day, but typically not events in the bedroom that took place during the dream (e.g., not recall what the bed partner said during the dream). Those hallucinating may not have a clear memory for all the events, but what they remember often includes conversations with their bed partner.

If the distinction between nighttime hallucinations and REM sleep behavior disorder is unclear, monitoring overnight in a sleep laboratory will usually sort this out.

NIGHTTIME CONFUSION

Dementia sometimes occurs in advanced PD. For people with impaired thinking, the most troublesome time is often during the night. During the waking day, they may be fairly well compensated and the cognitive impairment may not be too troublesome. However, these same people may become very confused in the middle of the night and their antics may disrupt the sleep of everyone in the household. Why do these problems seem to surface during the night? There are multiple reasons, including the following.

- External stimulation is less during the night; the lights are out and the room is quiet.

- Awakening from a deep sleep may have a disorienting effect.

- Medications taken at bedtime may contribute.

- Mental fatigue from a long day may accrue and culminate in the late evening.

Treatment depends on the extent of the problem. If the confusion goes beyond simply being mixed up, but with hallucinations (seeing things that are not there) or delusions (imagining bizarre things), specific medications may be necessary (chapter 24). For treatment of simple nighttime confusion, consider the following.

- A night light and familiar surroundings help people stay oriented. Dark rooms and strange bedrooms (e.g., hotel rooms) can be disorienting after awakening from sleep. Sleeping in the old familiar bedroom with the furniture arranged as always helps orientation.

- Sedating medications taken in the evening may need to be reduced or discontinued. A sleep medication may initially induce sleep, but the persistent sedation may contribute to confusion during the night when awakened.

- Focus on strategies that reduce the likelihood of awakening during the night, including the following.

  A quiet bedroom and comfortable bed and bedclothes may facilitate sleeping through the night.

  Alcohol should be avoided, since it may initially induce sleepiness but increase the likelihood of waking up in the middle of the night.

  Adequate levodopa coverage during the night will reduce the chance that parkinsonism will cause awakening, as discussed above. Occasionally, bedtime carbidopa/levodopa increases nighttime confusion but usually facilitates sleep and reduces nighttime problems.

  If all else fails, try a sleep-inducing medication. As mentioned, it may exacerbate the nighttime confusion, and if that occurs, it can be stopped. A low dose of trazodone (50 mg) would be a reasonable choice.

  For those with a reversed sleep–wake cycle, take measures to prevent sleeping during the day. A single nap of an hour or less is okay after lunch, but avoid napping beyond this, especially after supper.

Two factors determine how aggressively nighttime confusion is treated: (1) potential injury risk to someone wandering in a confused state and (2) disruption of the family's sleep (especially sleep partner). If neither is a problem, treatment of nighttime confusion may not be necessary.

NIGHTTIME HALLUCINATIONS AND DELUSIONS

Nighttime confusion may be compounded by hallucinations or crazy ideas. Hallucinations may be of people or creatures. Sometimes these are frightening; the entire household may be awakened as an illusory intruder is chased. However, the hallucinations may also be simple curiosities, such as a dog in the bedroom or a relative at the bedside. Delusional thinking (literally defined as false beliefs) often has paranoid themes such as:

- An intruder is in the house.

- Your spouse is conspiring against you.

- The police are watching.

- A family member is trying to steal your money.

Such hallucinations and delusions may be confined to the nighttime or may intrude into the daytime, as well. Seeing or imagining things that aren't there goes beyond simple confusion and requires unique treatment strategies. We discuss these in detail in chapter 24.

NIGHTTIME SWEATING (NOCTURNAL DIAPHORESIS)

Occasionally during sleep, the transition from a levodopa on-state to an off-state is accompanied by profound perspiration that soaks your bedclothes. Not only are you immersed in sweat-soaked sheets and pajamas, but also you're stiff and immobile from loss of the levodopa effect. The most effective treatment strategy is to improve levodopa coverage during the night, as outlined above; however, this may not be consistently effective, since complete elimination of levodopa off-states is often impossible.

Supplemental drugs have been used to reduce these bouts of perspiration, although with inconsistent success. This includes propranolol, with bedtime doses between 10 and 60 mg (or slightly higher if the long-acting formulation is used). Propranolol lowers the blood pressure; since those with PD are prone to a low blood pressure when standing, this could be a potential problem if awakening during the night to go to the bathroom. Hence, check the standing blood pressure. The anticholinergic drugs we previously discussed have also been tried for nighttime sweating, including trihexyphenidyl, with a bedtime dose of 2–5 mg. These drugs do not lower the blood pressure but do have other side effects: memory impairment (occasionally frank confusion), constipation, dry mouth/eyes, and difficulty urinating. However, for the person with a frequent need to urinate, an anticholinergic drug may be helpful because it dampens urinary urgency.

Supplement 20.1.

Guidelines for Carbidopa/Levodopa Therapy for Insomnia

Photocopy this page and have your physician check the appropriate boxes.

☐ Take a dose of carbidopa/levodopa in the evening, which will allow you to be comfortable in bed as you are trying to fall asleep.

Dose: _____

Time: _____

☐ Take a dose of sustained-release carbidopa/levodopa (Sinemet CR) just before you fall asleep, allowing you to stay asleep longer. Take this at the last minute before sleep, just as your head is hitting the pillow.

Dose: _____

Time: _____

☐ If you awaken in the middle of the night, you may take a dose of *immediate-release* carbidopa/levodopa, providing this is at least four hours after the Sinemet CR bedtime dose. This should allow you to get back to sleep. Have the pills on your nightstand with a glass of water. Alternatively, take the same carbidopa/levodopa dose as the new orally disintegrating form (Parcopa).

Dose: _____

You may repeat with another nighttime dose of *immediate-release* carbidopa/levodopa (or the orally disintegrating form), provided that at least _____ hours elapse since the last dose.

21

◆ ◆ ◆

Dizziness and Orthostatic Hypotension

Three Categories of Dizziness

"Dizziness" is a common word in our vocabulary and is often used by those with Parkinson's disease (PD) to describe one of their symptoms. However, the term dizziness has more than one meaning. There are three basic types of dizziness and each may be experienced by those with PD. It is crucial to distinguish these since the causes and treatments are quite different. The three categories of dizziness are:

- Imbalance

- Vertigo

- Faintness due to low blood pressure (hypotension)

The concepts behind these dizziness subtypes are summarized in table 21.1. To avoid confusing these terms, let's consider each type of dizziness in detail.

IMBALANCE

The word "dizziness" may be used to describe feeling unsteady—a tendency to fall or lose balance. This imbalance is not associated with lightheadedness, faintness, spinning sensations, wooziness, or other head sensations. The head is clear. To distinguish this from the other two major forms of dizziness, your

Table 21.1.   The Word "Dizziness" Has Three Meanings

Type of Dizziness	Description	Cause
Imbalance	Unsteadiness; head is clear.	Parkinsonism or other process affecting brain balance centers.
Vertigo	Sense of spinning in head; if mild, is experienced as head wooziness. Often provoked by certain head positions or quick head movements.	Most often due to non-worrisome problems affecting inner ears (vestibular system); not caused by PD or medications, but common with aging.
Orthostatic hypotension	Low blood pressure when standing or walking (orthostatic = standing; hypotension = low blood pressure). Symptoms are lightheadedness, faintness.	Due to problems in the autonomic nervous system plus medications.

physician may ask if the dizziness is experienced in the head or the body. If the head is clear but there is a sense of unsteadiness, then imbalance is being described.

Imbalance is a symptom of parkinsonism. Typically it is not prominent during the initial years of PD, although it may become troublesome after many years. Medications that cause sedation, such as sleep aids or antianxiety drugs, may also induce imbalance. However, the usual drugs for PD do not cause unsteadiness. Those with parkinsonism-plus syndromes, such as progressive supranuclear palsy or multiple system atrophy, may experience marked imbalance early in the course (see chapter 6).

If imbalance is a problem in someone with PD, more aggressive treatment with levodopa or one of the other antiparkinsonian drugs may help. Unfortunately imbalance is one of the most difficult PD symptoms to treat.

VERTIGO

Many seniors occasionally experience vertigo, another type of dizziness. This is not a symptom of PD. However, since many with PD are senior citizens, they are susceptible to this disorder because of age. Occasionally younger people also develop vertigo.

Vertigo implies a sense of spinning or movement in the head. When mild, it is experienced as a sense of head wooziness (swimming in the head). Those with vertigo typically complain that certain head positions or quick head movements will transiently provoke these symptoms. If the vertigo is severe, then a sense of imbalance may also be experienced. Obviously this is different from the person who is simply unsteady, but with a clear head, as described above.

Most of the time, vertigo originates from problems within the inner ear. Our inner ears contain sensors that inform the brain about our head position. These sensors monitor the speed and direction of head movements. Each ear has such a sensing apparatus. If signals from the right ear mirror those from the left, the brain is able to interpret this. However, problems occur if one ear malfunctions and the right and left signals don't match. When the brain receives two different signals, vertigo results.

These inner ear sensors may malfunction for a variety of reasons but most are not worrisome. As mentioned, it is common with aging. Often it develops for no identifiable reason. Such vertigo developing out of the blue and provoked by quick head movements or head positions has been termed benign positional vertigo or benign positional paroxysmal vertigo. Ear infections may also provoke vertigo. Only rarely is vertigo a sign of a brain disorder.

A less common cause of vertigo is Ménière's syndrome. This is associated with severe attacks of vertigo plus hearing loss and ringing in the ears. The medications used to treat PD do not induce vertigo. Vertigo neither improves nor worsens with treatment of Parkinson's disease.

Vertigo usually does not require much testing. If the neurological and ear examinations are normal, it may then be appropriate to simply observe, without any testing. If there are concerns, a brain scan may be performed to exclude other than the usual inner ear problems.

For very troublesome vertigo, an ear specialist should be consulted. For many with typical position-related vertigo, specific rehabilitation techniques may effectively treat this. These are termed canalith-repositioning maneuvers.

From our perspective, it is important that the common symptom of vertigo not be confused with dizziness due to low blood pressure, which we will consider next.

FAINTNESS DUE TO HYPOTENSION

This third type of dizziness is due to low blood pressure. The physician's term for low blood pressure is hypotension. It is important to recognize, since it, unlike the other two, can result in fainting. The symptoms are lightheadedness or a feeling that one might pass out. Other symptoms often accompany this faint feeling including lethargy, general weakness, and blurring or graying of vision. The lower the blood pressure, the more severe the symptoms; if the blood pressure drops very low, then actual fainting occurs. Spinning in the head (vertigo) is not a symptom of hypotension. Similarly, simple imbalance or fear of falling is not reflective of hypotension.

Among seniors, in general, the two most common causes of hypotension are medications and abnormal heart rhythms. First, medications prescribed to treat hypertension (high blood pressure) occasionally will make it too low, resulting in faintness. Sometimes drugs used to treat other problems will likewise do this. Second, sudden faintness may be due to a very irregular, a very slow, or an extremely rapid heartbeat. This results in inefficient pumping of blood and a corresponding drop in blood pressure.

People with PD, however, are especially likely to experience hypotensive symptoms for two quite different reasons: (1) dysfunction of the autonomic nervous system and (2) medications used to treat parkinsonism. These two factors make people with PD especially prone to low blood pressure symptoms. In PD, the low blood pressure is primarily in the upright (standing/walking) position, termed orthostatic hypotension, which was briefly touched on in previous chapters. We will now focus on this problem, including accurate detection and appropriate treatment.

Orthostatic Hypotension

Orthostatic hypotension implies a low blood pressure when on your feet (orthostatic = upright). In contrast to the upright position, the blood pressure is typically normal or near normal when sitting or lying down. Thus the symptoms of orthostatic hypotension are primarily or exclusively experienced when standing or walking. Unless severe, orthostatic hypotension will be relieved by sitting and always by lying down. People experience a lightheaded sensation (a faint feeling), generalized weakness, and sometimes graying of vision (but not spinning/vertigo). Orthostatic hypotension may also result in a chronic fatigue state.

If the blood pressure drops very low, loss of consciousness will occur. Typically, such loss of consciousness is brief if the person collapses to the ground; this is because the blood pressure and blood flow to the brain are reestablished in the collapsed (lying) position.

Orthostatic hypotension may be missed with routine blood pressure testing. Blood pressure recordings are conventionally checked in the seated position, where it may be normal. Thus your blood pressure should be checked in both the seated and standing positions if you have PD.

PREDISPOSITION DUE TO PROBLEMS IN THE AUTONOMIC NERVOUS SYSTEM

Dysfunction in the autonomic nervous system sets the stage for orthostatic hypotensive symptoms, as explained in previous chapters. The autonomic nervous system is the internal network of nerves that controls function of many internal organs. It modulates blood vessel diameter, heart rate and pumping function, sweating, bladder and bowel activity. Degenerative changes occur in the autonomic nervous system in those with PD, similar to what happens in the substantia nigra in the brain.

Normally blood pressure is kept stable by the autonomic nervous system, which appropriately modulates blood vessel diameter (resistance) and heart function. In normal humans, the blood pressure is regulated so that it is approximately the same whether one is lying, sitting, or standing. If not for the autonomic nervous system, blood would tend to pool in the blood vessels of our feet and legs whenever we stand up, pulled there by gravity. Normally, when we stand, blood vessels in our lower body constrict under the direction of the autonomic nervous system. In effect, this squeezes the blood up to our heads and maintains a constant blood pressure throughout our body, regardless of position.

When the autonomic nervous system malfunctions in PD, the internal reflexes that keep the blood pressure constant do not work properly. A failing autonomic nervous system will result in pooling of blood in the vessels of our feet and legs when standing. In this upright position, the brain does not receive enough blood. A mild reduction in blood flow to the brain will result in lightheadedness. If it is severe, a faint occurs.

PD MEDICATIONS AND ORTHOSTATIC HYPOTENSION

Typically in PD, the autonomic nervous system malfunction is not so severe and by itself would not result in lightheadedness or faintness. Medications, however, add to this problem. Ironically, the medications used to treat PD symptoms tend to cause orthostatic hypotension. This combination of factors may result in symptoms of this condition. All of the major drugs used to treat PD predispose to orthostatic hypotension. This includes carbidopa/levodopa and the dopamine agonist drugs (pramipexole, ropinirole, pergolide, and bromocriptine). For the majority with PD, this is not a problem. However, there is a distinct minority of people who need to have this addressed.

The tendency of these drugs to reduce the blood pressure is roughly in proportion to their potency in treating PD symptoms. Lower doses are less likely to provoke orthostatic hypotension than higher doses. Less efficacious drugs are less likely to lower the blood pressure than the more potent medications.

Are the dopamine agonist medications less likely to provoke orthostatic hypotension? No. Although a dopamine agonist drug may be tolerated in low doses, once the dose is raised into the therapeutic range, it will provoke orthostatic hypotension, just like carbidopa/levodopa.

Certain of the drugs used as supplements to levodopa therapy may not cause orthostatic hypotension when prescribed alone; however, they will exacerbate the tendency of levodopa to do this. This includes entacapone, tolcapone, amantadine, and selegiline.

What is the best strategy for treating PD in the face of orthostatic hypotension? First, be aware of this potential problem. Routinely check standing blood pressure when starting or adjusting medications. If the pressure is low, take measures to raise it before instituting more aggressive treatment of PD (see below). If orthostatic hypotension is a major problem, you should probably treat your PD symptoms with carbidopa/levodopa alone. Adding a dopamine agonist drug to carbidopa/levodopa may complicate management when orthostatic hypotension is prominent. Although levodopa will exacerbate low blood pressure, there are a variety of measures you can take to offset this, as we will subsequently discuss.

NON-PD DRUGS THAT LOWER BLOOD PRESSURE

A myriad of medications other than those for PD can lower blood pressure and aggravate orthostatic hypotension. Hence, a review of the medication list is appropriate at the first sign of this problem. Unnecessary medications can then be discontinued. The most common offenders are in the following categories.

- *Antihypertensive medications (blood pressure–lowering drugs)*. Sometimes high blood pressure treatment started years ago may no longer be necessary. This category includes many drugs from a variety of classes.

- *Diuretics (water pills)*, including furosemide (Lasix), hydrochlorothiazide (Hydrodiuril), triamterene (Dyrenium), hydrochlorothiazide plus triamterene (Dyazide, Maxzide), metolazone (Zaroxolyn), indapamide (Lozol), spironolactone (Aldactone), amiloride (Midamor), torsemide (Demadex), bumetanide (Bumex), and ethacrynic acid (Edecrin). These are used for a variety of problems including swelling of the legs, blood pressure reduction, and heart failure.

- *Certain heart medications*. Not all heart drugs aggravate orthostatic hypotension but a few may do this, such as the nitrate drugs used to treat angina.

- *Beta-blockers*. These are used for a variety of problems including heart conditions, hypertension, tremor control, and migraine. They include propranolol (Inderal), nadolol (Corgard), metoprolol (Lopressor, Toprol), atenolol (Tenormin), timolol (Blocadren), and Pindolol (Visken).

- *Calcium channel blockers*. These are used for various conditions including hypertension, cardiac problems, and migraine. These include verapamil (Calan, Isoptin, Verelan), diltiazem (Cardizem, Tiazac, Dilacor), nifedipine (Adalat, Procardia), amlodipine (Norvasc), felodipine (Plendil), isradipine (DynaCirc), and nicardipine (Cardene).

- *Certain prostate drugs*. These are used to treat an enlarged prostate and include tamsulosin (Flomax), doxazosin (Cardura), and terazosin (Hytrin).

- *Certain antidepressant drugs*, especially those from the triptyline class (also called tricyclics). These include amitriptyline (Elavil), nortriptyline

(Pamelor), protriptyline (Vivactil), imipramine (Tofranil), and desipramine (Norpramin). Three other antidepressants may also aggravate orthostatic hypotension: doxepin (Sinequan), mirtazepine (Remeron), and trazodone (Desyrel).

- *Male impotence medications.* These drugs include sildenafil (Viagra), vardenafil (Levitra), and tadalafil (Cialis).

Some of the medications on this list are for serious medical conditions. Your physician needs to advise whether any of these medications may be safely discontinued in the setting of orthostatic hypotension.

ORTHOSTATIC HYPOTENSION: OTHER FACTORS

In the setting of PD, a low standing blood pressure is almost always due to a combination of an abnormal autonomic nervous system plus the effect of medications. However, there could be other factors. Low blood pressures can also be caused by anemia and, rarely, metabolic problems. When orthostatic hypotension is first detected, it is usually appropriate to do limited routine blood tests, including a complete blood count and a chemistry profile.

The Basics of Blood Pressure

SYSTOLIC AND DIASTOLIC READINGS

Blood pressure measurements are recorded using two values, which relate to the two cycles of the heart. The first value is termed the "systolic" blood pressure and is the peak pressure generated by the pumping action of the heart. The second value, the "diastolic" blood pressure, relates to the low point of the heart pumping cycle. Thus, blood pressure readings are expressed as the systolic over the diastolic, for example, 120/80. The units of measurement are given in millimeters of mercury (mm Hg). This relates to the pressure required to raise a column of mercury in a tube. Although we now only rarely use columns of mercury to measure blood pressure, this system has survived as the unit of measurement.

HOW MUCH CAN THE BLOOD PRESSURE DROP WITHOUT CAUSING PROBLEMS?

Faintness and other symptoms of low blood pressure do not occur unless the reading drops below a certain level; in other words, there is a threshold. Readings above this threshold do not cause faintness. Values slightly below this threshold may result in lightheadedness. If much below this threshold, the lightheadedness increases and there is a risk of fainting. In other words, the drop in blood pressure from sitting to standing can be profound, but if the standing blood pressure does not drop below a certain threshold level, symptoms will not occur.

So what is the threshold value? This varies between people, but we can provide some general guidelines. It is simplest to focus on the systolic (upper) blood pressure value (e.g., the number, 120, from a blood pressure reading of 120/80). A general rule of thumb is: *A systolic blood pressure that is always above 90 is adequate and will not result in low blood pressure symptoms.* Extrapolating from that rule of thumb, consider the following examples.

> Mrs. Stone has a sitting blood pressure of 180/90, which drops to 110/70 when standing; since the systolic value of 110 is still well above 90, no symptoms result. This is despite a drop in the systolic blood pressure of 70.

> Mr. James has a sitting blood pressure of 110/70 that drops to 80/40, which results in faintness. Here, the drop in blood pressure is sufficient to reduce the pressure below threshold and cause symptoms.

The blood pressure threshold for faintness is around 90. A systolic blood pressure of 90 or higher provides adequate blood flow to your brain. Values below this may result in faintness, which is especially likely if much below 90. This is not to say that if your blood pressure drops below 90 you will feel faint. If slightly below and if your body is used to this, you may feel fine. However, the risk of faintness starts at about that level. As a corollary to this rule: *Dizziness experienced when the systolic blood pressure is above 90 is not due to low blood pressure.* In that case, consider some other explanation for your dizziness. It is important to emphasize, however, that this is valid if the blood pressure reading was taken when you are dizzy. This rule is not appropriate if the blood pressure reading was taken after feeling dizzy. Here is a scenario illustrating this mistake:

> Mr. Thomas walked across the living room and felt dizzy. He sat down and his wife measured his blood pressure. It was perfect at 120/80. They concluded that his dizziness was not due to low blood pressure.

What was wrong in reaching this conclusion? Once he sat down, his blood pressure likely reverted to normal. If he has orthostatic hypotension, it could be very low when standing/walking, but return to normal when he sits. His wife should have checked it in the standing position. Thus, if you are feeling dizzy, check the blood pressure when you are dizzy (assuming you are not so dizzy that you will faint).

BLOOD PRESSURE MAY VARY DRAMATICALLY: IMPORTANCE OF TIMING

The tendency to orthostatic hypotension often fluctuates throughout the course of the day. This variation is especially related to the transient effect of medica-

Table 21.2. Factors Predisposing to Fluctuations in Your Standing Blood Pressure

Factor	Effect on Standing Blood Pressure (BP)
Carbidopa/levodopa	Will tend to lower BP for 2–6 hours after each dose
Dopamine agonist medications (pramipexole, ropinirole, pergolide, bromocriptine)	Will tend to lower BP
Supplemental drugs: selegiline, COMT inhibitors (tolcapone, entacapone)	Will increase the tendency of levodopa to lower BP
Meals	Will tend to lower BP for a couple of hours
Night's sleep	Will tend to lower morning BP
Hot environments, such as hot tub	Heat will tend to dilate blood vessels and lower BP

tions and, in particular, carbidopa/levodopa. Thus, the low pressures will occur when the levodopa effect is most prominent, within a few hours after the last dose. On the other hand, when the levodopa effect has worn off, the blood pressure often reverts back to normal or even high.

Other factors may also contribute to orthostatic hypotension and play a role in its variability (see table 21.2). Meals tend to exacerbate orthostatic hypotension due to diversion of blood to the gut plus circulating factors released in the digestive process. Hence, those with orthostatic hypotension tend to experience symptoms after meals.

The tendency to orthostatic hypotension is also increased by a night's sleep. Thus it tends to be more of a problem in the morning than later in the day. Finally, a very hot environment, such as soaking in a hot tub, will tend to lower the blood pressure. This is because heat causes our blood vessels to dilate (expand). Because of these factors, the blood pressure of someone with PD may be normal at one time in the day and very low at another time. Hence, a single blood pressure reading is insufficient to draw any conclusions.

When will blood pressure be lowest? Usually right after breakfast. The combined effects of a recent night's sleep, a meal, and medications (first dose of carbidopa/levodopa taken before breakfast) will converge and may provoke orthostatic hypotension. Hence this is a good time to routinely check the standing blood pressure.

General Principles in Treating Orthostatic Hypotension

In orthostatic hypotension, the blood tends to pool in blood vessels of the legs when standing. There are two general strategies for increasing the standing-up blood pressure.

- Increase the volume of blood in your blood vessels. If you can add fluid to the blood supply, the pressure within these blood vessels increases.

- Constrict your blood vessels with medications or compressive stockings.

Both strategies are used to treat orthostatic hypotension.

INCREASING YOUR BLOOD VOLUME

How can you increase the volume of blood in your bloodstream? Simply drinking more water might seem like the appropriate treatment; however, this alone is insufficient. The kidneys regulate your water balance and extra water is usually rapidly excreted (into the urine). However, a crucial element that effectively holds the water in the circulation is sodium—salt (sodium chloride). Salt is the primary source of sodium. In general, the more water held in the bloodstream by sodium, the higher the blood pressure. This drawing of water into the bloodstream by sodium occurs by osmosis, the process that we studied in high school biology (but may have forgotten). Thus, adding salt to one's diet is often an initial step in treating orthostatic hypotension.

Ingesting salt may fail to adequately raise the blood pressure. Again, this is because of the kidneys. The kidneys tend to excrete extra salt into the urine. Sometimes this tendency can be overcome by administering large amounts of salt, in the form of salt tablets. Also, the tendency for the kidneys to remove salt from the bloodstream can be countered with a medication, fludrocortisone (Florinef). Fludrocortisone administration specifically causes the kidneys to retain sodium (salt). Hence this medication is often used to treat orthostatic hypotension.

The over-the-counter anti-inflammatory medications used for pain relief also tend to cause sodium retention. These are the so-called nonsteroidal anti-inflammatory drugs (NSAIDs), such as ibuprofen (Advil) and naproxen (Aleve); there are also a variety of prescription drugs from this class. However, the effect on blood pressure is slight and these have not been very effective in treating the orthostatic hypotension of PD.

COMPRESSIVE STOCKINGS

The tendency for blood to pool in the vessels of the legs can be offset by compressive stockings. Tight-fitting compressive stockings that go up to thigh or waist level are often effective treatments. These must be specifically fitted to match the size of your legs. Unfortunately, there is a major hassle factor with these compressive stockings; they are hard to put on and some people find these uncomfortable and hot in the summertime. They must be washed carefully with gentle detergents in cold water to avoid damaging the compressive elastic. Also, they are expensive since they must be custom fit to the leg size. Despite the efficacy of compressive stockings, many people discontinue using these because of the expense, discomfort, and inconvenience. In my practice, it is rare for someone to tolerate these beyond a few months.

MEDICATIONS TO CONSTRICT BLOOD VESSELS

Certain adrenaline-like medications will also raise the blood pressure. Some of these are available as over-the-counter drugs, such as ephedrine or phenylpropanolamine. However, the over-the-counter drugs also stimulate the heart and may cause too rapid a heart rate. The prescription drug midodrine (ProAmatine) raises the blood pressure by a similar adrenalin-like effect but spares the heart; it raises the BP primarily by constricting blood vessels.

OTHER MEASURES

As mentioned above, those with orthostatic hypotension will tend to have lower blood pressure in the morning. Elevating the head of the bed by about six inches may partially offset this. You can put bricks or blocks under the bedposts at the head of your bed.

Large meals contribute to orthostatic hypotension. If you frequently experience low blood pressure symptoms after eating a big meal, do the obvious: eat smaller meals. High-carbohydrate foods seem to be especially problematic at aggravating orthostatic hypotension and reducing carbs may additionally be helpful. Alcohol dilates blood vessels. Those with significant orthostatic hypotension should avoid alcoholic beverages.

WHAT SHOULD I DO IF I FEEL FAINT?

The measures noted above address prevention of orthostatic hypotension. If you do feel faint due to orthostatic hypotension, there are no medications that will immediately reverse your symptoms. However, there are some commonsense strategies to avoid faints.

In orthostatic hypotension, the blood pressure is low when you are on your feet. So what should you do? Sit down. If there is prominent faintness, don't try to tough it out or you might pass out. Usually sitting is adequate; however, if you still feel faint when sitting, lie down. Also, let your family know that if you start to faint they should not try to prop you up. This is a common error when someone starts to pass out; well-meaning friends or family often pull them back up to standing or sitting. If you are about to faint, the appropriate strategy is to lay you down. Why? Because it's a lot easier for the blood to flow from your heart to your brain when the heart doesn't need to pump upwards against gravity.

If orthostatic symptoms develop, how long will they persist? Typically they are time-locked to the effect of your carbidopa/levodopa dose; when it wears off, the blood pressure will rise again.

PRELUDE TO TREATMENT: NEED FOR FREQUENT BLOOD PRESSURE CHECKS

Blood pressure monitoring is imperative to adequately treat orthostatic hypotension. If you have orthostatic hypotension, purchase a home blood pressure testing device. When buying a blood pressure testing instrument, don't necessarily choose the cheapest; some of the less expensive instruments may not be calibrated for accurate readings in low ranges. If no one in the household has experience in taking blood pressures, have the nurse in your doctor's office instruct you.

Once you start checking your blood pressure, remember to check both the sitting and standing values. A common mistake is to record only the sitting pressure, which obviously misses the crucial readings when you have orthostatic hypotension.

When is the best time to check the blood pressure? As we discussed, the lowest readings will typically be in the morning after breakfast. This is a good time for one of your measurements. A second reading in the afternoon, after lunch, may also be helpful to determine if low readings persist. Once measures are taken to elevate the blood pressure, a third reading while lying in bed at the time you retire is appropriate. This is to make certain the readings don't go too high with treatment.

Be certain that blood pressure readings are taken within a couple of hours after a levodopa dose. Blood pressures may vary greatly between the levodopa on-state (when levodopa is working) and the levodopa off-state; it will typically be much lower when there is a good levodopa effect. In fact, it is often only low during levodopa on-states.

TREATMENT TARGETS: BLOOD PRESSURE RANGE

When treating orthostatic hypotension, it is difficult if not impossible to consistently achieve perfectly normal blood pressures. Hence, we will need to accept that. An occasional aberrant reading should not be cause for alarm unless it is some very extreme value.

The standing-up systolic blood pressures should be brought up to at least 90. This will provide adequate blood flow to your brain. What if your systolic blood pressure is occasionally 80 (e.g., 80/50)? This is acceptable if you don't feel faint and if most of the readings are higher than that.

Table 21.3.   Treatment of Orthostatic Hypotension: Blood Pressure Targets

Blood Pressure	Value	Position to Detect These Readings*
Too low?	If less than 90 systolic	Standing
Perfect	Systolic = 100–120 Diastolic = 60–80	
Too high?	If the systolic is over 160 or the diastolic over 95	Lying down

*The lowest readings will occur when standing and the highest, lying down. Hence these are the positions to assess the extremes.

What is the optimal blood pressure? In a perfect world, we would shoot for a systolic blood pressure of between 100 and 120. Similarly, the diastolic readings would be between 60 and 80. However, those with autonomic dysfunction cannot control the pressures precisely, so anticipate substantial deviations, even with the best of treatment. Again, we will not shoot for perfection, but rather target a broader range of blood pressures that are acceptable.

What is high blood pressure? As mentioned, we would like systolic blood pressures between 100 and 120. However, anticipate that our efforts will result in some higher readings. I typically will accept systolic values up to 160 and even a little higher than that if not frequent. We would like the diastolic blood pressures to be below 95. Since the highest blood pressures are found lying down, this is a good position to monitor for excessive values (see table 21.3).

Is it dangerous to have high blood pressure? Yes, but not for brief periods unless it is dramatically elevated. The primary problem with high blood pressure is that it contributes to hardening of the arteries—atherosclerosis—which leads to heart attacks and strokes. Atherosclerosis is basically a buildup of plaque inside artery walls. This occurs with aging and high blood pressure contributes prominently. If this plaque builds up and narrows the lumen, blood flow will be restricted. If blood flow to the heart muscle is restricted, a heart attack occurs. If blood flow to an area of the brain is restricted, this results in a stroke. However, this buildup of plaque inside artery walls is a slow, insidious process, occurring over years. Hence occasional, brief blood pressure elevations are not dangerous unless extremely high. What is an extremely high blood pressure that requires immediate attention? This varies depending on your usual blood pressure. However, systolic readings over 220 or diastolic readings over 120 that persist for more than a few hours should be brought to your physician's immediate attention.

Occasionally, when orthostatic hypotension is a problem during the day but high blood pressure is a problem at night, a short-acting blood pressure lowering drug may be added at bedtime. If this strategy is employed, however, be cautious to avoid low blood pressures during the night that might lead to faints when going to the bathroom.

REMINDER: HEART RHYTHM PROBLEMS MAY ALSO CAUSE FAINTNESS

Faintness developing in someone with PD is most often due to orthostatic hypotension. However, don't forget that heart rhythm irregularities are also a cause of faintness. If the heart beats too fast or too slow, the blood pressure may plummet. In contrast to the symptoms of orthostatic hypotension, faintness due to heart irregularities occurs in any body position and is not linked to standing. Heart rhythm spells tend to be infrequent and occur haphazardly. If faints or near faints develop in the seated or lying positions, heart irregularities should be considered.

If you think this might be the cause of your spells, learn to feel your pulse or have your spouse learn to do this. Then if symptoms develop, you can assess whether your heartbeat is very irregular, very slow, or very fast. This information could be very helpful to your physician.

Specific Treatment Strategies for Orthostatic Hypotension

My approach to treatment of orthostatic hypotension is based on several premises. First, it makes the most sense to do the simplest things first. Second, those strategies that are theoretically effective but which often fail in practice will not be emphasized. An example is treatment with an NSAID (e.g., ibuprofen, indomethacin). Third, those treatments that are rarely tolerated will also not be emphasized. An example of this is the use of compressive stockings, which can be very effective but are often not tolerated. Finally, it is important to continue to monitor the blood pressure (sitting and standing; also occasionally in bed in the evening); these readings are necessary to make the correct treatment decisions.

The general strategy that I use can be organized into a series of steps. Again, the target is a standing systolic pressure that is consistently at least 90, and frequent blood pressure checks are necessary. The order in which I do things is as follows (also summarized in table 21.4).

First, review your medication list as discussed above. Sometimes drugs of marginal benefit may be contributing to low blood pressure and can be eliminated. Occasionally, some with PD have been hypertensive, but no longer require blood pressure lowering drugs. Simply stopping offending medications may be a sufficient treatment.

Second, increase the salt in your diet. Often senior citizens are instructed to maintain a low salt diet, since high blood pressure is common in the general population. The head of the bed may also be elevated by 4–6 inches, although this makes a minor contribution to effective treatment. It does, however, help avoid high blood pressure when you sleep.

Table 21.4.   Maintaining an Adequate Blood Pressure (BP)

Target = Consistent Systolic Readings of at Least 90

Strategy *(Doing Simplest Things First)*	*Comment*
1. Review medication list	Physician to eliminate unnecessary drugs that lower BP
2. Exclude other causes of low BP, including blood tests	A complete blood count and chemistry profile may reveal other causes of low BP, such as anemia
3. Increase salt in diet*	Will also need to increase fluid intake (6–10 tall glasses of water, juice, soda pop daily)
4. Elevate head of bed	Raise head of bed 4–6 inches
5. Use salt tablets*	One tablet 2–3 times daily
6. Add fludrocortisone (Florinef)*	Dose of one tablet daily to two tablets twice daily. Induces the kidneys to retain salt rather than excreting it into the urine
7. Add midodrine (ProAmatine)	BP is raised for about 3–4 hours after each dose. Start with low dose, and raise as necessary

Note: Waist- or thigh-high compressive stockings, specially fitted to the leg size, can be a very effective treatment, if tolerated.

*If severe heart, kidney, or liver failure, salt is typically restricted and this must be discussed with your physician.

Third, if increasing the salt (sodium chloride) in the diet is insufficient, then the use of salt tablets is appropriate. These are available over the counter; one common brand is Thermotabs, but any brand is acceptable. Start with one salt tablet twice daily and increase to three times daily if necessary. It is often tolerated best if taken with or right after meals, but this isn't mandatory.

For salt supplementation to be effective, you need adequate intake of fluids. The salt (sodium) in your bloodstream draws in water, and you need adequate fluid intake to allow this. Water per se isn't mandatory; juice, soft drinks, and so on, are just fine. How much fluid is required? About six to ten tall (10-ounce) glasses daily should satisfy this fluid requirement. Don't go overboard on drinking fluids. You don't need more than about ten glasses daily. If you drink milk, recall that this is a protein drink and the protein may block levodopa passage to the brain (hence restrict milk to mealtimes).

Are there any reasons that increasing dietary salt or taking salt tablets might be a bad idea? Those with heart, liver, or kidney failure should not do this. If any serious heart, liver, or kidney problem is present, a careful review by a physician is required. If the above treatment results in shortness of breath, discuss this with your physician.

Increasing salt intake may also lead to mild swelling in your legs. This is usually not a serious problem. However, if it becomes very pronounced, talk with your physician. For leg swelling, elevating the legs is often an effective treatment. When you are sedentary, watching TV, reading the newspaper, and so on, rest your legs on a footrest that is about chest level. This helps gravity draw off the fluid, returning it to the circulation where the kidneys can excrete it. Remember that water pills (diuretics) are not an appropriate treatment for leg swelling in this situation. They will lower the blood pressure and increase orthostatic hypotension.

High salt intake may be associated with increased calcium excretion in your urine. The calcium concentrations in the bloodstream are very tightly regulated by internal mechanisms. To make up for dumping of calcium into the urine, calcium may be pulled out of bones to keep the blood concentrations of calcium at the ideal level. Extra dumping of calcium into the urine is not important if only for days or weeks. However, if this continues for years, this may lead to bone weakening (osteopenia/osteoporosis). Consequently, if a high salt intake is maintained, make certain that you are consuming enough calcium in your diet. For men and premenopausal women, 1200 mg of elemental calcium daily is necessary; for postmenopausal women, 1500 mg of daily elemental calcium is required. This calcium intake should be maintained when on high salt diets. Over-the-counter calcium supplements may be necessary. This is discussed further in chapter 30.

At this point, if you are not making progress, consider compressive hose. They can be very effective in controlling orthostatic hypotension. Admittedly, however, they are hard to put on, hot, and expensive, and few people in my practice are willing to put up with them. If you think you might tolerate them, see the section later in this chapter on compressive hose.

Fourth, if the above adjustments are inadequate, your physician can then prescribe fludrocortisone (Florinef). The starting dose is one 0.1 mg tablet daily. It takes about a week to appreciate the response. If insufficient, it can be raised to one 0.1 mg tablet twice daily. Higher doses may subsequently be administered; I usually push the dosage up to two 0.1 mg tablets twice daily before moving to the next step. Remember that fludrocortisone works by causing your kidneys to retain salt (sodium). Hence you need to continue the salt supplements (and fluid intake) for this to be effective.

The blood (serum) potassium level should be checked a week or two after starting fludrocortisone; it can cause loss of potassium into the urine. If the blood level of potassium is low, a potassium supplement should be given. Fludrocortisone is more effective when there are normal potassium concentrations in the blood.

Fifth, if the above measures fail, then midodrine (ProAmatine) is the appropriate next step. It is more expensive and a little more complicated to use than the other measures, so I usually save this medication for last. Note that it is used in conjunction with the above measures, not in place of these. In other words, you need to continue the salt supplements, fluids, fludrocortisone, and so on, and add midodrine to this program. Let's discuss some general facts and principles relating to midodrine; we will address dosing in the next section.

Midodrine will elevate the blood pressure for about 3–4 hours following each dose. This is just right for offsetting the blood pressure–lowering effect of levodopa. As we previously discussed, carbidopa/levodopa will lower the blood pressure for up to a few hours after each dose. Thus, if midodrine and carbidopa/levodopa are taken together, the blood pressure effects should cancel out (if the midodrine dose is high enough to do this).

Midodrine is usually started in a low dose and then raised, guided by the blood pressure readings. Because this drug works for only a few hours, doses will need to be repeated throughout the waking day.

Some people only have problems with low blood pressure in the morning, with salt, fluids, and fludrocortisone controlling blood pressures at other times. For this group, a single dose of midodrine in the morning is adequate. Sometimes a second dose in the late morning (3–4 hours after the first) is also required. Thus, it is important to check your standing blood pressures over the course of the day to document your needs.

Midodrine is taken only when you are up and about. Do not take it before bed. Obviously we do not want too high a blood pressure and taking midodrine before lying down may cause this. Recall that with orthostatic hypotension the blood pressure is low when on your feet; it is not low when lying in bed. Taking midodrine before you lie down could cause your blood pressure to go from normal to high.

Midodrine is an expensive medication. If money is an issue, you may reconsider compressive stockings at this juncture. Although they are not cheap, they don't cost anything after the initial investment. See the section later in this chapter on compressive hose.

A summary of these steps for treating orthostatic hypotension is attached at the end of this chapter, supplement 21.1. Photocopy this and have your physician check the boxes appropriate to your needs. You can then use this for quick reference.

SPECIFIC INSTRUCTIONS FOR MIDODRINE (PROAMATINE)

Midodrine can be very effective, but only if properly used. You need to follow these guidelines to obtain the desired effect and avoid side effects.

- Check the sitting and standing blood pressure at least twice daily. This should include readings in the morning, after breakfast, and again in the afternoon, after lunch. If only the morning systolic blood pressures are frequently below 90 (standing), then afternoon doses of midodrine will not be necessary.

- Do not take midodrine within 3 hours before going to bed at night. Also, avoid taking this before long daytime naps. Since the blood pressure will rarely be low when lying down, you don't need this before naps or bedtime and taking it then may cause the blood pressure to go from normal to high.

- The effect from midodrine lasts 3–4 hours; do not take it at intervals less than this. If taken at too brief intervals, the effects will overlap and summate.

- Midodrine can be taken with carbidopa/levodopa and often works best this way. The tendency for levodopa to lower the blood pressure can then be offset by midodrine.

- If carbidopa/levodopa is taken at intervals of less than three hours, then don't take midodrine with every carbidopa/levodopa dose, since the midodrine effects will overlap. In this case, it may work to take midodrine with every other dose of carbidopa/levodopa, recognizing that the midodrine effect lasts up to about four hours. Thus, if carbidopa/levodopa is required at 2-hour intervals, midodrine taken with every other dose will work out perfectly. You simply need to do the arithmetic, remembering that the midodrine response will last 3–4 hours.

- When starting midodrine, check the standing blood pressure 1–2 hours after each dose. After just a few readings, it will become apparent if the dose of midodrine is adequate. If the systolic blood pressure is still frequently below 90, then the dose can be raised, as often as every two days.

- Avoid overshooting with midodrine. The goal is to achieve standing systolic blood pressure readings of 90 to 120 and to avoid sitting or lying pressures much higher than 160/95. However, it is difficult to achieve perfection and occasional deviations that are not too far out of line may be accepted.

- Midodrine comes in three tablet sizes, 2.5 mg, 5 mg, and 10 mg. I usually begin with a dose of 2.5 mg, using 1/2 of a 5 mg tablet. Since the effect lasts for 3–4 hours, it is taken at this interval, unless only required in the morning. Usually the 2.5 mg dose is too low to substantially increase the blood pressure and further increments are required. The dose may be raised every few days with careful blood pressure monitoring. It can be increased by 1/2 tablet increments, using this 5 mg tablet until acceptable blood pressure readings are achieved. For example, if doses of 1/2 and then 1 of the 5 mg tablets are insufficient, then 1 1/2 tablets (7.5 mg) can be tried. Low blood pressures can typically be controlled with doses between 5 and 15 mg. How many doses each day are required depends on how many hours per day you are up and about (and whether you need coverage after the morning). The first dose of midodrine should be taken with the first dose of carbidopa/levodopa in the morning. If carbidopa/levodopa is taken at 3–6 hour intervals, subsequent midodrine doses can be taken with each of these carbidopa/levodopa doses. If carbidopa/levodopa is taken at less than 3-hour intervals, you could then consider taking midodrine with every other carbidopa/levodopa dose or simply taking midodrine at 4-hour intervals. The rule of thumb is that the midodrine effect lasts 3–4 hours and if taken at intervals of much less than this, the effect may overlap and summate.

- If the morning and afternoon blood pressure readings are both low (i.e., frequently less than 90 systolic), then midodrine is taken throughout the waking day (but not right before going to bed at night). However, if only the morning blood pressure is low, midodrine can be taken just in the morning.

The midodrine dosing instructions in supplement 21.2 at the end of this chapter incorporate these principles. This is divided into instructions for those requiring only morning treatment and for those who will require midodrine throughout the waking day. Photocopy this to guide you.

TREATMENT EXAMPLES

Although the treatment of orthostatic hypotension can get complicated, careful attention to these guidelines should allow control. Let us illustrate this with a couple of examples.

> Mrs. Thomas frequently feels faint and this problem recurs throughout the waking day. Blood pressure readings when standing are often around 80/50 and sometimes lower. However, when her levodopa effect has worn off, the blood pressure returns to normal. She takes carbidopa/levodopa every 3 hours (six doses a day, with the last at bedtime). Salt supplementation and fludrocortisone have only partially been helpful and she could not stand wearing compressive stockings. What to do?

This is an appropriate situation for midodrine. I would begin with 1/2 of a 5 mg midodrine tablet with each of her first five doses of carbidopa/levodopa. She should not take midodrine with her last carbidopa/levodopa dose, since this is at bedtime. As she continues taking blood pressure readings, she will learn whether these doses are sufficient (2.5 mg doses are usually insufficient). Since the effect of midodrine is almost immediate, it doesn't take many doses to determine the effect; this will be apparent in a few days at most. If she still runs pressures of around 80/50, then she could raise the dosage to 1 and subsequently 1 1/2 of the 5 mg tablets five times daily. After a few more days, if the readings are still low, and if she is still experiencing faintness, she could then raise the midodrine to two 5 mg tablets with her first five carbidopa/levodopa doses. Occasionally, up to three tablets each dose may be necessary (i.e., three 5 mg tablets five times daily).

Mr. Peterson has an almost identical story, but he takes carbidopa/levodopa every two and a half hours. When his levodopa effect is present ("on"), he runs low blood pressures and feels faint. If it wears off, the readings normalize. However, he is careful about taking his carbidopa/levodopa and he rarely is in an off-state. Simpler measures have not been adequate and he is ready to start midodrine. How should he do this?

First, we should ask him whether his blood pressures are low all day or only in the morning. If the latter, then only morning doses of midodrine are necessary. Let's assume, however, that the pressures are low all day long. Recall that midodrine has a 3–4 hour effect, yet his carbidopa/levodopa doses are at an interval (2 1/2 hours) that doesn't fit precisely. There are two options. One is to take a midodrine dose with every carbidopa/levodopa dose and monitor the blood pressures to make certain that with this small overlap the blood pressures don't go too high. The other option is to take the midodrine every 3–4 hours on a separate schedule from carbidopa/levodopa. However, this is more complex and it may be difficult to stay on time with two different dosing schemes.

Mr. Peterson now complains that he is also experiencing wearing-off of his levodopa effect with the 2 1/2 hour carbidopa/levodopa intervals; that is, a little before each dose of carbidopa/levodopa, he develops tremor and walking problems. This is in addition to the low blood pressures.

There is an easy solution. First, have him reduce the interval between his carbidopa/levodopa doses to every two hours (this will counter the wearing-off problems). Second, have him take a dose of midodrine with every other dose of carbidopa/levodopa. Thus he will be taking carbidopa/levodopa every two hours and midodrine every 4 hours.

PYRIDOSTIGMINE TREATMENT OF ORTHOSTATIC HYPOTENSION

Recent preliminary reports suggest that the drug used to treat myasthenia gravis, pyridostigmine (Mestinon), improves orthostatic hypotension. Doses of one-half to one 60 mg tablet elevate the standing blood pressure for a few hours. The effect parallels the time course of midodrine and hence could similarly be taken with each carbidopa/levodopa dose to offset levodopa blood pressure effects. Side effects are not serious, but include loose stools, sweating, or urinary urgency. Since I have not had personal experience with pyridostigmine for this purpose, I will not comment further in this chapter.

When Treatment Is Insufficient

If you have done all of the above and you are still experiencing unacceptable symptoms of orthostatic hypotension, we are then ready to reconsider compressive hose. As mentioned, most people have trouble tolerating these. However, when all else fails, these may be the answer.

Compression of leg veins with tight-fitting hose can be quite helpful in treating orthostatic hypotension. They prevent the pooling of blood in the lower extremities. This, in effect, helps squeeze blood upwards towards the brain.

These should be a first-line treatment of orthostatic hypotension, but they do have a few practical drawbacks that often dissuade people from using these. They are:

- Tight and hot

- Hard to put on, especially for someone with PD

- Expensive (and multiple pairs are required)

- Harder to wash than your regular hose (requires washing by hand with gentle detergents to avoid damaging the elastic)

- Specially fitted, requiring measurements of calf, thigh, and foot to ensure proper fit

Nonetheless, if simpler measures fail, or if the medications noted prove insufficient or not tolerated, these are an option. In fact, if you think you will be able to tolerate them, go ahead and try them as a first option rather than last resort. Here are a few things you need to know about compressive hose for orthostatic hypotension.

- They must be thigh-high or waist-high to be useful for treating orthostatic hypotension. Knee-high hose do not work. Knee-high stockings may help reduce leg swelling but they need to be higher to counter low blood pressures. The waist-high hose work a little better than the thigh-high.

- They need to be fitted according to your leg size. There are specific sites on your legs to take the measurements. You will need to refer to instructions from the stocking company or the medical supply store advising exactly how to do this. This is best done by the person waiting on you in the medical supply store or a physical therapist (physical therapists are knowledgeable about these stockings).

- There are two standard pressures, 20–30 mm Hg (millimeters of mercury, a measurement of pressure) and 30–40 mm Hg. The 30–40 mm Hg stockings are a little more effective (squeeze a little tighter) but are also a little harder to get on. You might start with the 20–30 mm Hg stockings and see if they are adequate.

- Pay close attention to the washing instructions, since very hot water and certain harsh detergents may damage the elastic and make these baggy and useless.

- An abdominal binder can supplement these hose, available from medical supply companies. Binders fit around your waist and help squeeze blood up toward your brain. You will need to try one of these on before you purchase them to make sure they will be tolerated when sitting. They come in different lengths. You can adjust the pressure using Velcro fasteners.

- Often physiatrists and physical therapists can assist and advise about these garments.

- Put the hose on before you get out of bed. Often blood pressure is lowest early in the morning and faintness may be a risk on your way to the bathroom.

You will probably want to purchase two pairs of hose—one to wear and one to wash. However, you may not tolerate these, so defer buying more than two in the beginning. Additional pairs can later be purchased.

Avoid any tight bands around your legs, such as rubber bands or stockings with an elastic band that cuts into your leg. Compressive hose facilitate the flow of blood out of your legs because of the widespread pressure gradient. However, narrow bands around your legs may do the opposite; they may block the flow of blood and may even lead to a blood clot in your leg (thrombophlebitis).

There are tricks for putting these on. The manufacturer often provides helpful tips and may also supply simple devices for assisting. Some people find that these go on more easily if they wear rubber gloves to get a better grip. The rubber gloves sold for dishwashing are adequate as long as they fit tightly.

TRICKS FOR QUICKLY RAISING YOUR BLOOD PRESSURE

If you are about to faint, sit down; if very faint, lie down. However, there are a few things you can do when the faintness is not too severe and sitting is not possible. When standing, cross your legs and squeeze your thigh muscles together. This muscle contraction state helps squeeze the blood upstream. Bending forward as if you are tying your shoe may also help counter faintness. Squatting may additionally be effective. If you need to do a few tasks in the kitchen, you can buy some time by placing one leg up on a chair while you work. Remember, however, if you feel very faint, you need to sit and, if necessary, lie down.

RECORD YOUR BLOOD PRESSURE READINGS

Remember that it is very important to record your blood pressure readings. You and your physician need this data to make therapeutic decisions. At the end of this chapter is a blood pressure record that you may photocopy for this purpose (supplement 21.3).

Supplement 21.1.

Instructions for Treating Orthostatic Hypotension

Photocopy and use for quick reference. Your physician may check the appropriate boxes. Blood pressure readings below 90 systolic are too low.

☐ Check your sitting and standing blood pressure _____ times per day, including after breakfast. Also check your blood pressure if you feel dizzy.

☐ Increase the salt in your diet.

☐ If the standing blood pressure readings are frequently below 90 systolic, purchase salt (sodium chloride) tablets and take one tablet twice daily. If the systolic blood pressures are still often less than 90 in the standing position, increase this to one tablet three times daily.

☐ If salt tablets are started, adequate calcium intake via diet or supplements is necessary to prevent weak bones. Men and premenopausal women require 1200 mg of elemental calcium daily; postmenopausal women require 1500 mg of elemental calcium daily. A daily multivitamin will provide the necessary vitamin D for calcium absorption.

☐ Check your blood pressure in the evening in the lying position to make certain that these measures do not raise it too high. Readings less than 160/95 are desirable. If the systolic readings are frequently much higher than these values, bring this to the attention of your physician.

☐ Elevate the head of your bed about six inches.

☐ If the standing blood pressure readings continue to be less than 90 systolic, despite the above, start the medication fludrocortisone (Florinef). Begin with the single 0.1 mg tablet once per day. After one week, if the systolic blood pressure readings in the standing position are still frequently less than 90, increase this to one tablet twice per day. It may be increased as high as two of these tablets twice daily, but do this only if your physician directs. Remember that you still need to have salt plus adequate liquids in your diet for the fludrocortisone to work.

If the above treatment strategies prove inadequate, start midodrine (ProAmatine). See the guidelines for use on the separate midodrine instruction sheet.

Supplement 21.2.

Midodrine (ProAmatine) Instructions

Photocopy and have your physician check the appropriate box below.

- Each dose of midodrine will elevate your blood pressure for about 3–4 hours.

- Check the sitting and standing blood pressures at least twice daily (after breakfast and after lunch).

- Systolic blood pressure target: at least 90 standing (accept occasional deviations).

- Midodrine should be taken only during the waking day; do not take within 3 hours of going to bed. If a prolonged nap in the middle of the day, skip the dose of midodrine before the nap.

- Midodrine offsets the blood pressure lowering effect of carbidopa/levodopa, and these drugs may be taken together to offset that effect.

If your standing systolic blood pressure readings are less than 90 only in the morning, then only morning doses are required. If your systolic blood pressures are less than 90 all day long, then you will need it throughout the day. Have your physician check the box appropriate for you.

☐ *For those with a low standing blood pressure only in the morning:* Start with 1/2 of a 5 mg tablet of midodrine with the first dose of carbidopa/levodopa in the morning. Don't go back to bed. Check your sitting and standing blood pressure 1–2 hours later and continue to do that on successive days.

- After 4–5 days, if the standing blood pressure (systolic) is still less than 90, raise the midodrine dose to 1 tablet (5 mg).

- After 4–5 days, if the standing blood pressure (systolic) is still less than 90, raise the midodrine dose to 1 1/2 tablets (7.5 mg).

- After 4–5 more days, if the standing blood pressure (systolic) remains less than 90, then raise the midodrine dose to 2 tablets (total of 10 mg).

- After 4–5 more days, if the standing blood pressure is still less than 90 (systolic), then raise the midodrine dose to 2 1/2 tablets (total of 12.5 mg).

- After 4–5 more days, if the standing blood pressure continues to be less than 90 (systolic), then raise the midodrine dose to 3 tablets (15 mg).

If your schedule calls for a late-morning dose of carbidopa/levodopa, also check your standing blood pressure about 1–2 hours after that. If this is low (less than 90 systolic), then also add a second dose of midodrine with this carbidopa/levodopa dose (use the same dose you took earlier in the morning). In general, an occasional systolic reading between 80 and 90 is acceptable as long as most are above 90.

☐ *For those with a low standing blood pressure throughout the waking day:* The number of midodrine doses you take will depend on how often you take carbidopa/levodopa; your physician should check the appropriate box below corresponding to your carbidopa/levodopa dosing schedule.

   ☐ If carbidopa/levodopa is taken every 3–8 hours, then midodrine can be taken with each carbidopa/levodopa dose.

   ☐ If carbidopa/levodopa is taken every 2 hours, then midodrine can be taken with every other carbidopa/levodopa dose.

   ☐ If carbidopa/levodopa is taken at less than 2-hour intervals, then midodrine should be scheduled at about 4-hour intervals, starting at the time of the first carbidopa/levodopa dose of the day.

Start with 1/2 of a 5 mg tablet of midodrine for each dose. Continue to check your sitting and standing blood pressure 1–2 hours after both a morning and afternoon dose.

- After 4–5 days, if most of the standing blood pressures are still less than 90 (systolic), raise the midodrine doses to 1 tablet (5 mg).

- After 4–5 days, if most of the standing blood pressures are still less than 90 (systolic), raise the midodrine doses to 1 1/2 tablets (7.5 mg).

- After 4–5 days, if most of the standing blood pressures remain less than 90 (systolic), raise the midodrine doses to 2 tablets (10 mg).

- After 4–5 days, if most of the standing blood pressures are still less than 90 (systolic), raise the midodrine doses to 2 1/2 tablets (12.5 mg).

- After 4–5 days, if most of the standing blood pressures continue to be less than 90 (systolic), raise the midodrine doses to 3 tablets (15 mg).

In general, an occasional systolic reading between 80 and 90 is acceptable as long as most are above 90.

Supplement 21.3.

Blood Pressure Chart

Photocopy and record your blood pressures to guide you and your physician.

Date and Time	Symptoms (if present)	Sitting BP	Standing BP	Lying BP

22

◆ ◆ ◆

Depression

Depression is a mental state. It is synonymous with feeling blue, unhappy, sad, gloomy, hopeless, melancholy, and so on. It is a perceptual state: the glass is always half-empty rather than half full. One sees only the dark side of things. It is tied to daily activities; it sabotages motivation and saps energy. It affects the most basic elements of life, causing insomnia, loss of appetite, and sexual dysfunction. Sometimes it's linked to obsessive worry and rumination, always anticipating and expecting the worst to happen.

Why Do People Become Depressed?

We all encounter things in life that eat at our souls. Who would not be depressed when a loved one dies or illness strikes the family? If you have Parkinson's disease (PD), the prospect of a chronic disease is discouraging in and of itself. If you have had to restrict your lifestyle because of PD, that is all the more reason to become discouraged. Hence depression is a part of the normal human existence and is appropriate during times when things are going very badly. Depression becomes pathological when it is prolonged, severe, or out of proportion to events. Although depression may be triggered by major life trauma, it sometimes comes out of nowhere.

When depression becomes pathologic and disabling, it presumably is associated with changes in brain chemistry. Deficient activity of such brain neurotransmitters as serotonin, norepinephrine, and dopamine are believed to underlie depressive states. PD predisposes to this by virtue of the neurodegenerative process also affecting these systems. In PD, the same process that causes degeneration of the dopamine-containing neurons in the substantia nigra leads to degeneration of brain neurons containing serotonin, norepinephrine, as well as other dopamine systems. Hence it's not surprising that people with PD are predisposed to depression. On the other hand, the recognition of the biochemical substrates of depression has opened the door to medical treatment.

How Do I Know If I Am Depressed?

It may be difficult to be objective about one's emotional state. Reading your own psyche in an unbiased manner is not something most of us are good at doing. Am I just a little discouraged by a few of life's downturns or has this blue outlook reached pathological proportions? It is helpful to discuss this with a loved one, your physician, clergy, or a professional psychologist or psychiatrist. The typical symptoms are summarized in table 22.1.

You will note from this table that PD causes symptoms that look like depression. Your spouse may notice that you don't smile anymore but that may reflect the facial masking of PD. You may have scaled back your activities, but perhaps that has to do with the reduced energy that is part of PD. Similarly, some of the signs that psychiatrists use as indicators of depression, such as reduced appetite, insomnia, and reduced libido, may be due to PD, your PD medications, or both.

The decision to treat your depression may be made by your family physician, internist, neurologist, or a psychiatrist. If the problem is straightforward, your primary physician may feel comfortable initiating treatment.

"But I'm Not Depressed!"

There is typically a tendency to resist and deny a diagnosis of depression. Some people view this as a sign of weakness: "I should be able to deal with this on my own!" Being stubborn about this, however, may deprive you of experiencing life's pleasures once again; this might be right around the corner with appropriate treatment. In most cases, the treatments are effective and well tolerated; they should be welcomed. Years ago there was stigma tied to a diagnosis of depression. Now, with celebrity lives made public by the media, we have grown accustomed to seeing our favorite and most respected public figures treated for depression and related disorders. Like stomach ulcers and asthma, depression is now recognized for what it is, a bona fide medical illness. This is even more apparent in the case of PD; depression is typically caused or exacerbated by changes in brain chemistry as part of the underlying neurodegenerative process.

Table 22.1.   Symptoms of Depression*

Symptom	Comment
Sadness, tearfulness, feeling blue	
Loss of interest	
Reduced activities and energy (but sometimes agitation)	But PD also reduces energy levels
Rumination and worry	
Everything seems bleak and hopeless	
Focus on the negative; failing to see the positive	
Poor self-esteem, guilt, worthlessness	
No longer smiling	But hard to tell when PD causes masking
Loss of appetite (sometimes increased appetite)	Poor appetite could be due to medications
Insomnia	But often is due to PD (which responds to PD drugs, as discussed in chapter 20)
Sleeps excessively	But this may be related to medications, or the effects of PD on sleep patterns (see chapter 20)
Reduced libido	But may have other causes such as age, drugs, as well as PD (see chapter 28 on sexual functioning)
Thoughts of death, suicide	Suggests urgent attention necessary

*Considered significant when depressed mood and other symptoms interfere with daily functioning and persist beyond two weeks.

Suicide

Depression may make life seem not worth living. "I would rather be dead." If depression reaches these proportions, objective thought is often no longer possible. In fact this is what depression often does. It may produce thoughts so twisted and dark that perceptions of the world are turned inside out. Everything is evil and worthless, especially me. Why live in this world?

If depression is sinking to these depths and leading to thoughts of suicide, it is critical to cry out for help. You will not be able to work through this type of a depressive illness when suicidal thoughts are becoming prominent. Call your doctor, and when you meet in the office, be open about the depths of the depression. If you have contemplated suicide, this must be put on the table. Your doctor will know what to do.

Origins of Depression in PD

PD predisposes to depression for a variety of reasons.

- It may be a reaction to the disability of PD. Such depression may improve simply with treatment of your parkinsonism.

- It may relate to the dopamine deficiency state. For example, some with fluctuating motor responses note that depression coincides with their levodopa off-states; this lifts when the levodopa response kicks in. Appropriate treatment is the same as for the motor symptoms of PD.

- It may relate to a deficiency of the brain neurotransmitter serotonin, caused by the PD neurodegenerative process. This can be adequately treated with drugs that enhance serotonin activity within the brain. Drugs from the medication class called selective serotonin reuptake inhibitors (SSRIs) are often effective. Theoretically these may aggravate parkinsonism, but in practice they typically are well tolerated by those with PD.

- Other brain chemistry problems linked to PD may also play a role in depression. For example, the PD neurodegenerative process also affects brain systems containing the neurotransmitter norepinephrine. Deficient activity of this neurotransmitter is known to cause depression, and antidepressant drugs are available that target norepinephrine.

Pseudo-dementia

People who are depressed may seem dull and uninterested to the point of seeming demented. In other words, depression can affect your ability to think and remember. Physicians call this pseudo-dementia and recognize that this possibility must be considered when evaluating people with impaired thinking. The good news is that this is treatable; once depression is controlled, memories and thoughts flow once again.

Treatment of Depression

As you might surmise, the treatment needs to fit the problem. The therapeutic strategies differ depending on the severity, the cause(s), the family, and other support systems. The basic elements of the treatment approach start with the following.

- Treat the symptoms of PD. Unless the depression is quite severe, I typically do this first. Sometimes the improvement in gait, tremor, and mobility are sufficient to improve one's outlook and reverse depression.

- Treat insomnia. Although insomnia may be a symptom of depression, it may also be a cause of depression, if sleep deprivation is marked. Many people with PD require levodopa therapy at bedtime or during the night to attain a good night's sleep (refer back to chapter 20).

- Make a conscious effort to be active. It's easy to sit back on the couch in front of the TV if you're not feeling 100 percent. However, this feeds into the depressive process. If you are physically able to be up and about, force yourself, little by little, to engage in social and recreational activities.

Your physician will need to decide with you when to start an antidepressant drug; this decision is based on the severity of your problem and the likelihood that these simple measures will be sufficient. The medications we have for treating depression are usually effective, easy to use, and well tolerated; hence doctors usually have a low threshold for starting one of these drugs.

One important thing to keep in mind about all drugs used to treat depression is that they are slow to work. They don't produce a high. Rather, they gradually, over weeks, change the brain chemistry to give you a more positive outlook on life. The benefits never happen suddenly. It is often several weeks later that you realize you are feeling much better. Those who are always worrying about every small incident begin to appreciate that these ruminations are slowly fading away. Given the insidious and slow responses with these medications, you need to be patient. Anticipate that it may take 6–8 weeks or so for the benefits to become apparent.

Table 22.2 lists the medications commonly used to treat depression. The middle column lists the " typical starting dose" for each drug. In many cases, this is too low to be consistently effective. However, the medication is started conservatively to make certain that it is tolerated before escalating to doses more likely to be effective. Often the starting dose is maintained for one to two weeks and then raised. The last column, "usual dose range," provides the doses that are typically employed on a long-term basis. If the starting dose is tolerated after one to two weeks, then it can be raised to correspond with the lower dose in the last column. That should be maintained for several weeks to determine if this dose is effective. Your physician could then recommend a higher dose if necessary.

This list in table 22.2 is long and not all of these drugs are appropriate for every person. Some of these medications are sedating and some have an opposite effect. They differ in terms of other potential side effects as well. Physicians usually have a few favorites that they have found effective and well tolerated; they then tend to stick with them. Let's consider each of these drug classes.

Table 22.2. Medications Commonly Used to Treat Depression

Class of Drug/Medication	Typical Starting Dose	Usual Dose Range
SSRI		
Fluoxetine (Prozac)	10 mg each morning	10–50 mg each morning
Sertraline (Zoloft)	25 mg each morning	50–150 mg each morning
Paroxetine (Paxil)	10 mg each morning	10–40 mg each morning
Paroxetine sustained release (Paxil CR)	12.5 mg each morning	25–50 mg each morning
Fluvoxamine (Luvox)	50 mg at bedtime	100 mg once at bedtime–300 mg daily in 2 divided doses
Citalopram (Celexa)	10 mg once daily (A.M. or P.M.)	20–40 mg once daily (A.M. or P.M.)
Escitalopram (Lexapro)	10 mg once daily (A.M. or P.M.)	10–20 mg once daily (A.M. or P.M.)
Tricyclics		
Amitriptyline (Elavil)	10–25 mg at bedtime	75–150 mg at bedtime
Desipramine (Norpramin)	10–25 mg at bedtime	75–150 mg at bedtime or divided into 2 daily doses
Doxepin (Sinequan)	10–25 mg at bedtime	75–150 mg at bedtime
Imipramine (Tofranil)	10–25 mg at bedtime	50–150 mg at bedtime
Nortriptyline (Pamelor, Aventyl)	10–25 mg at bedtime	50–150 mg at bedtime or divided into 2–3 daily doses
Protriptyline (Vivactil)	5 mg once to twice daily	5 mg 3–4 times daily
Trimipramine (Surmontil)	25 mg at bedtime	50–150 mg daily as either a bedtime dose or divided into two daily doses
Clomipramine (Anafranil)	10–25 mg at bedtime	75–150 mg at bedtime

Others

Bupropion (Wellbutrin)	75–100 mg each morning	100 mg two to three times daily
Bupropion sustained-release (Wellbutrin SR)	150 mg each morning	150 mg once to twice daily
Maprotiline (Ludiomil)	25 mg–75 mg once daily	50 mg–150 mg as a single dose or divided doses
Mirtazapine (Remeron)	15 mg at bedtime	15 mg–45 mg at bedtime
Nefazodone (Serzone)	100 mg at bedtime	100 mg–200 mg twice daily
Trazodone (Desyrel)	50 mg at bedtime	50 mg–200 mg twice daily
Venlafaxine (Effexor)	25 mg twice to three times daily	25 mg–75 mg three times daily
Venlafaxine sustained-release (Effexor XR)	37.5 mg–75 mg once daily	75 mg–225 mg once daily
Duloxetine (Cymbalta)	20 mg once to twice daily	20–30 mg twice daily (or 60 mg once daily)

SSRI Medications

The SSRI drugs are favored by many physicians as initial treatment of depression; these are listed first in table 22.2. SSRI stands for selective serotonin reuptake inhibitor. Serotonin is a brain neurotransmitter. We have known for some time that it is found in brain circuits linked to affective states, that is, states of elation and depression. Brain serotonin activity is low in at least some people with depression. Moreover, brain serotonin levels are reduced among people with PD due to the underlying neurodegenerative process that also damages brain serotonin neurons. The SSRI drugs increase the activity of brain serotonin systems. They do this by blocking the reuptake of serotonin.

What is reuptake? Neurons containing serotonin use this neurotransmitter to signal the next neuron in the brain circuit. The neuron releases tiny amounts of serotonin into the synapse, activating the receptor on the adjoining neuron. If the released serotonin remains in the synapse, the receptor will continue to be activated. The signal is terminated by sucking the serotonin back into the cell that released it. This is termed reuptake. When this process is blocked by the SSRI drug, serotonin remains in the synapse longer and continues to stimulate the serotonin receptor. Thus SSRI drugs increase the activity of brain serotonin.

Among the SSRI drugs listed in table 22.2, no one stands out as superior. They are all quite effective, although if one fails, that does not mean that another may not work. These drugs typically do not make people sleepy (with the exception of fluvoxamine: Luvox). They are simple to use, requiring only one dose daily, although fluvoxamine is often administered twice a day.

My usual medication choice for treatment of depression is a drug from this SSRI class. They are usually effective, easy to use, and have few side effects.

INSOMNIA AND SSRI DRUGS

The SSRI medications may induce insomnia if taken later in the day (except for fluvoxamine, which is sedating); hence, they are usually administered in the morning. If insomnia is a problem, it may be appropriate to add a low dose of one of the sedating antidepressants at bedtime. Typically the drug chosen for that purpose is trazodone. Trazodone in a dose of 50 mg, taken a little before bedtime, is usually adequate to induce sleep. If ineffective, the dose can be raised to 100 mg.

CAN SSRI DRUGS CAUSE OR WORSEN PARKINSONISM?

There have been a number of published reports of SSRI medications inducing parkinsonism. However, in my experience, this is extremely rare. It is also very rare for one of these SSRI medications to worsen parkinsonism in someone with PD. I have been involved in the care of hundreds of people with PD who have been treated with an SSRI medication and almost never see any problems of this type. Hence I regard this as a safe class of drugs for people with PD. If you experience a problem, however, you can switch to another medication from table 22.2.

Tricyclic Medications

The tricyclics, the second class of drugs shown in table 22.2, are so named because of their chemical structure (three chemical rings). They are the oldest class of antidepressants and were the primary medications used for years, prior to the development of the SSRI drugs. They have more side effects than the newer drugs and now are prescribed less often for that reason. Except for protriptyline, they tend to be sedating; however, this is often not a problem since they are usually administered as a single bedtime dose (beneficial in some cases). They also tend to have anticholinergic side effects, which include constipation, dry mouth, visual blurring, and rarely mild memory impairment. They tend to dampen the urinary flow, which may be advantageous if you are experiencing urinary urgency but problematic if you have trouble starting your stream.

Other Medications for Depression

The last category of drugs shown on table 22.2 ("Others") is a heterogeneous group of newer drugs that are fairly well tolerated and effective. Some physicians may choose one of these as their favored initial medication for treatment of depression. The exception is trazodone, which is used only rarely to treat depression but frequently to treat insomnia. Mirtazapine and nefazodone tend to be sedating and sometimes are prescribed for people who are agitated or can't sleep in addition to being depressed.

Blocking Reuptake of Other Brain Neurotransmitters

Most of the drugs listed in table 22.2 block the reuptake of serotonin. However, deficiencies of two other brain neurotransmitters have also implicated in depression—norepinephrine and dopamine. Some of these drugs block reuptake of these neurotransmitters, either selectively or in addition to serotonin.

Brain dopamine is deficient in PD, and you might think that an antidepressant blocking dopamine reuptake might be effective when depression develops. Bupropion selectively blocks reuptake of dopamine, but it doesn't seem to have any unique benefit in management of depression in PD. However, no clinical trial has compared bupropion head to head with any of the

SSRI drugs in depressed people with PD. It is a reasonable choice for depression treatment in PD, as are many of the other drugs. Bupropion is also used for smoking cessation (Zyban).

Desipramine (Norpramin) selectively blocks norepinephrine reuptake, whereas venlafaxine (Effexor) and duloxetine (Cymbalta) block reuptake of both norepinephrine and serotonin. Intuitively, you would expect this to confer some very unique properties, but in fact differences compared to the SSRI drugs are not striking.

Talk Therapy

For some, an appropriate medication for depression, plus the simple strategies described above, may be sufficient to turn the corner. For others, there may be things weighing on their minds. Without doubt, people who are depressed benefit from talking to someone. Occasionally someone other than a psychiatrist or psychotherapist may be appropriate. Clergy or family may serve in that capacity (although the family member needs to be patient, nonjudgmental, and more willing to listen than talk, which may be difficult). Usually your personal physician with a busy practice is not in a position to be a good listener because of time constraints. However, he or she could direct you to a counselor, psychologist, or psychiatrist.

Electroconvulsive Therapy (ECT)

Electroconvulsive therapy or ECT has been used for many years to treat depression resistant to simpler forms of therapy. It is a last resort. Only infrequently is it required to treat depression in the context of PD, but when employed in that situation it often works well. In fact, for a brief time (days to weeks) after the ECT treatment, parkinsonian movement symptoms are improved. This is most apparent the day of the treatment and may require a reduction of carbidopa/levodopa on that treatment day. ECT involves administering an electrical shock to the brain. It briefly convulses the brain and in doing this seems to wipe it clean of bad thoughts and memories. For a day or a few days memory may be impaired, but when it then comes back, it tends to return without the baggage of all the ruminations and dark thoughts that had been plaguing that person.

Usually ECT is initially performed in a hospital. However, once things are stabilized, it can be done in an outpatient clinic. For people with the most severe and disabling depression that has defied all other forms of treatment, this can be life saving.

23

◆ ◆ ◆

Thinking, Memory, and Dementia

Parkinson's disease (PD) is primarily a disorder affecting movement, but memory, judgment, and thinking may become impaired in some cases. The physician's term for thinking, judgment, and memory is cognition. When impairment of cognition is substantial, irreversible, and interfering with activities of daily living, we term this dementia.

Dementia may complicate otherwise typical PD, representing progression of the disease process. When this has been assessed in PD clinics, it is found in a minority of patients and usually late in the course. Thus, just because you have PD does not mean that you are destined to become demented. Moreover, not everyone with PD who complains of memory impairment is demented. There are other reasons why thinking and memory may be affected. Let's consider this in more detail.

Normal Aging and Memory

Like the rest of the body, the brain ages and memory declines with age. Those over seventy typically have occasional difficulties recalling names and phone numbers. If you fall into this age class and this is your problem, you may consider this part of the normal aging process.

Bradyphrenia: Slowed Thinking

People with PD experience slowed movements, termed bradykinesia (brady = slow). Similarly, they also may experience slowness of thinking, termed bradyphrenia. Those with bradyphrenia can arrive at the right answer; it just takes longer. The checkbook still balances but the answers come more slowly and deliberately. Bradyphrenia should not be interpreted as an early sign of dementia.

Treatment of bradyphrenia is the same as bradykinesia. Just as levodopa therapy or dopamine agonist drugs improve your movements, they also tend to speed up the thought process. It may not get back to your normal level but can improve if your PD medications are optimally adjusted.

Pseudo-dementia: Depression

People with prominent depression become apathetic. They seem dull, lose interest in their normal activities, have impaired memory, and are unable to make decisions. They may even say things that don't make much sense, not because they are confused, but because they don't care. As such, severe depression may occasionally be mistaken for dementia. This is an important distinction to make since depression is a very treatable disorder.

Diagnosing depression and gauging the severity can be difficult in PD; many of the clues pointing to depression are also signs of parkinsonism. The facial masking of PD makes people appear depressed. People with PD may restrict their social and recreational activities, not because of depression but because it simply is harder to do these things. Appetite loss may not be a sign of depression but could be due to PD medications or PD-related problems of the digestive system (chapter 26). Insomnia, another sign of depression, is also a product of PD.

To determine whether depression is masquerading as dementia sometimes requires consultation with a psychiatrist. This is usually supplemented with formal testing of intellectual function (psychometric testing).

Poor Sleep and Cognition

If you're sleep deprived, it's hard to think straight. Those who are severely and chronically deprived of sleep may function like someone in the early stages of dementia. Sleep deprivation should be obvious; after all, we know if we are not sleeping. However, it could also be occurring in a subtle fashion, due to disordered breathing during sleep (sleep apnea) or repetitive leg jerks while asleep (so-called periodic leg movements of sleep). In such cases, you perceive that you slept through the night and probably did. However, *deep* sleep will not have been achieved due to the arousing effects of breathing difficulties or movements recurring throughout the night. If this sufficiently disrupts deep sleep, thinking will be affected. This was discussed in chapter 20.

Medication Effects on Thinking and Memory

Certain medications may compromise your memory and occasionally lead to confusion. This is more likely if you are:

- A senior citizen
- Experiencing mild memory problems even before these medications
- Taking multiple drugs that get into your brain (see below)
- Experiencing other significant medical problems that are less than optimally controlled (e.g., congestive heart failure, chronic lung disease, etc.)

If you have experienced a decline in memory and thinking, review your medication list with your physician to make certain that drugs are not contributing. Medications that may affect your cognition are listed in table 23.1. If you are only rarely taking one of these drugs (e.g., a drug for diarrhea a couple of times a month), don't worry about this. The drugs on this list are not necessarily the cause of cognitive problems but are included because they have the potential to do this in at least some people. This is not an all-inclusive list; for example, drugs used to suppress the immune system of organ transplant patients and cancer drugs are not listed.

This potential for a medication to impair cognition must be balanced against the benefit. For example, a heart drug, amiodarone, occasionally causes one of a variety of neurological problems, including cognitive impairment. However, it is perhaps the most effective drug for controlling life-threatening cardiac rhythm problems. Even though there might be concern that it is causing side effects, it may be necessary to continue it. These are issues that you would need to have your physician address.

One clue that a medication may be at fault relates to the time the cognitive problem developed. If confusion developed on the heels of a newly prescribed medication, this raises suspicions. This is especially likely if the onset was rather sudden and pronounced; dementia develops insidiously.

Medical and Neurologic Problems May Impair Cognition

It's easy to blame everything on PD. If you've had PD for a number of years and now are experiencing problems with thinking and memory, PD could be

Table 23.1. Medications That May Contribute to Memory Impairment or Confusion

Medication Classes	Commonly Prescribed Medications in These Classes
Anticholinergic drugs for controlling the bladder	Oxybutynin (Ditropan), tolterodine (Detrol), hyoscyamine (Levsin, Levsinex, Cystospaz)
Anticholinergic drugs for PD	Trihexyphenidyl (Artane), benztropine (Cogentin), procyclidine (Kemadrin), biperiden (Akineton)
Anticholinergic drugs for loose stools, irritable bowel	Atropine, hyoscyamine, scopolamine (ingredients in a variety of anti-diarrheals), propantheline (Pro-Banthine), clidinium (ingredient in Librax), dicyclomine (Bentyl)
Antianxiety drugs	Alprazolam (Xanax), diazepam (Valium), clorazepate (Tranxene), lorazepam (Ativan), clonazepam (Klonopin), hydroxyzine (Atarax, Vistaril)
Muscle relaxants, antispasticity drugs	Cyclobenzaprine (Flexeril), tizanidine (Zanaflex), orphenadrine (Norgesic, Norflex), carisoprodol (Soma), baclofen (Lioresal), chlorzoxazone (Parafon Forte)
Narcotics	Codeine (in Tylenol #3), hydrocodone (in Vicodin, Lortab), oxycodone (in Percodan, Oxycontin, Roxicet), propoxyphene (Darvon, Darvocet), fentanyl (Duragesic patch)
Certain nonnarcotic prescription pain relievers	Tramadol (Ultram), butalbital (used in headache preparations)
Seizure drugs	Phenytoin (Dilantin), carbamazepine (Tegretol), phenobarbital, zonisamide (Zonegran), gabapentin (Neurontin), lamotrigine (Lamictal), oxcarbazepine (Trileptal), primidone (Mysoline), topiramate (Topamax)
Nonprescription antihistamines	Diphenhydramine (Benadryl)
Longer-acting sleep medication	Flurazepam (Dalmane)
Heart rhythm medication	Amiodarone (Cordarone, Pacerone)
Tricyclic drugs for depression	Amitriptyline (Elavil), nortriptyline (Pamelor), desipramine (Norpramin), imipramine (Tofranil), doxepin (Sinequan), trimipramine (Surmontil)

the reason. However, there are other medical and neurological problems that could be superimposed, causing or contributing to cognitive problems. These are likely if the cognitive problems developed over minutes, days, or weeks. The dementia of PD evolves over months to years.

Examples of medical conditions that could affect cognition include thyroid disease, severe anemia, or major liver or kidney problems. Sometimes this will be obvious but not always. Thus the evaluation of cognitive problems in those with PD should include a review of the general medical state plus the blood tests that internists and family physicians typically order for routine medical screening (see below).

Other disorders affecting the brain may also occur in people with PD. If cognitive impairment develops suddenly, then strokes, brain hemorrhages, or seizures need to be considered. Much less commonly, more diffuse conditions may affect the brain such as infectious (e.g., Lyme disease, HIV) or inflammatory (e.g., lupus or other autoimmune disease); they evolve over days, weeks, or a few months. Even very slow development of cognitive impairment may be from some other brain condition such as a tumor or chronic blood clot (subdural hematoma).

TESTING

Testing is clearly appropriate when confusion has developed. This includes a review of your general medical state and your medications, plus (1) brain scan (MRI or CT) and (2) blood work, usually a complete blood count, sedimentation rate, thyroid, vitamin B-12, and a chemistry profile. The chemistry profile typically includes sodium, potassium, calcium, glucose, creatinine, AST, alkaline phosphatase, albumin, and bilirubin. This assesses basic elements circulating in your bloodstream, plus liver and kidney function. Your doctor may add other blood tests depending on your history.

A spinal fluid examination may also be a part of this workup in certain cases. It is usually not done if dementia is long-standing, such as present for more than two years. Your brain floats in spinal fluid, and any infectious or inflammatory process affecting the brain will generate spinal fluid abnormalities. This test is performed by inserting the collection needle into your low back region and puncturing the sac containing the spinal fluid (skin deadened with a local anesthetic). Tests run on the collected spinal fluid include a cell count plus measurement of the glucose, protein, and inflammatory proteins (immunoglobulin studies). If these are normal, it is unlikely that an inflammatory or infectious condition is causing the confusion.

Dementia

If cognitive problems are substantial and persistent, interfering with your activities of daily living, and if other causes have been excluded, this fits the general criteria for dementia. Does this mean that this is a part of the PD process? Probably, but not necessarily. Let's consider dementia in the broader perspective.

DEMENTIA AND AGING IN THE NORMAL POPULATION

Dementia occurs in seniors, irrespective of PD. The likelihood of dementia in the general population rises after the mid-seventies. This jumps dramatically after ninety, when another 5–6 percent become demented each year, mostly due to Alzheimer's disease. Thus all of us are at some risk of dementia if we live long enough, regardless of whether we have PD.

THE RISK FOR LATER-DEVELOPING DEMENTIA AMONG THOSE WITH PD

Those with PD are at a higher risk for dementia than the general population. This has been assessed in multiple studies with various degrees of risk reported. When dementia has been assessed among large groups of people seen in PD clinics, the frequency has ranged from 11 percent to 29 percent. In other words, among a few hundred people coming to a given PD clinic, 11 percent to 29 percent are found to be demented. However, this might underestimate the true risk, since perhaps the most severely affected people will not be seen in these clinics, especially if they reside in nursing homes.

Investigators have also gone directly into well-defined communities and identified not only everyone with PD but also those with PD and dementia. This is a more representative number. The prevalence of dementia among these community-based PD patients has ranged from 12 percent to 41 percent.

Age interacts with PD to increase the risk of dementia. Younger people with PD tend not to experience substantial thinking and memory problems. Although there are no accurate assessments to allow us to estimate the risks according to age, the general experience among doctors treating PD is that the dementia risks are relatively low among those under sixty-five.

To summarize, those with PD are at increased risk for developing dementia, but in any community, the majority of those with PD are not demented. Furthermore, the risk is quite low for those under sixty-five with PD.

PROBLEMS EXPERIENCED BY THOSE WITH DEMENTIA AND PD

When dementia occurs in PD, the onset is insidious and the progression is slow. Those affected may be able to function in most respects and not have to rely on their families for a number of years. Memory is compromised, but typically less than in Alzheimer's disease, where it may be severely impaired. Judgment may be affected, which may affect business decisions. Complex concepts become difficult. Conceptualizing things in three-dimensional space may be especially challenging, explaining why those affected often get lost in slightly unfamiliar surroundings. Personality may change. Previously meticulous people may become sloppy and oblivious to hygiene. They may become a little inappropriate in conversations, saying things that in the past would have embarrassed them.

People with PD and dementia often experience hallucinations and delusions, which we will consider in more detail in the next chapter. Hallucinations imply seeing or hearing things that are not there. In the dementia of PD the hallucinations are almost always visual. Schizophrenics hear voices warning them or telling them to do things. Those with PD and dementia usually do not hear these voices, but rather see imaginary people, animals, or other things. The medications for PD tend to exacerbate hallucinations.

Delusions imply false beliefs. They may be paranoid, accusing friends or family of devious acts. They often focus on the spouse, frequently suspecting an affair. Like hallucinations, delusions may be provoked by medications to treat PD; also like hallucinations, they can be treated (discussed in the next chapter).

CAUSE OF DEMENTIA IN SOMEONE WITH PD

When dementia occurs, it often surfaces after many years of levodopa-responsive PD. Why does this evolution to dementia occur? The precise cause is not known, just as we do not know what causes PD in the first place. Apparently the same process that causes typical PD becomes more widespread, affecting broader areas of the brain, including cognitive regions. When dementia develops, the Lewy body degenerative process is no longer primarily confined to the substantia nigra (plus a few other brain regions). Rather, the neurodegenerative process extends to other regions including the cortex, which is the seat of intellectual function.

Who is destined to become demented? Besides age, no other strong risk factors have been identified. Obviously many with PD never evolve to this state.

In chapter 6, I briefly discussed diffuse Lewy body disease, also known as Lewy body dementia. That disorder is primarily defined by the nearly simultaneous development of parkinsonism and dementia—the parkinsonism and dementia develop around the same time. How does that differ from PD followed years later by dementia? The brain appearance is essentially the same; there are widespread Lewy body neurodegenerative changes in both cases. Whether these reflect the same condition is debated.

Medications for Improving Memory

The available drugs for restoring memory and thinking are only mildly effective. These drugs work by enhancing the activity of the neurotransmitter acetylcholine. Acetylcholine is contained in brain memory circuits, and raising acetylcholine levels mildly improves recall. By the same token, drugs that block brain acetylcholine tend to worsen memory; these are the so-called anticholinergic drugs discussed in prior chapters.

Medications that increase brain acetylcholine activity are termed procholinergic and are shown in table 23.2. These medications work by blocking the breakdown of acetylcholine. They block the enzyme acetylcholinesterase, which degrades acetylcholine.

These procholinergic drugs should not be administered to people with very slow heart rates or major heart rhythm problems without physician scrutiny. They can slow the heart rate, although this is not a problem unless predisposed.

My choice for a procholinergic medication for those with PD and memory impairment is donepezil (Aricept). Compared to the other medications in this class, it is the easiest to use and has the fewest side effects. It is initiated as a single 5 mg tablet taken in the morning or bedtime. Give this at least six weeks to work. If this isn't beneficial or if you are seeking an even better effect, you may increase this to 10 mg once daily (two 5 mg tablets or one 10 mg tablet). Side effects are few, with occasional people experiencing nausea, diarrhea, or insomnia. This is an expensive drug and if you don't appreciate any benefit, you could ultimately discontinue it.

If you don't respond to donepezil, should you try another medication from table 23.2? My own practice is to try donepezil and not go beyond that. The other medications in this group (table 23.2) are much more likely to cause side effects and there is no conclusive evidence to suggest they are more effective than donepezil. Nausea, vomiting, and diarrhea are more common with rivastigmine (Exelon) and galantamine (Reminyl). The last medication listed in table 23.2 is tacrine (Cognex). Tacrine was the first drug of this type released for prescription use. However, it has potential for serious liver toxicity. It is still prescribed but requires blood test monitoring of liver enzymes (ALT/SGPT). This drug may also cause nausea, vomiting, and diarrhea. For those with PD and cognitive impairment who have failed donepezil, there seems to be no compelling reason to try tacrine.

ANTICHOLINERGIC DRUGS TO AVOID IF POSSIBLE

Table 23.1 shows medications that may contribute to memory impairment or confusion, including some commonly prescribed anticholinergic drugs. In general, anticholinergic drugs are best avoided in the face of cognitive impairment, unless they are so useful in other respects that the benefits offset these potential side effects. Note also that the tricyclic drugs (last entry in the table) have variable degrees of anticholinergic properties. Occasionally I encounter people who are taking both a procholinergic drug for memory (e.g., donepezil) and also an anticholinergic drug for some other purpose (e.g., oxybutynin, for bladder problems). Since these tend to work in opposite directions, they may have offsetting effects. It makes sense to use either one or the other, but not both.

Table 23.2. Medications to Enhance Memory

Medication	Brand Name	Tablet/Capsule Sizes	Starting Dose	How to Raise the Dose	Highest Dose
Donepezil	Aricept	5 mg, 10 mg	One 5 mg tablet daily	After about 6 weeks, consider raising to two 5 mg tablets or one 10 mg tablet daily	10 mg daily
Rivastigmine	Exelon	1.5 mg, 3 mg, 4.5 mg, 6 mg	One 1.5 mg capsule twice daily with meals	If tolerated, raise the dose every 2–4 weeks to: 3 mg twice daily, then 4.5 mg twice daily, then 6 mg twice daily	6 mg twice daily
Galantamine	Reminyl	4 mg, 8 mg, 12 mg	One 4 mg tablet twice daily with meals	If tolerated, increase every 4 weeks to: 8 mg twice daily, then 12 mg twice daily	12 mg twice daily
Tacrine	Cognex	10 mg, 20 mg, 30 mg, 40 mg	One 10 mg capsule 4 times daily	If tolerated, increase every 4 weeks to: 20 mg 4 times daily, then 30 mg 4 times daily, then 40 mg 4 times daily	40 mg, 4 times daily

DO PD MEDICATIONS IMPAIR MEMORY?

Carbidopa/levodopa, dopamine agonist drugs, selegiline, and the COMT inhibitors (entacapone, tolcapone) do not cause confusion or memory impairment but may provoke or exacerbate hallucinations or delusions. Hallucinations and delusions are a separate issue from dementia, although they are much more likely among those with cognitive problems. Among drugs for PD, only the anticholinergic medications, such as trihexyphenidyl, impair memory. Rarely amantadine will provoke a confusional state.

VITAMIN E

In a single large clinical trial of Alzheimer's disease patients, high doses of vitamin E (1000 units twice daily) seemed to slow disease progression. On the other hand, people with uncomplicated PD studied in another trial did not benefit from two years of vitamin E (same dose). Based on these results, vitamin E supplementation was often recommended for cognitive impairment, although not for PD in general. The doses employed in these studies, 1000 units twice daily, appeared to be harmless. However, a recent composite analysis of all controlled vitamin E trials suggested otherwise; doses over 400 units daily were associated with a small, but significant increase in mortality. Consequently, vitamin E supplementation is no longer recommended.

MEMANTINE (NAMENDA)

Recently memantine (Namenda) was introduced as symptomatic treatment for Alzheimer's disease. This drug is very similar to the PD drug amantadine, which we considered in chapter 10. Both these medications mildly and partially block the brain neurotransmitter glutamate. Memantine is much more expensive than amantadine, however. Whether memantine has any role in the treatment of PD dementia is unknown. It is also unclear whether the same benefits (and side effects) might be obtained with amantadine.

Sundowning (Nighttime Confusion)

Those with dementia often have more problems at night, which has been termed sundowning. There are probably multiple reasons why this occurs. With darkness, some of our visual orienting influences are lost, especially in the middle of the night. Also, the cumulative mental fatigue from a long day may contribute. In addition, there may be something about our internal biological clocks that predisposes to cognitive problems at night. Finally, those with dementia often have reversal of their day–night cycle, compounding this problem; they sleep during the day and are awake at night. Sedating medicines administered in hopes of inducing sleep have a paradoxical effect with increased nighttime confusion.

Sundowning may be a major source of upheaval for the spouse or family, disrupting everyone's sleep. Treatment strategies tried for sundowning include the following.

- Attempt to establish a normal day–night cycle. Minimize naps during the daytime (allow one after lunch but no others). Encourage exercise during the day. Establish a consistent daily routine. Do relaxing things in the evening and arousing things earlier in the day. The intent is to entrain the sleep cycle with everyone else.

- For those with PD, nighttime sleep may require adequate doses of levodopa therapy, as discussed in chapter 20.

- To entrain sleep at night, you could consider a sleep medication (see chapter 20). However, in some cases, it may increase the confused state.

- Avoid the medications listed in table 23.1 as much as possible, especially in the evening.

- For those awakening during the night, a night-light may help with orientation. Otherwise the total darkness of night may add to the disorientation.

- If sundowning includes hallucinations or delusions, then special medications can be used for that purpose (discussed in the next chapter).

Note that sundowning must not be confused with REM sleep behavior disorder, which we considered in chapter 20. With this phenomenon, people talk in their sleep or act out without fully waking up. This is common among those with PD, including those with no cognitive problems. It often requires no treatment.

Financial, Legal, and Safety Issues Relating to Dementia

Those with PD typically have led active and fulfilling lives, which they continue for many years, despite PD. In the advent of dementia, however, certain life changes are necessary. You obviously want to avoid unfortunate business, professional, or financial decisions. It is important to recognize your limitations and restructure business and financial dealings so that responsibilities are appropriate to capabilities.

Home safety issues also need attention in cases where dementia is prominent. Operation of power machinery, cooking (with potential for fire), and similar activities may need to be limited. Driving may need to be prohibited.

Nutrition is also of concern in some individuals with dementia. PD is often associated with weight loss, and this may be exacerbated in those with dementia. Forgetting to eat and loss of appetite frequently accompany dementia and may be further exacerbated if depression is present. If weight loss develops, this should be brought to your physician's attention. A structured diet from a dietitian, food supplements, and a daily multivitamin may be appropriate (addressed further in chapter 30).

24

◆ ◆ ◆

Crazy Ideas, Visions, and Behavior: Hallucinations, Paranoia, Delusions, and Hypersexuality

Hallucinations: Seeing Things That Aren't There

Most people with Parkinson's disease (PD) do not experience hallucinations. However, they do develop in a distinct minority, usually later in the course of PD. These are not necessarily reflective of dementia and if they develop, this does not necessarily imply that you are becoming demented. Medications for PD may be responsible in some cases. Most importantly, they are treatable.

THE CHARACTER OF HALLUCINATIONS

Hallucinations experienced by people with PD are varied. In the mildest and simplest form, they are spots, dots, lines, or other small shapes in your field of vision. More troubling are hallucinations of people, animals, bugs, and so on. Hallucinations that I have commonly heard described include the following:

- Animals in the yard
- Children playing outside the window
- Family, friends, or strangers sitting in the living room
- Bugs crawling on the refrigerator (or countertop, floor, etc.)

There are countless variations on this theme. Usually they are not perceived as frightening or threatening. The person experiencing them may have insight or may not recognize them for what they are. These may be fleeting or may last for minutes or hours.

Hallucinations experienced by those with PD are almost always visual; they are seen and rarely heard. When the hallucinations are people, they typically don't talk back or answer questions. This is an important distinction from certain primary psychiatric disorders, such as schizophrenia, where hallucinatory voices issue commands or denigrate the psychotic patient.

It may take awhile for the person with PD or family members to figure out the problem. People who lack insight respond to what they see. If the hallucinations are bugs, bug killer may be compulsively sprayed and the area scrubbed. If children are seen in the bedroom, they may be asked to play outside; when they don't leave, the conversation may get more interesting (hallucinated people usually don't listen). Sometimes hallucinated people are incorporated into the day's activities. I recall one senior lady who fixed a large dinner for her friends, only to realize as she sat down to eat that her "friends" were all illusory.

WHAT CAUSES HALLUCINATIONS IN PD?

Two primary factors underlie these hallucinations. First are medications. All the drugs we use to treat PD may induce hallucinations. This doesn't happen in most cases, but the likelihood increases as the PD medication list grows longer; as we prescribe more drugs, the risk of hallucinations rises. Other medications may also contribute, specifically drugs passing into the brain such as narcotics for pain, muscle relaxants, tranquilizers, or sedatives.

The second factor responsible for hallucinations is the brain itself, specifically brain perception circuits that are affected by the underlying parkinsonian process. Areas of the brain that interpret visual images may have some inherent instability due to PD. Presumably this is due to the same neurodegenerative process that causes the tremor and movement symptoms of PD. Some people continue to experience hallucinations despite discontinuing all medications.

WHO EXPERIENCES HALLUCINATIONS?

Fortunately most people with PD do not experience hallucinations. However, some are predisposed. They are more likely with:

- Dementia

- Advanced age

- Long durations of PD

- Multiple medications for PD (especially certain drugs; see below)

- Other serious medical illness (e.g., pneumonia or other major infections, liver or kidney failure, advanced lung disease)

- Anesthesia for surgical procedures (transiently after the surgery)
- Blindness
- Severe insomnia with sleep deprivation

Dementia is by far the greatest predisposing factor. Most people with PD and dementia experience at least occasional hallucinations. On the other hand, hallucinations are uncommon in younger people with PD, and are distinctly rare early in the course of PD.

ARE HALLUCINATIONS DANGEROUS?

Hallucinations are not necessarily a sign of dementia and they don't mean that your PD has necessarily taken some terrible turn for the worse. However, they certainly may interfere with your life and for that reason require attention.

If you experience only fleeting hallucinations, you may not need to do anything. If you see a few bugs in the periphery of your vision on rare occasions, you may choose to ignore them. However, if hallucinations are more substantial and have the potential to interfere with your activities, then you need to do something.

In some circumstances hallucinations are particularly worrisome, and this includes such situations as driving a car or operating power machinery (e.g., table saws, farm equipment). Clearly, if you are experiencing hallucinations, you should avoid these activities until they are completely controlled.

HALLUCINATIONS: WHAT TO DO FIRST

Hallucinations typically can be abolished with appropriate medical treatment. The first step is usually not adding a new drug, but subtracting. The drugs used to treat PD can all induce hallucinations. Are all of these necessary? How much is each helping? Are you taking drugs for other purposes that could also be provoking hallucinations? Did the hallucinations start within a few weeks of starting one of the medications from our list?

A practical strategy starts with listing all your medications that could be contributing to hallucinations, with the intent of eliminating those drugs that are otherwise unnecessary. This elimination process is usually done one drug at a time. Choose first the medication from that list that is providing the least benefit and taper off that.

Table 24.1 lists the drugs we use to treat PD and the risk of hallucinations. Some drugs are more critical to the control of parkinsonism than others, and the order shown in the table reflects that. For example, if someone is taking selegiline, I generally eliminate that first (it is the first drug listed). Unless amantadine has been dramatically helpful in reducing dyskinesias, I typically will eliminate that next (the second drug listed). Obviously most people will not be taking all these drugs; however, table 24.1 provides a rough idea how

Table 24.1. Drugs for PD: Risk of Hallucinations and Delusions

Medication	How Likely to Cause Hallucinations?	Comment	How to Discontinue*
1. Selegiline (Eldepryl)	Uncommon when used alone, but more frequent in combination with other drugs	Has only mild benefit and often can be eliminated without substantial deterioration	May be stopped abruptly (long duration of action that slowly dissipates over weeks)
2. Amantadine	Mild-moderate risk when used with other drugs	Primary role is to reduce levodopa-dyskinesias; if not a problem, this may be tapered off	Reduce by one 100 mg tablet weekly
3. Anticholinergic drugs: trihexyphenidyl (Artane), benztropine (Cogentin), procyclidine (Kemadrin), biperiden (Akineton)	Mild-moderate risk when used with other drugs	Has only limited role in treating PD: reduces tremor and dystonia. Most people can eliminate without major decline	Reduce each week by 1/2 tablet, but go more slowly if you are experiencing problems**

4. COMT inhibitors: entacapone (Comtan), tolcapone (Tasmar)	When added to levodopa therapy, increases the risk	Potentiates the levodopa response; usually can be eliminated without major deterioration	May be stopped abruptly
5. Dopamine agonists: pramipexole (Mirapex), ropinirole (Requip), pergolide (Permax), bromocriptine (Parlodel)	Three times as likely to provoke hallucinations as levodopa therapy	In low doses, probably won't be missed. Substantial benefit in higher doses	Refer to chapter 13
6. Carbidopa/ levodopa (Sinemet)	May cause hallucinations in those predisposed	By far the best drug we have for treating PD	Taper this last and not below the level that allows you to walk and function

*The tapering schedules shown are a bit arbitrary and your physician may suggest a different scheme. In general, the longer you have taken a medication, the longer to taper off. If you just started one of these drugs in the past week, you could stop it abruptly.

**Some people taking an anticholinergic drugs for many years find it difficult to discontinue, unless done very slowly.

to prioritize your drug elimination scheme. Some drugs should not be stopped abruptly and require tapering; strategies for doing this are shown in the table, but you should also have your physician advise.

Drugs besides those used to treat PD may also contribute to hallucinations. Any drug that crosses the blood–brain barrier could be playing a role. Table 23.1 lists the major medications of this type; these same drugs could also contribute to hallucinations. If you are taking drugs listed in that table and can do without them, consider elimination. In fact, you may wish to do this before reducing any of your PD drugs. Your physician should advise how to taper off these medications.

In general, I eliminate only one medication at a time. However, if your hallucinations are very troublesome and if there are many contributing drugs, you may need to reduce a couple of these immediately. Your physician should advise.

DON'T ELIMINATE CARBIDOPA/LEVODOPA

Carbidopa/levodopa is the foundation of symptomatic treatment of PD. Unless your parkinsonian symptoms are extremely mild, you will not want to eliminate levodopa therapy. Taper off everything else if necessary, but not this drug. You will need this to control your parkinsonian symptoms.

What about reducing carbidopa/levodopa? If hallucinations haven't responded to elimination of other drugs, you could try getting by with a slightly lower carbidopa/levodopa dose. However, there is no need to sacrifice control of your parkinsonism, since we have drugs to reduce hallucinations.

QUETIAPINE

If subtracting unnecessary drugs has not helped, we then start a medication for abolishing hallucinations. My first choice for this purpose among those with PD is quetiapine (Seroquel). Quetiapine appears to have negligible potential for worsening parkinsonism, unlike most other drugs in this class.

There are a variety of strategies for arriving at the optimum dose of quetiapine. The approach I take to control hallucinations is shown in table 24.2. Quetiapine is started in a low dose of one 25 mg tablet taken in the evening. It can cause sleepiness and is started just before bedtime. How rapidly the dose is raised depends on the degree of urgency. Typically, I recommend raising the dose by 25 mg (one tablet) increments every week until the hallucinations are controlled, as illustrated in table 24.2. For those with PD, low total daily doses of 25–100 mg daily are usually sufficient; occasionally slightly higher doses are necessary, perhaps up to 200 mg daily. Rarely, even higher doses, up to several hundred milligrams daily, are required.

I try to get by with a single evening dose; at that time, any drug-induced sleepiness is not a problem. However, the conventional dosing scheme is twice daily, and if a single evening dose isn't providing coverage during the day-

Table 24.2.   How to Start Quetiapine (Seroquel) to
Control Hallucinations and Delusions
(Raise the dose until hallucinations have been controlled)

Week*	Dose: Number of 25 mg Tablets*	Total Daily Dose (mg)
1	One in the evening	25
2	Two in the evening	50
3	Three in the evening	75
4	Four in the evening**	100
5	One in the morning and four in the evening	125
6	Two in the morning and four in the evening**	150
7	Two in the morning and five in the evening	175
8	Two in the morning and six in the evening	200

Note: Higher doses, up to several hundred milligrams per day, may be administered if necessary and tolerated.

*Your physician may choose to administer more or less of your total daily dose in the morning.
**A single 100 mg tablet may be substituted for four of the 25 mg tablets.
(Photocopy this table and put it on your bulletin board to guide you.)

time, a second dose in the morning may be required. Quetiapine comes in both 25 mg and 100 mg tablets.

Quetiapine may cause orthostatic hypotension—a drop in the standing blood pressure. This should not be a major problem as long as you are aware of this tendency. As we have discussed in prior chapters, people with PD tend to be prone to orthostatic hypotension. Check your sitting and standing blood pressure before and after starting quetiapine to make certain it is okay. As long as your standing systolic blood pressure is at least 90, you should not experience any problems (recall that the systolic reading is the upper number, 120 in the reading 120/80). If it starts to drop below this, then you will need to refer back to chapter 21, which discusses treatment of orthostatic hypotension.

In the scheme I just outlined, quetiapine is started after medications that could be contributing to the problem are eliminated. However, is it necessary to wait until we have done this? After all, it may take a few weeks to taper off these other drugs one by one. What if the hallucinations are threatening? In that case, it would be reasonable to start the quetiapine while the other drugs are being tapered off. Later, if it seemed likely that it is no longer necessary, it could be slowly tapered off.

HOSPITALIZATION

Usually hallucinations can be managed outside the hospital. However, if these problems are disruptive and pose a danger to the person or family, these medication adjustments should be done in the hospital. Most communities have a mental health hospital that is well equipped to deal with these types of problems, keeping the person safe and relatively comfortable as treatment proceeds.

THESE DOSES OF QUETIAPINE HAVEN'T CONTROLLED THE HALLUCINATIONS; NOW WHAT?

It is unusual for hallucinations to require quetiapine doses beyond 200 mg daily among those with PD. However, if that occurs, one strategy is to continue to raise the dose, provided that it isn't making you too sleepy or causing other side effects. In fact, much higher doses are used to treat schizophrenia, and we are not close to the maximum allowable dosage with the scheme outlined in table 24.2.

CLOZAPINE

A more effective drug for treating hallucinations in PD is clozapine (Clozaril). Unfortunately it also has more side effects. It is even more sedating than quetiapine and at least as likely to cause orthostatic hypotension. More important, however, is the potential for clozapine to occasionally cause a dramatic reduction in the white blood cell count (agranulocytosis). This is rare but very serious. The white count may drop so low that there is a risk of life-threatening infection (white blood cells are critical to fighting infections). Fortunately this is reversible and the white blood count will return to normal when the drug is stopped. However, close vigilance is required when this medication is used. The U.S. Food and Drug Administration has mandated that if clozapine is prescribed, a white blood cell count must be done weekly for the first six months and less frequently thereafter. Pharmacists may only dispense a week's supply at a time, so that low white counts are not overlooked. With clozapine therapy, there is also a very small risk of seizures or potentially serious heart inflammation (myocarditis). This is a highly effective drug for controlling hallucinations and related problems, but is reserved for the most refractory situations.

If used to treat hallucinations in someone with PD, clozapine is typically started with 1/4 of a 25 mg tablet in the evening. It can be very sedating and that is the reason for starting with such a small dose. It can be raised by 1/4 tablet increments weekly until the hallucinations have been controlled. Usually it is given as a once daily or twice daily dose. Because of the sedation, most of the total daily dose is given in the evening. For those with PD, low doses are usually sufficient to control the hallucinations, on the order of 12.5–100 mg daily, or occasionally slightly higher. Compare this to treatment of schizophrenia with clozapine, where the typical dose is 300–400 mg daily.

OLANZAPINE

Olanzapine (Zyprexa) may be tolerated by those with PD when prescribed in low doses. The effective range of doses is 5–15 mg daily, but doses above

5 mg daily may worsen parkinsonism. It is not as effective in treating hallucinations as quetiapine or clozapine in my experience, especially in lower doses. It is acceptable to try this drug if quetiapine is not tolerated; however, monitoring of parkinsonism is necessary to make certain it does not deteriorate. If the parkinsonism worsens (i.e., worsening gait, tremor, increased slowness), then olanzapine may not be a good alternative. Like quetiapine, it may induce sedation and orthostatic hypotension. It is taken once daily, with a starting dose of 1/2 to one 5 mg tablet. It is typically raised at one or two week intervals by 1/2 increments until hallucinations are controlled, up to 15 mg daily (a dose that could worsen parkinsonism).

DRUGS THAT SHOULD NOT BE USED TO TREAT HALLUCINATIONS

Drugs used in the treatment of schizophrenia reduce hallucinations, but most should not be used in those with PD (the exceptions were discussed above). These drugs tend to block dopamine receptors in the brain. It is the dopamine receptor that we are trying to stimulate with our PD treatments, levodopa, and dopamine agonists. If we block the dopamine receptors, the parkinsonism will worsen and levodopa will stop working. Drugs from this class to avoid are listed on table 6.1 (chapter 6).

OTHER DRUGS

Two newer drugs for treating hallucinations have only mild potential to block dopamine receptors, ziprasidone (Geodon) and aripiprazole (Abilify). Although the dopamine receptor blockade is relatively mild, these drugs may still exacerbate parkinsonism and are generally not a good choice if you have PD.

Q: Do you think a sedative would help Dad's hallucinations?

A: Family members sometimes inquire if a sedating medication (e.g., Valium) might calm down a loved one who is experiencing hallucinations. This may backfire, leading to increased confusion and perhaps even more hallucinations.

Q: I saw pink elephants after my surgery; should I worry?

A: Sometimes seniors experience confusion and hallucinations after major surgery. This is even more likely among seniors with PD. Presumably, this is the consequence of the anesthetics and metabolic factors linked to the surgery or illness. Being in a strange room (hospital) is also a little disorienting. Often no treatment is necessary and this subsides in a few days. This is not necessarily a harbinger of such problems in the future.

If postsurgical confusion develops, make certain that your surgeon is reminded that you have PD and he or she should avoid prescribing medications that block dopamine receptors. The forbidden drugs listed in chapter 6 (table 6.1) are among those typically prescribed for postoperative hallucinations and confusion.

Delusions and Paranoia

The same factors that cause hallucinations may also provoke delusions and paranoia. We treat this exactly as we do hallucinations. The key is to recognize them for what they are.

Delusions are absurd beliefs or ideas that have no basis in fact. In PD, they often involve the spouse, such as suspecting infidelity. Delusions may have financial implications, with a conviction that some preposterous business idea will be profitable.

Paranoia refers to delusions that are marked by extreme suspicion and a sense of persecution. The paranoid ideation often involves family or friends, perhaps imagining that they are conspiring to steal your money. It may be quite outlandish, such as the suspicion that the police are spying on you.

DELUSIONS AND PARANOIA: WHO NEEDS TREATMENT?

Probably all of us have had some thoughts at times that others might regard as a little paranoid or delusional. Most basketball and football games I watch, I'm convinced the referees are favoring the opponent; although a little paranoid, at least I have insight into this. We don't want to label people as delusional or paranoid when they think differently from us or simply need some reality testing. Just because we don't agree doesn't indicate that one of us should be on medical treatment.

Treatment is appropriate when one's ideas and thoughts become bizarre or markedly inappropriate, and interfere with activities and interactions. Here are a few examples from my own practice (names changed to preserve anonymity).

Mr. Petersen had PD for a dozen years with his symptoms quite well controlled on several medications. He and his wife recently celebrated their eightieth birthdays and their golden wedding anniversary. In recent weeks, Mr. Petersen started accusing his wife of seeing other men and checked on her incessantly. She related this tearfully in the office when they came for his appointment.

Mr. Smith was a retired businessman with PD who was enrolled in one of our drug treatment protocols. His wife called for an urgent appointment. He became fixated on plans to construct a large raft to sail on Lake Michigan, big enough for a hundred people. This was going to be a commercial party boat and he would make money selling beverages on board. He had already contacted the bank, potential business partners, and shipbuilders.

Mrs. Herman had PD for over ten years and was beginning to experience mild memory impairment. Her husband requested an appointment because of "strange thinking." She accused him of being an impostor; she was convinced he was not her real husband, despite the fact they had been married for over thirty years. Mrs. Herman had no explanation for how or why the switch occurred; she was simply convinced that this was some other guy.

Mrs. Thomas was a homemaker, wife, and community volunteer. When PD of many years sapped her energy levels, she started to reduce her activities, but she remained outgoing with many friends. However, one spring day her husband brought her to my office noting that she had become extremely suspicious. She thought the FBI was tapping their phones and watching their house. Sometimes she would awaken during the night to peer out the window to see if she could identify the FBI agent behind the telephone pole. Of course, this was a little absurd, given their status as pillars of the community in a small town.

All these people developed delusions that were seriously interfering with their lives. Clearly delusions of this type demand that something be done.

If delusions do not pose any danger, they can be managed outside the hospital. However, someone who is extremely paranoid or is quite delusional is usually best treated initially in the hospital.

HOW DELUSIONS AND PARANOIA ARE TREATED

The treatment of delusions and paranoia is the same as for hallucinations. This starts with a review of current medications and eliminating unnecessary drugs. This may require tapering off PD medications, one by one, leaving only carbidopa/levodopa. If this fails, quetiapine could then be started and adjusted, just as described above. Let's consider one example of how we might handle such a problem.

Mr. King is seventy-six years old and has had PD for ten years plus troublesome low back pain. In the last few months he has frequently awakened during the night thinking a burglar was downstairs. Twice he has called 911, bringing the police to the house; no burglar was found. During the daytime, he worries constantly about people looking in the windows. He accused his brother of stealing money. His wife is tearful as she describes this dramatic personality change. Mr. King takes only three prescription medications: carbidopa/levodopa, ropinirole, and Tylenol #3 for his troublesome low back pain. (Tylenol #3 contains codeine, a narcotic.) He also takes an over-the-counter sleep aid at bedtime.

Doing first things first, review Mr. King's medications. All of his drugs could be contributing to his paranoid state. I would start by eliminating his narcotic, Tylenol #3, and substituting another pain medication for his lumbar problems. Senior citizens, in general, are sensitive to narcotic drugs and may become confused or hallucinate when these are administered. I would also consider eliminating his sleeping drug; anything that makes you drowsy can add to confusion and delusions. If his paranoia didn't improve within a week or so, I would then begin to reduce his ropinirole. Dopamine agonist drugs are more likely than carbidopa/levodopa to provoke delusions as well as hallucinations. This might require managing his parkinsonism with carbidopa/levodopa alone. If necessary, quetiapine could subsequently be initiated. Finally, it should not be forgotten that with situations like this, the home should be made as safe as possible. Guns should be removed and, if appropriate, car keys should be locked away.

Should spouse or family confront the person with delusions or paranoia? Should they try to explain reality to them? Generally you cannot reason with someone in the throes of a psychotic belief. The family or spouse should be reassuring but not confrontational or argumentative.

Hypersexuality

On rare occasions, the medications we use in the treatment of PD may provoke a fixation on sexuality with the development of a ravenous sexual appetite. This is a problem developing almost exclusively in men. It is out of character, and the spouse or family will emphasize that "he's never done anything like this before." The usual story starts with a frantic phone call from a wife reporting that her husband has started demanding sex several times a day. She can't keep him satisfied and typically is at wit's end.

Fortunately this problem is uncommon. When I've encountered this, it has often been linked to starting a new medication, such as one of the dopamine agonist drugs. If that is the case, the treatment is straightforward; simply taper off the new drug. If it can't be easily linked to a particular drug, I would review the medications in table 24.1 and start to taper off any unnecessary drugs, just as we discussed for hallucinations or delusional behavior. As with treatment of hallucinations, it may be necessary to manage parkinsonism with carbidopa/levodopa alone. Similarly, quetiapine is the initial drug of choice using the strategy we just described. If the hypersexuality is a major problem, hospitalization could be considered and quetiapine could be started as the initial step. Although such hypersexuality can be extremely challenging to families, it has not led to any felonious behavior among people I have treated.

Another strategy for hypersexuality is administering one of the SSRI antidepressants. These SSRI drugs were discussed in chapter 22 on depression (table 22.2). Besides treating depression, they sometimes reduce libido. Hence an SSRI drug could be prescribed to tame an overactive sex drive.

UNEQUAL SEX DRIVE

Not all sexuality is bad, but it may seem that way to a partner who has no interest in sex. On occasion, I have heard a spouse complain that her husband was making inappropriate advances. For example, Mr. Jones had been immobile for several years due to undertreatment of his parkinsonism; once he was adequately medicated and regained his mobility, he rediscovered his libido. Mrs. Jones had grown accustomed to celibacy and was not very happy when their potential sex life resurfaced. Counseling may be the best treatment in that situation.

Compulsive Gambling

With the proliferation of casinos, it has now become apparent that on rare occasions, PD medications may provoke compulsive gambling. When it occurs, it is important to recognize, since it can be effectively treated with medication adjustments. The scenario in my practice has been the person who never or rarely gambled becoming obsessed with gambling after starting a dopamine agonist drug, mainly pramipexole. If I encounter someone with this problem who is taking a dopamine agonist medication, I taper off this drug over two to three weeks, or at least markedly reduce the dose. If this continues, I may then reduce or discontinue other PD medications until I am left with carbidopa/levodopa alone. Typically, this strategy should be sufficient, although counseling or psychiatric consultation may also be necessary in some cases.

25

◆ ◆ ◆

Problems with Swallowing,
Saliva, and Speaking

Trouble Swallowing

"Dysphagia" is the physician's term for difficult swallowing. This is rarely a major problem early in the course of PD. Even after many years, significant swallowing problems may never develop. If dysphagia is an early and prominent symptom, this may be a red flag for a condition other than PD (see chapter 6).

Dysphagia in PD is typically due to slowness and hesitancy initiating the act of swallowing. This is analogous to the general slowness of body movement that occurs in PD. Food and liquid tend to pool in the mouth.

Severe dysphagia may lead to pneumonia (infection of the lungs). Normally swallowed food or liquid passes down the tube-like esophagus to the stomach. However, the passageway to the lungs (trachea) is right in front of the esophagus. If swallowing is impaired and food or liquid goes down the wrong pipe, it ends up in the lungs. This usually triggers coughing, which is a protective reflex that tends to expel this material out of the lungs. Hence frequent coughing during eating is often a sign of aspiration—food or liquid passing into your lungs.

Physicians are able to observe the swallowing function via X ray techniques. They can administer a liquid that shows up on X ray, such as barium. Once swallowed, a series of X rays can trace the passage from the mouth into the throat and down the esophagus. If it passes inappropriately into the trachea, this can be seen on the X ray.

TREATMENT OF DYSPHAGIA

Among those with PD, the most effective drugs for dysphagia are the same ones we use to treat other aspects of parkinsonism. The most potent is carbidopa/levodopa, and adjusting the dose may be the best strategy for improving swallowing problems. You may wish to refer back to the discussion of medication adjustments in previous chapters. Dysphagia may not fully respond to medications, however. A few simple strategies can also help improve swallowing:

- Sit upright when eating or drinking.

- A slight downward tuck of your head may help the food go down the right pipe. In other words, try to keep your chin down as you swallow.

- Don't take large bites or huge gulps. This is especially important when eating food that could get stuck, such as meat; if a big chunk of meat is inadvertently swallowed into the windpipe, it could obstruct breathing.

- Slow down your eating.

- If solids are more of a problem than liquids, you could wash down small bites with a little water.

- Choose foods that are easy for you to swallow. For example, pureed fruits, certain puddings, and creamed dishes are swallowed more easily compared to tough-textured foods such as steaks or dry, crumbly foods like pretzels. Sometimes sticky foods are a problem, such as peanut butter or mashed potatoes.

- Experiment with different temperatures of liquids. For example, most people find that ice-cold liquids are easier to swallow than those that are lukewarm.

- If water and soda tend to go down the wrong pipe (i.e., the trachea), you could substitute thicker liquids, such as milkshakes or eggnog, or add a thickener. Thickeners are available under brand names such as Thick-it; they can be added to juices, and so on, to increase the consistency. Recall, however, that milk products contain protein, so milkshakes and eggnog are not good choices to wash down your carbidopa/ levodopa.

If dysphagia is a major problem, you may wish to consult a swallowing specialist, who might be a speech pathologist or physiatrist (physical medicine and rehabilitation specialist).

Rarely, swallowing is so severely impaired that nutrition is compromised. In my experience, this is distinctly rare in PD but does occur in the parkinsonism-plus disorders discussed in chapter 6. In that case, a feeding tube may be considered when simpler measures have failed. This often requires only minor surgery with the tube extending from your abdomen; this is inconspicuous when covered by a shirt or blouse.

TROUBLE SWALLOWING CARBIDOPA/LEVODOPA

If swallowing carbidopa/levodopa is difficult, you might switch to the new orally disintegrating formulation (Parcopa). The pill sizes and colors are the same as with the immediate-release formulation of carbidopa/levodopa; the doses are interchangeable. These pills dissolve in your mouth on your tongue; however, the dissolved ingredients still must be swallowed with your saliva. They are considerably more expensive, however, than generic carbidopa/levodopa (see chapter 12).

Drooling

Drooling (sialorrhea) is common in PD. It has nothing to do with increased saliva output but is caused by reduced frequency of swallowing. Normally saliva is constantly secreted and swallowed automatically. However, automatic movements are generally impaired in PD, such as arm swing, gesturing when talking, or facial animation. Thus swallowing frequency, like other automatic movements, is reduced in PD.

What's the best treatment for drooling? It is the same medications we use to treat other movement problems, especially levodopa therapy. Just like improvement of arm swing with levodopa treatment, the frequency of swallowing returns, and drooling stops or is reduced.

What about medications that dry the mouth? Certain drugs, specifically drugs from the "anticholinergic" class, reduce saliva output. They have also been used in the treatment of parkinsonism, as discussed in earlier chapters. These drugs include trihexyphenidyl (Artane) and benztropine (Cogentin); a longer list of anticholinergic drugs is shown in table 23.1. However, most people do not like the cotton-mouth feeling associated with inhibiting saliva output.

BOTULINUM TOXIN TREATMENT OF DROOLING

If drooling proves refractory to simpler solutions, botulinum toxin injections may be administered. Typically, botulinum toxin injections are used to relieve muscle spasms, such as occur in dystonia. However, they are also useful in reducing the output of saliva. For this purpose, botulinum toxin is injected into the parotid glands (in front of the ears). Saliva output drops a few days after the injection, and this lasts up to a few months. Botulinum toxin is available in two forms, botulinum toxin A (Botox) and B (Myobloc); the latter is more effective in reducing saliva. It is rare that these injections are necessary in PD, but may be appropriate in the parkinsonism-plus disorders that we discussed in chapter 6.

Speech and Voice Problems

Speaking may be affected by PD. First, the precision of your speech (articulation) may suffer. This may give it a garbled quality. Second, the volume of your voice may decline; people may comment that they can't hear you because you're speaking too softly. Making matters worse for seniors with PD is that spouses and friends may be hard of hearing (the hearing loss that accompanies normal aging).

TREATMENT OF SPEECH AND VOICE PROBLEMS

Although speech therapy often has a role in treatment (see below), optimizing your medications is usually the first step to improve your speaking voice. Speaking involves muscle movement just like walking. When you speak, you are using your lips, tongue, and palate to form words and sounds. Similarly, the muscles of breathing play an important role in the volume of your voice. These muscles of articulation and breathing may be compromised by parkinsonism, similar to the muscles of your limbs. Just as your limb muscles may be slow and stiff, the same may occur with these speaking muscles. Adequate doses of medications, including carbidopa/levodopa, may be necessary to improve your speaking voice. Thus the same medication principles we discussed in earlier chapters to improve walking or tremor apply to speech.

OTHER SIMPLE THINGS TO TRY

A consultation with a speech therapist may also be helpful. The general principles that apply to the speech problems of PD include the following.

- Speak more slowly. Simply slowing down the rate of speech is often helpful in improving speech intelligibility.

- Speak deliberately. As you slow down, concentrate on precise articulation. Although normal speech is generated without consciously thinking about it, if you concentrate, you can improve the precision.

- Take a deep breath before speaking. This will help ensure that you will have a large volume of air to push past your vocal cords.

- Purposely try to speak more loudly than you think is appropriate. People with PD often inappropriately perceive that they are shouting, when simply speaking loud enough to be heard. In other words, feedback of your own voice may cue you to speak too softly.

- Practice your speech in front of a mirror, reciting or reading familiar text while raising your voice. Shout this out so that someone in the next room could easily hear you with the door closed. Do this to develop a habit of "thinking loud" whenever you speak. For this to be consistently effective, you must practice this on a daily basis; otherwise you tend to fall back to your old speaking habits.

There are other practical considerations to improve your intelligibility and communication:

- If your spouse has impaired hearing, as frequently occurs with normal aging, purchase a hearing aid.

- For conversations, seek out quiet rooms. If the TV or stereo is playing in the background or if others are speaking, this competition from other sounds may drown you out. This is especially likely if your friends or spouse are hard of hearing. Note that hearing aids tend to amplify every sound; if other sounds are present in the room, the hearing aid will also make them louder.

- Face your friends during conversations and hold your head up. Often cues from your lips and face, as well as hand gestures, may help the communication.

LEE SILVERMAN VOICE THERAPY

Where the measures cited above prove insufficient, consider consulting with a speech therapist who is familiar with Lee Silverman voice therapy. This technique incorporates some of the above principles into a rigorous program of speech rehabilitation designed to raise the volume of your speech. This has proven beneficial in controlled clinical trials.

26

◆ ◆ ◆

Managing Digestive Problems and Constipation

Autonomic nervous system dysfunction makes a substantial contribution to the symptoms of Parkinson's disease (PD). We previously considered one such problem, orthostatic hypotension. Now we will address impairment of bowel movement and digestion caused by autonomic malfunction.

Normal Stomach Function

Digestion starts with the breakdown of food in the stomach. This food is attacked by stomach enzymes, which chemically cut it into smaller components that can subsequently be absorbed by the small intestine. Fluids are necessary to keep things mobile and flowing. A valve between the stomach and the small intestine controls the exit of food. As the stomach fills, this valve reflexively opens, allowing food products to pass into the small intestine where absorption into the body begins (see figure 26.1).

Delayed Stomach Emptying

In PD, the stomach may be slow and hesitant to empty its contents into the small intestine. This may result in a sense of bloating, or even nausea. This delayed emptying of the stomach may also delay the levodopa response in some cases. Levodopa is not absorbed in the stomach; it must pass to the small intestine where absorptive mechanisms can transport it into the bloodstream. If the stomach is slow to release levodopa, it may take a full hour to respond to immediate-release carbidopa/levodopa and two hours for the sustained-release pill.

Normal Function of the Colon and Bowel Movements

The absorption of dietary nutrients and medications takes place in the small intestine. What is unused and left over then passes into the colon (large intestine), as illustrated in figure 26.1. Feces collect in the rectum and are expelled as a bowel movement.

Passage of the food contents through the small and then the large intestine is by peristalsis. This is a coordinated contraction of the intestines to propel the

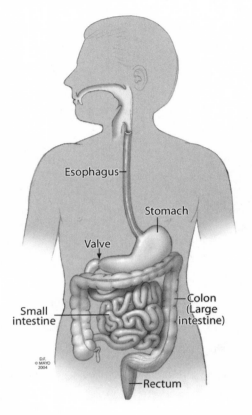

26.1 Digestive system. Digestion starts in the stomach, with subsequent passage to the small intestine. Absorption of nutrients is primarily from the small intestine. What is left over accumulates as feces in the colon (large intestine), which terminates in the rectum.

contents downstream. The intestines are like a flexible hose whose walls can be stretched. Within these walls are small muscles that can contract and squeeze down; their activity is coordinated and regulated by the autonomic nervous system. When the intestine fills and the walls are stretched, internal reflexes are activated. This triggers wall muscles to contract in sequence along the length of the intestine, pushing the food contents along. Ultimately the residua collects in the rectum as feces and similar reflexes result in a bowel movement.

Slowed Colon Function in PD: Constipation

People with PD tend to have impaired colon reflexes resulting in slowed and dampened peristalsis. The feces accumulate but don't stimulate the internal reflexes that ultimately result in bowel movements. This is the essence of constipation. Stool backs up in the colon.

Imaging the Colon

For most with PD who are constipated, there is no sinister cause, such as cancer. However, the general rule of thumb is that if there has been a substantial change in your stool habits, the colon should be visualized. This can be done by either colonoscopy or a barium enema combined with proctoscopy.

Colonoscopy and proctoscopy involve putting an instrument into your rectum, which allows the doctor to see inside. Colonoscopy reveals the entire colon, whereas proctoscopy only visualizes the near end; hence proctoscopy is combined with a barium enema to image all the colon.

Barium comes in liquid form and shows up on X ray. It outlines the contours of the colon when introduced by enema. It is not as sensitive as colonoscopy for visualizing small tumors.

Medications That May Slow Stomach Emptying and Cause Constipation

Although the autonomic nervous system is primarily responsible for the digestive problems of PD, medications may contribute. Certain drugs slow stomach emptying and cause constipation by inhibiting peristalsis. They do this by influencing the neurochemical signals that regulate gastrointestinal activity. If constipation or slowed gastric emptying is a problem, review your medication list. Specifically focus on drugs that

- Block the effects of acetylcholine
- Activate opioid receptors (i.e., narcotics)
- Stimulate dopamine receptors

Drugs with these properties may cause constipation and slow down the gastrointestinal system. Let's consider this in more detail and identify the specific drugs.

Drugs Blocking Acetylcholine

The autonomic nervous system uses neurotransmitters for signaling, just like brain circuits. One key neurotransmitter in the gastrointestinal system is *acetylcholine*. We have examined acetylcholine in earlier chapters since it is an important brain chemical in the basal ganglia. Drugs that block acetylcholine may improve tremor.

Table 26.1.   Common Drugs That Block Acetylcholine
(may induce constipation or slow stomach emptying)

Class of Drug Used For:	Drug
Parkinsonian tremor	Trihexyphenidyl (Artane) Benztropine (Cogentin) Procyclidine (Kemadrin) Biperiden (Akineton)
Urinary urgency	Oxybutynin (Ditropan) Tolterodine (Detrol) Hyoscyamine (Levsin, Levsinex, Cystospaz)
Antidepressants	Amitriptyline (Elavil) Nortriptyline (Pamelor) Desipramine (Norpramin) Imipramine (Tofranil) Doxepin (Sinequan) Trimipramine (Surmontil)
Diarrhea or irritable bowel*	Atropine (may be an ingredient in a variety of antidiarrheals) Hyoscyamine (ingredient in a variety of antidiarrheals) Scopolamine (ingredient in a variety of anti-diarrheals, as well as motion sickness patch) Propantheline (Pro-Banthine) Clidinium (ingredient in Librax) Dicyclomine (Bentyl)

*Loperamide (Imodium) is not strictly an anticholinergic drug, but it slows peristalsis by another mechanism.

In the gastrointestinal system, acetylcholine released by autonomic nerves induces the stomach and intestines to contract (stimulates peristalsis). Drugs that block acetylcholine slow stomach emptying, reduce intestinal peristalsis, and tend to cause constipation. This class of medications includes those for parkinsonian tremor, drugs used to slow the bladder (reduce urinary urgency), and some of the older drugs used to treat depression. Also, some drugs used to treat diarrhea and the loose stools of irritable bowel syndrome block acetylcholine. These drugs are listed on table 26.1. If you are taking one of these medications and if constipation, bloating, or other signs of delayed peristalsis are a problem, you may wish to consider whether it can be discontinued; discuss that with your doctor.

Narcotics and the Gastrointestinal System

Narcotic medications for pain are notorious for causing constipation. They are not used to treat PD; however, pain is a common human experience and hence you may be taking one of them. If constipation overshadows your pain, you may consider using a nonnarcotic drug for pain control. Narcotics commonly used for chronic pain in pill form include:

- Codeine (Tylenol #3)
- Hydrocodone (Lortab, Vicodin, Vicoprofen)
- Oxycodone (Oxycontin, Roxicet, Roxicodone, Percocet, Tylox)
- Hydromorphone (Dilaudid)
- Fentanyl (Duragesic patch)
- Propoxyphene (Darvon, Darvocet)

This is not an exhaustive list of narcotic drugs. If you are unsure if one of your medications is a narcotic, your pharmacist can answer that question. Note that narcotic pain relievers are often formulated with aspirin, acetaminophen (sometimes abbreviated APAP; Tylenol), or ibuprofen.

Dopamine and the Gastrointestinal System

Dopamine is also a neurotransmitter in the gastrointestinal system and works opposite to acetylcholine. Hence drugs that stimulate dopamine will tend to slow down the gastrointestinal system. This is not as profound an effect as blocking acetylcholine. Although levodopa and the dopamine agonist medications tend to slow peristalsis, this is not a prominent effect. In my experience, they make constipation mildly worse. However, for those with PD, stopping these medications is not an option, so we won't worry further about this.

By the same token, drugs that block dopamine are also used to stimulate peristalsis, such as metoclopramide (Reglan) or prochlorperazine (Compazine). However, this class of drugs can worsen parkinsonism and should not be used in those with PD.

Delayed Opening of the Stomach as a Cause of Nausea or Bloating

If the stomach does not empty properly, people experience bloating, nausea, or early satiety. Thus in PD, not all nausea is due to levodopa or dopamine agonist drugs. Another cause should be considered if nausea develops long after the levodopa and dopamine agonist doses have been stabilized. Gastroenterologists sometimes do special tests to specifically evaluate these problems.

Medications commonly used to improve stomach emptying may not be tolerated if you have PD. This includes metoclopramide (Reglan), which blocks dopamine receptors and may exacerbate parkinsonism. However, modification of your eating habits may help. Fatty foods, oils, or foods in heavy, rich sauces tend to slow down stomach emptying. Spicy foods, especially tomato sauces, trouble some people. Alcohol or caffeine may also contribute to slowed stomach emptying. You can try eliminating such foods and beverages one by one, and observe your response.

Delayed Medication Responses

Another consequence of slowed stomach emptying is a delay in your levodopa response. How to speed this up? Recall that filling the stomach triggers internal reflexes that open it. Hence, one way to facilitate passage of levodopa into the small intestine is to drink adequate fluids along with your pills. This actually helps in two ways. (1) Fluids tend to expand the stomach and this expansion will tend to stimulate stomach opening. (2) For the carbidopa/levodopa pill to be absorbed, it must first be dissolved, and fluids are necessary for this to occur. Food may also help open the stomach but must be nonprotein if ingested with levodopa. Thus dry bread or soda crackers may be tried.

Treating Constipation

The majority of people with PD are constipated. The primary problem is the impairment of the autonomic nervous system, but with a contribution from their parkinsonian medications. Compounding this still further is the normal aging process that also tends to cause constipation. With all of these factors converging, it is not surprising that the constipation experienced by those with PD often requires maximal therapy.

In medical school, doctors are taught to use simple, natural measures to treat constipation and avoid laxatives when at all possible. This is correct for the public at large and reasonable as the first attempt at treating the constipation in PD. However, if this fails, more aggressive therapy may be required and is appropriate, including frequent use of laxatives.

Basic Principles in Managing Constipation

Let's start with the elementary principles of managing constipation.

- Drink adequate fluids, which is about eight to ten eight-ounce glasses daily.
- Make certain that your diet includes liberal portions of fruits and vegetables, both cooked and raw.

- Your diet should include fiber sources on a daily basis. This includes whole grain cereals or whole grain snacks. Also, a variety of high-fiber products are sold as "bulk-forming laxatives" (e.g., Metamucil, Citrucel, Fibercon). These contain fiber ingredients such as psyllium, ispaghula husk, methylcellulose, polycarbophil, bran, and barley malt extract. You could ask your druggist about them.

- Prune juice may be especially helpful. One strategy is to heat a cup of prune juice in the microwave, similar to heating coffee or tea. Drinking the heated prune juice will tend to stimulate peristalsis.

- Get adequate exercise.

Stool softeners, such as docusate sodium (Colace), are benign and may also be considered an elementary component of constipation management. A 100 mg capsule of docusate sodium twice daily may help with mild constipation.

More Aggressive Constipation Management

If the above general principles are inadequate, we then employ more aggressive strategies. But first, what should we accept as an adequate number of bowel movements? As a general rule, if you have a well-formed stool at least once every two days, that is acceptable. If you frequently go more than two days without a bowel movement and are uncomfortable from this, additional measures may be appropriate.

There are many different drugs and strategies for managing difficult constipation. The following discussion is not an exhaustive list of drugs or methods; it is intended to provide you with several that are commonly used to treat constipation in those with PD. Your physician may have other suggestions as well. As with any medical treatment, common sense is necessary. If more aggressive therapy causes diarrhea, cramping, or other gastrointestinal side effects, then don't continue.

Saline and Osmotic Laxatives

Agents in this class pass into the colon undigested and draw water from the intestinal wall (by osmosis). This water expands the colon content, stimulating internal reflexes leading to peristalsis. It also liquefies the stool.

One form of osmotic laxative suitable for frequent use is lactulose (Cephulac, Chronulac, Duphalac). This comes as a liquid in a typical concentration of 10 grams per 15 mL (milliliters) of syrup. You may take 1–2 tablespoons (15–30 mL) daily, perhaps mixed with fruit juice. Additional doses may be necessary, up to 4–6 tablespoons per day (40–60 grams, but not all at once). A powdered form (Kristalose) is also available in 10 and 20 gram packets. This can be mixed in water or juice, starting with 10 grams once daily and increasing up to 40–60 grams daily, if necessary (in divided doses). The primary side effects are stomach cramping and occasionally nausea; these are not dangerous but could be distressing. Some of these lactulose preparations contain sugar, so if you are diabetic, discuss this with your doctor.

Another commonly used osmotic laxative contains magnesium. You will undoubtedly recognize this by the name, milk of magnesia (magnesium hydroxide). The standard dose is 1–3 tablespoons per day (1 tablespoon = 15 mL). This is an acceptable laxative for frequent use, provided that you do not suffer from any major problems with your kidneys or congestive heart failure.

Stimulant Laxatives

There are several laxatives that stimulate the muscles of the colon walls to contract (peristalsis). They also stimulate the passage of water into the colon. Side effects are similar to lactulose, with potential for stomach cramping or nausea. If frequently used, they do have the potential to irritate the lining of the intestinal system. Common over-the-counter drugs of this type include the following:

- Bisacodyl (Dulcolax) comes in 5 mg tablets. If 1-2 tablets are taken at bedtime, a bowel movement is likely to occur the following morning. It also comes in a 10 mg rectal suppository, which will often result in a bowel movement in 15–60 minutes.

- Senna is the active ingredient in Senokot. One to two Senokot tablets (or 1–2 teaspoons of the syrup) at bedtime should produce a bowel movement the following morning. If necessary, this dose may be doubled. It also comes in a double-dose form, marketed as SenokotXtra. Senna may discolor urine to brownish or pink-red hues.

Enemas

Enemas flush the stool out of the colon. Enema kits may be purchased from your drug store. Those with prepackaged small volumes of enema fluid, such as the small Fleets enema, may not be sufficient if the constipation is long-standing. Chronic constipation may result in stool being backed up in your colon for long distances. You then will need a larger amount of fluid to flush it out.

Enemas are necessary if you have gone many days without an adequate bowel movement. In that case, the stool may have become hard and impacted in your colon. This may prevent even stimulant laxatives from working. In fact, the peristalsis induced by stimulant laxatives may cause severe abdominal cramps if impacted stool is blocking the colon.

Paradoxically, some people with severe constipation experience watery fecal discharge (not due to laxatives). Sometimes, when hard stool becomes stuck in the colon, only watery feces can pass around it. For this problem, a high volume, cleansing enema is necessary to clear the colon.

My Strategy for Managing Constipation

I always make certain that the basic principles listed above are followed (i.e., fluids, fiber, fruits and vegetables, exercise, and perhaps prune juice). If this is insufficient to produce a bowel movement at least once every two days, I then accept the fact that we may need to use laxatives on a frequent basis. Here is the scheme that I often use when people are troubled by constipation that does not respond to simple measures.

- If you are starting this scheme with severe constipation and no bowel movement for several days, it is wise to begin with a thorough cleansing enema. Bowel cleansing allows the laxatives to subsequently work appropriately and without cramping.

- If you go two days without a bowel movement, it is appropriate to use a laxative (go an extra day if it doesn't bother you).

- Allow a day for the laxative to work. If no bowel movement, then use an enema.

- Repeat the cycle.

27

◆ ◆ ◆

Urinary Symptoms

PD may cause problems with urination. Typically, this is not an early symptom and may never be a problem. However, when such symptoms develop, there are appropriate tests, consultations, treatments, and caveats to consider.

Anatomy of the Urinary System

When urinary symptoms develop in PD, they reflect problems in the bladder and structures connected to the bladder. Although the kidneys make the urine, kidney problems do not cause difficulties passing urine. The kidneys essentially filter the blood, extracting water and other products that need to be excreted. As the kidneys produce urine drop by drop, it passes down tubes to the reservoir that stores the urine. That reservoir is the bladder. The conduits from kidneys to bladder are called the ureters. When urine is released, it passes from the bladder through another conduit, the urethra. This anatomy is illustrated in figure 27.1. Normally urine is stored in the bladder until the brain is signaled that it is time to urinate.

The act of urination entails contraction of muscles within the walls of the bladder that squeeze the urine out. Coinciding with this is opening of outlet valves that permit the urine to pass into the urethra.

Aging and the Urinary System

Simply getting older may produce problems with urination, irrespective of PD. Aging affects the urinary systems of men and women differently.

Women often develop urinary incontinence in middle age or beyond, primarily due to child bearing. The process of delivering a baby may damage the bladder outlet. In later life this predisposes to incompetence of the outlet valve. The typical symptoms are leakage of small amounts of urine when coughing, sneezing, or laughing. Because the bladder outlet valve is poorly competent, urine is pushed out when the abdominal wall muscles suddenly contract during coughing or straining. This is termed stress incontinence. If troublesome, the bladder outlet can be surgically corrected.

Men have a different problem, which relates to the prostate. The urethra passes through the middle of the prostate gland. In young men, the prostate does not compress the urethra and urine passes easily. However, with aging, the

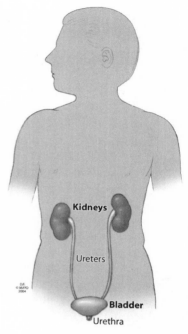

27.1 Urine is made in the kidneys and stored in the bladder. It is excreted via the urethra.

prostate tends to enlarge, sometimes constricting the urethra passing through it and impeding the urine flow. This enlargement of the prostate is a typical aging effect and is not necessarily a sign of prostate cancer.

Normal aging may also result in more general dysfunction of the bladder control system, which tends to operate less efficiently as we get older. This may add to the urinary problems unique to men and women.

The Neurogenic Bladder of PD

The autonomic nervous system controls bladder function, and this may be impaired in PD. In a properly functioning system, contraction of the bladder and opening of the valves to expel urine is regulated via internal reflexes; it only tends to occur when the bladder is full and only when we allow it to happen. When autonomic control of the bladder malfunctions, this is termed a neurogenic bladder.

The challenge in PD is to sort out whether the urinary symptoms are due to a neurogenic bladder or structural problems of the urinary system due to aging (or some other cause). These have different treatments.

Autonomic urinary dysfunction in PD may result in several different symptoms, which vary from person to person. They relate to problems of bladder contraction, opening of the outlet valves, or aberrant signals from bladder nerves to the brain. Let's consider each of these symptoms individually.

Hesitancy

Urinary "hesitancy" is a medical term implying that it is difficult to initiate urination. You may sense the need to urinate but can't get it started as you sit on the toilet or stand at the urinal. Once the urinary stream is started, the flow may be very slow and emptying your bladder may seem to take forever.

Hesitancy is typical of male prostate problems where the enlarged prostate compresses the urethra, preventing flow. However, it can also be a symptom of damaged bladder reflexes from autonomic nervous system dysfunction. In that case, signals from the full bladder, which should induce contraction of the bladder muscles, result in insufficient bladder emptying. Consequently the bladder tends to fill up and stay full. If there is an incompetent outlet valve, urine may slowly leak out when the bladder becomes fully distended and can't hold any more (overflow incontinence).

Incomplete Emptying

When urinary hesitancy becomes pronounced, it is often associated with a bladder that never fully empties. In other words, after passing urine at the toilet, there is still a substantial amount left in the bladder. This can be problematic in at least a couple of ways:

- Stagnant urine that doesn't get expelled may predispose to a urinary tract infection.
- If the bladder is very full and unable to empty, it can be uncomfortable or even painful.

In men, autonomic problems causing hesitancy may be additive with the prostate symptoms of aging.

Urgency

Urinary urgency implies a heightened need to urinate. This is the feeling that we all experience if prevented from getting to the bathroom when we need to urinate (e.g., a car trip when no gas stations are in sight). Urgency implies an abnormal sense of urination. Abnormal urge is not linked to a full bladder but rather reflects false signals to the brain that the bladder is distended. It may also be experienced by those with urinary tract infections (see below).

In one sense, urgency is opposite to hesitancy, although the same person may experience both. Urgency is often reflective of increased bladder reflexes, the so-called overactive bladder. There is an exaggerated reflex as the bladder is filling, which stimulates the bladder muscles to contract long before the bladder is full. This may result in an urge at very short intervals, recurring perhaps 30–60 minutes after previously urinating.

When urgency is due to heightened bladder reflexes (overactive bladder), this is treated opposite to hesitancy. A hesitant bladder requires a stimulus to contract, whereas an overactive bladder needs to be dampened. This may be problematic when these symptoms occur in the same person.

Incontinence

Urinary incontinence implies inappropriate leakage of urine (peeing in your pants). There are several ways this may happen. First, incontinence may occur if the normal bladder outlet has been damaged, such as by childbirth or following certain pelvic surgeries. Second, those with PD and autonomic nervous system dysfunction may have a hesitant bladder with reduced contraction of bladder muscles; this lazy bladder may fill beyond the capacity, spilling urine. This is termed overflow incontinence. Third, autonomic dysfunction may result in an overactive bladder with increased bladder reflexes that expel urine. This is termed urge incontinence.

Nocturia

If the bladder fills to capacity during sleep, we awaken with an appropriate urge to urinate. The need to urinate during the night is termed nocturia. Having to do this once or perhaps twice a night is common among seniors. However, this may be exacerbated by the bladder dysfunction of PD, disrupting sleep.

The tendency for nocturia is increased in poor sleepers. People who sleep soundly tend to unconsciously suppress the urge to urinate until it becomes prominent; only then do they awaken. Light sleepers are easily awakened by the slightest stimuli, in this case, from the bladder. People with PD who sleep poorly because of insufficient PD medications may be especially susceptible to this problem (see chapter 20).

Enuresis

Enuresis (bed-wetting) is not a common problem among those with PD and is rare early in the course. When it occurs, it is often associated with cognitive problems that may develop later. However, there are exceptions and obviously enuresis sometimes develops among seniors who do not have PD. Sedating medications may contribute to this problem.

Dysuria and Urinary Tract Infections

Dysuria is a medical term meaning painful urination. Typically, this is experienced as a painful burning sensation and suggests a urinary tract infection. Stagnant urine pooling in a lazy, neurogenic bladder is prone to infection. If it hurts to urinate, you should have a urinalysis and a urinary culture performed. The urinalysis includes examining your urine under the microscope. If bacteria and inflammatory cells (white cells) are present, this indicates infection. A urine culture is also routinely done to identify the strain of bacteria and guide the choice of antibiotic. This is less critical if it is your first urinary infection or at least the first in many years. However, those with repeat urinary infections often harbor bacteria that are resistant to many antibiotics.

A sense of urinary urgency may also be a symptom of a urinary tract infection. Occasionally the symptoms of urge incontinence will resolve simply with treatment of an infection.

Are These Urinary Problems Inevitable?

Not necessarily; not everyone with PD has difficulty with urination, and when it does occur, it often is much later in the course. Furthermore, when urinary symptoms develop, they may be limited; however, it is important to sort them out and employ proper treatment.

How to Assess

The workup of any urinary problem starts with a routine urinalysis and gram stain (looking for bacteria under the microscope), plus a urine culture if positive. If an infection is found, it is treated with antibiotics. Bladder symptoms beyond a simple infection may require consultation with a urologist. They are in the best position to characterize a neurogenic bladder and distinguish other factors, such as prostate or age-related female stress incontinence. Urological tests that they may consider include the following:

- If substantial urinary hesitancy is present with suspicion of incomplete emptying, a catheter may be inserted into your bladder after urinating, to measure the volume of residual urine. Normally you should almost completely evacuate your bladder with urination.

- Cystoscopy is usually performed to look inside the bladder. This is done through a tiny scope that allows the urologist to see the bladder wall and passages. If there are pockets of infection, bladder wall cancer, or certain types of obstruction to the normal flow of urine, this can be detected.

- Neurologic function of the bladder is assessed by urodynamics. Urodynamic studies involve inflating the bladder with water or carbon dioxide and then assessing the neurologic reflexes. For example, normal bladders do not contract until they have filled to a certain volume and then contract with a measurable force. These recorded outcomes can be compared to known normal values.

Urodynamic testing will identify whether the bladder is overactive or underactive. You might think that this could be accurately predicted from the symptoms; for example, hesitancy should suggest an underactive bladder and urge incontinence the opposite. However, experience has taught us that such assumptions are often incorrect. Hence it is often wise to define the problem with the appropriate tests before deciding about chronic therapy.

Anticholinergic Medications for an Overactive Bladder: Urgency, Urge Incontinence, or Urinary Frequency

A hyperactive bladder can be toned down with anticholinergic drugs, which block the neurotransmitter acetylcholine. It is released by nerves that signal the bladder muscles to contract. If this effect is inhibited, then the bladder contractions are reduced and symptoms of an overactive bladder are diminished (urgency, urge incontinence, and frequent urge to urinate).

Acetylcholine is found throughout the nervous system and drugs that block acetylcholine have widespread effects, as previously noted. Side effects include constipation, dry mouth and eyes, blurred vision, and exacerbation of glaucoma. They tend to cause mild memory impairment, which may be especially problematic in those with dementia. These drugs also reduce sweat output, which is important if exercising on a hot day; impaired perspiration may predispose to heat stroke. Pharmaceutical companies have tried to tailor bladder drugs to minimize these problems. Although the frequency of these side effects is less with these medications for the bladder, they still may occur.

As a general rule, it is wisest to take smaller doses of these bladder drugs, at least in the beginning; this will reduce the risk of side effects. Raise the dose only if necessary. Also, if your bladder symptoms are only a problem during certain times, such as at night, more limited treatment may be appropriate. For example, perhaps only a single dose of the short-acting (immediate-release) bladder drug just before bed might be sufficient if your symptoms are primarily during the night.

The most commonly prescribed drugs for an overactive bladder are oxybutynin (Ditropan) and tolterodine (Detrol). Other anticholinergic drugs occasionally prescribed include hyoscyamine (Levsin, Levbid, Levsinex, Cystospaz) and flavoxate (Urispas). We will focus on oxybutynin and tolterodine, in view of their common use. These two drugs are similar in potency. However, tolterodine is a little better tolerated and is perhaps the better choice among those with PD.

If overactive bladder symptoms are a problem both day and night, then the extended-release form of tolterodine (Detrol LA) may be prescribed. It is administered once daily. Start with the smaller dose of 2 mg taken once a day. If insufficient and if no side effects, it could be raised to 4 mg once daily. This pill comes in both 2 mg and 4 mg sizes.

An alternative is the extended-release formulation of oxybutynin (Ditropan XL), starting with 5 mg once daily. It can later be raised to 10 mg once daily if necessary. Both a 5 mg and 10 mg extended-release tablet are available. With both tolterodine and oxybutynin extended-release tablets, the smaller dose is almost as effective as the larger dose.

If your problem is primarily or exclusively at night (nocturia), a single dose of the immediate-release form of tolterodine or oxybutynin at bedtime could be tried. In the immediate-release form, tolterodine is clearly better tolerated, so that is the better choice of the two. A dose of 2 mg of tolterodine (immediate-release) could be taken at bedtime and increased to 4 mg if necessary (but most of the benefit will accrue with the smaller 2 mg dose). A single bedtime dose of 5 mg of immediate-release oxybutynin is an alternative.

Redundancy with Other Anticholinergic Drugs

Before starting a drug for overactive bladder, review your medication list to make certain that you are not already taking a drug from the anticholinergic class (listed on table 26.1). This includes anticholinergic medications for PD, loose stools, as well as certain antidepressant drugs. If you are taking one of these medications, then adding an anticholinergic bladder medication is redundant, with potential for side effects.

Treatment: Frequent Awakening to Urinate

Nocturia, frequent awakening to urinate, can disrupt sleep and secondarily result in daytime drowsiness. Four different factors can contribute to your nocturia.

1. Water balance:

   Drinking liquids in the evening

Taking diuretics (water pills) later in the day (e.g., hydrochlorothiazide, triamterene, furosemide)

Drinking coffee, tea, caffeinated soda, or alcohol in the evening (all have a diuretic effect)

2. Parkinsonism:

Poor control of parkinsonism during the night, resulting in light sleep

Taking selegiline in the evening

3. Light sleep having nothing to do with PD or bladder:

Chronic insomnia, independent from PD

Stress in your life

Depression

4. Bladder dysfunction:

Urinary tract infection

Overactive bladder

Prostate problems in men

If you experience nocturia, avoid drinking liquids after supper and empty your bladder just before bed. If you take any pills in the evening, have your physician confirm that none are diuretics. Selegiline can cause insomnia and stimulate a sensitive bladder; take this drug only in the morning.

If your parkinsonian symptoms are not controlled during the night, this can and frequently does result in very superficial sleep. Hence you will easily awaken with any stimulus (including the need to urinate). If you think this could be a contributor to your problem, review chapter 20.

Light sleep for any reason can make it easier for urinary symptoms to awaken you (see chapter 20). If you need a sleep medication, consider low dose amitriptyline (10–75 mg at bedtime); this not only is sedating but also tends to dampen the urge to urinate (anticholinergic properties). Also, recall that depression can result in disrupted sleep (chapter 22).

A routine urinalysis is appropriate to make certain no infection is causing nocturia. This can be followed up by a urologist.

Medications for Enuresis

For those with PD, bed-wetting during sleep may be difficult to treat with medications. The usual medications are these same anticholinergic drugs used for an overactive bladder. They will not be helpful, however, if an overactive bladder is not the primary cause. Your urologist needs to advise after doing the appropriate studies.

Drugs for enuresis include immediate-acting tolterodine or oxybutynin at bedtime; the doses were cited above. Amitriptyline is an alternative with both anticholinergic and sleep-inducing properties, as mentioned above. Sometimes imipramine is used for this same purpose; it is less sedating and is prescribed in the same dosage as amitriptyline. Either drug can be started in a dose of 10–25 mg at bedtime; if insufficient, it can be raised to 50 and then 75 mg at bedtime.

For the most troublesome enuresis, some physicians have prescribed a synthetic hormone that induces the kidneys to retain water. This results in less urine production and hence less urine passing to the bladder. The natural hormone with this property is vasopressin, and the synthetic drug used to mimic this effect is desmopressin. In seniors, however, desmopressin may upset the balance of fluids and electrolytes (i.e., sodium, potassium). Hence I generally avoid prescribing this drug. If it is prescribed, blood sodium and potassium levels should occasionally be checked.

Medications for Memory Have Opposite Effects

In chapter 23, I listed four drugs prescribed to enhance memory: donepezil (Aricept), rivastigmine (Exelon), galantamine (Reminyl), and tacrine (Cognex). They all work by enhancing the effect of acetylcholine in the brain. However, this procholinergic effect is not confined to the brain and potentially includes the bladder. This is opposite to the anticholinergic drugs used to treat urinary urgency. Surprisingly, these memory-enhancing drugs do not frequently exacerbate bladder problems, as you might predict. However, it seems irrational to prescribe both simultaneously, since the effects may offset each other.

Treatment of a Distended, Underactive Bladder with Symptoms of Hesitancy, Incomplete Emptying, Overflow Incontinence

Effective drugs to stimulate lazy, distended bladders have yet to be developed. Your urologist obviously needs to exclude the possibility of obstruction to urine flow, as might occur with an enlarged prostate. However, if no impediment to urine flow is present, drugs are unlikely to be helpful.

For most with this problem, the urologist employs other strategies. Urine left behind in the bladder has a tendency to become infected, and if this is a frequent occurrence, an antibiotic to keep the bacteria counts low may be prescribed on a chronic, preventive basis. The urologist may also instruct in the Crede maneuver, which involves squeezing down on the pelvis to help expel urine out of the bladder. Pads, such as Depends, may also be advised to catch urinary leakage.

If bladder emptying is extremely slow and incomplete, the urologist may suggest use of a catheter. Self-catheterization requires you to insert sterile, rubber-like tubing (catheter) into your bladder to allow it to drain. This can be done several times daily and allows you to stay one step ahead of incontinence due to overflow from a distended bladder. By catheterizing just before social and other activities, embarrassing overflow incontinence can be prevented. Obviously there is a major hassle factor with this strategy. Fortunately most people with PD do not need to resort to this.

Drugs for Male Prostate Problems: Be Wary of Low Blood Pressure

An enlarged prostate may obstruct the flow of urine out of the bladder, resulting in hesitant urination and incomplete bladder emptying. Drugs that block certain of the effects of adrenalin are often prescribed to reduce enlarged prostate glands. The three medications used for this purpose are:

- Tamsulosin (Flomax)
- Doxazosin (Cardura)
- Terazosin (Hytrin)

These drugs also lower the blood pressure. In fact, the last two were initially introduced primarily for that purpose. As noted in chapter 21, a low blood pressure when standing or walking (orthostatic hypotension) is common in PD. These three drugs may exacerbate this potential problem. Tamsulosin is the least likely to do this and may be the best choice of the three. However, if orthostatic hypotension is a major problem, these medications should probably not be used. If one of these drugs is prescribed for an enlarged bladder, the standing blood pressure should be checked before and after starting it.

Finasteride (Proscar) is also used to reduce the size of the prostate. However, this drug does not lower the blood pressure.

Caveat: Prostate Surgery

Men with markedly enlarged prostate glands may be offered a TURP, which stands for transurethral resection of the prostate. Essentially, the passageway for urinary flow is surgically cleared and expanded. This is routine surgery for a urologist and typically goes well. However, those with PD who undergo a TURP procedure are prone to urinary incontinence. This relates to loss of the normal valve function at the bladder outlet following this surgery. Urologists usually are aware of this potential problem and will factor this into a surgical decision. However, they may overlook it if they are not aware that you have PD; hence you must inform them.

28

◆ ◆ ◆

Sexual Dysfunction, Estrogen, and Menstrual Cycles

Male Sexual Dysfunction

For men in general, there are a variety of reasons for impaired sexual performance, including depression, anxiety, and medications. For men with PD, additional factors may play a role. Let's think about this in more detail.

IMPOTENCE IS UNIVERSAL

Impotence implies difficulty with sexual performance—problems achieving and maintaining an erection, which should lead to ejaculation. Before considering all the things that can disrupt sexual performance, we should recognize that occasional impotence is common. This is something that can and does happen to even the most macho guy.

AGE

Men are at their sexual peak during their teenage years and a little after. With passing decades, not only does the urge for sexual gratification decline but also the ability to perform. Hence, as men pass beyond the years when all they think about is sex, occasional impotence is fairly common. We need to accept this, just as we are stuck with the joint pains that never bothered us when we were young, or the middle-age requirement for reading glasses.

PSYCHOLOGICAL ISSUES

Any man who is depressed, anxious, worried, or distracted will be at an increased risk of impotence. Appropriate treatment of these problems is an important first step in treating impotence.

PERFORMANCE ANXIETY

Sexual acts come naturally. You cannot "will" an erection. In fact, if you try to do that, the erection is sabotaged. For men who have experienced impotence, this tends to become a focus during subsequent sexual engagements. "What if this happens again?" "I need to do something to avoid this embarrassment!" If this is the foremost thought in your mind as you begin sexual foreplay, you will be doomed. Like a quarterback who throws an interception, you can't take this mistake to your next play. Forget about it and move on. All men will experience this on occasion. You can't dwell on it. Unfortunately this is easy to say but hard to do.

MEDICAL CONDITIONS AND IMPOTENCE

A variety of medical problems (besides PD) can cause impotence. These problems become more common as we age.

First, any disorder that leads to atherosclerosis (hardening of the arteries) increases the likelihood of impotence. This is because blood circulation to the penis is a crucial component of erections; it is engorgement of blood within the penis that makes it firm and elongated. Disease or conditions that lead to atherosclerosis may impair circulation to the penis. Predisposing conditions include:

- Diabetes mellitus
- High cholesterol
- Smoking
- Uncontrolled high blood pressure
- Normal aging

These factors do not cause impotence directly or immediately; however, after years, they contribute to atherosclerosis, which may then be a factor in circulatory problems in the penis. Unfortunately, once atherosclerosis develops, it is difficult to reverse it; however, with attention to these risk factors, it may be stabilized. Occasionally limited reversal is possible.

Any major illness or disease of the internal organs may be associated with impotence. Thus liver, kidney, heart or lung failure, or major infectious illness (e.g., pneumonia, kidney infections) make sexual performance problematic. Endocrine disorders such as thyroid disease may also be associated with impotence.

Certain neurologic diseases besides PD are also associated with impotence, including multiple sclerosis, peripheral neuropathy, and spinal cord conditions. Also disorders resulting in chronic pain make sexual performance difficult.

Long-standing substance abuse may ultimately result in impotence. This is especially common among alcoholics.

TESTOSTERONE

The male hormone testosterone is crucial to male sexual performance. It is uncommon for this to be the primary cause of impotence, however. Furthermore, treatment with testosterone-like substances does not cure impotence except for those occasional men with measured low blood levels. Although you might think this would be a good treatment for problems with erections, it is inadequate unless your doctor identifies a deficiency. Furthermore, even when testosterone treatment is administered to those with low levels, impotence may not be cured since there often are other contributing problems.

If your testosterone blood levels are low, therapy with this male hormone may be considered. However, be aware of its potential to activate prostate cancer. Prostate cancer becomes increasingly common as men age. In fact, by the time men are in their seventies, the majority have some signs of cancerous changes in their prostate glands. Fortunately only the minority will experience spread of this cancer. However, testosterone and related male hormones increase the activity of these prostate cancer cells. Hence testosterone treatment runs the risk of encouraging the growth of prostate cancer that might otherwise have been indefinitely dormant. In fact, treatment of prostate cancer involves blocking the effects or release of testosterone. If you have ever been diagnosed with prostate cancer, you should not receive male hormone replacement therapy.

MEDICATIONS (OTHER THAN PD DRUGS) AND IMPOTENCE

All types of medications have the potential to cause impotence. The list is too long to enumerate here. Furthermore, many of the medications on this list will cause impotence only occasionally. The list includes a variety of medications to lower blood pressure, treat chronic pain, relax muscles, and treat cancer, as well as certain psychiatric conditions. Some or all of these may be critical to your health. However, it is appropriate to have your physician review your list to determine if any drug is particularly likely to be responsible. If such a drug is identified, your physician can tell you whether it is safe to stop it for a few weeks to determine if this was the offending agent. Sometimes the offending drug is obvious. If impotence only became a problem following treatment with a new drug, this medication may be the culprit.

The selective serotonin antidepressant medications (SSRIs) used to treat depression are sometimes blamed for reduced libido or impotence. This may be true in some cases, but in others, as they effectively treat depression, sexual function secondarily improves. Untreated depression blunts sexual desire and function. An antidepressant drug that has perhaps the least likelihood of causing problems with libido and sexual function is bupropion (Wellbutrin).

PD AND IMPOTENCE

Parkinson's disease may predispose to impotence. This is not to say that everyone with PD is impotent. However, PD increases this risk. PD is associated with autonomic nervous system dysfunction, which may result in bladder difficulties, constipation, or orthostatic hypotension. Since sexual functioning is also regulated by the autonomic nervous system, it also is susceptible.

PD MEDICATIONS AND IMPOTENCE

The drugs we administer for PD are sometimes blamed for impotence. But I suspect that the opposite is more often true: adequate treatment of parkinsonism may actually facilitate sexual performance. Undertreatment may be more likely to result in impotence, although this is an area that has not been adequately studied.

Interestingly, following the introduction of levodopa therapy, several physicians published reports of increased sexual function among those newly treated. Initially this was thought to represent a true aphrodisiac effect. However, it later became clear that most of these people were experiencing improved sexual performance simply as a consequence of better mobility and movement. Levodopa turned out to have no substantial aphrodisiac effect in men without PD.

Recently apomorphine has received publicity as treatment for male impotence. You may recall our consideration of this drug from chapter 18; its utility in PD is to rescue you from a levodopa off-state. It is a dopamine agonist medication that can be administered by injection. Apomorphine appears to be mildly helpful in treating male impotence in general; however, it's unlikely to be effective in treating impotence among men with PD for a couple of reasons. First, optimal treatment with carbidopa/levodopa will probably overshadow the effects of apomorphine on impotence. Second, the more substantial erectile problems of PD will probably require more potent agents than the mildly effective apomorphine. Controlled studies of apomorphine treatment of erectile dysfunction have not been done in men with PD.

There are rare cases of hypersexuality among men linked to one of the PD drugs (even less frequently among women). The hypersexuality resolves with reduction or discontinuation of the offending drug. Carbidopa/levodopa, dopamine agonists, selegiline, and amantadine have all been reported to do this, as noted in chapter 24.

SIMPLE STRATEGIES TO MAXIMIZE MALE SEXUAL PERFORMANCE

Although some of the factors that may sabotage sexual functioning are beyond our control, there are a variety of things we should consider that may enhance performance.

- Treat any psychological and psychiatric problems; if things are weighing heavily on your mind, performance will suffer.
- Learn to forget about past potency problems.
- Work with your physician to treat active medical problems.
- Do all the right "health" things:
    Exercise regularly.
    Get enough sleep.
    Drink enough fluids.
    Consume no more than modest amounts of alcohol (alcohol may affect potency).
    Avoid obesity. If you are in good physical shape, things that should come naturally (i.e., sexual function) are more likely to do exactly that.
- Have your physician review your medication list for drugs that could be contributing to impotence.
- Discuss with your physician whether there is any merit in measuring your blood (serum) testosterone levels.
- Treat your symptoms of PD adequately. Sexual performance may suffer if you are in a parkinsonian off-state.
- For PD treatment, add medications one at a time. If sexual performance declines after a new drug is started, at least you know the cause.
- Discuss any potency concerns openly with your partner, who may be able to supply additional stimulation techniques, and more patient expectations.
- Recognize and respect your partner's role changes with the advent of your PD. Your partner may be taking on added work and burdens that make it more difficult to find the time and energy to be sexually receptive.
- Engage in sex in a relaxed environment without time constraints. Set aside a period of time for this rather than trying to squeeze it in before work in the morning, or at other times when you are hurried. Also, things may go better if you don't defer it until late at night when you are starting to become tired.

Although this list is for male impotence, many of these commonsense strategies are relevant to women with PD as well.

WHEN SIMPLER STRATEGIES DON'T WORK: DRUGS FOR ERECTIONS

If you have done all the right things and failed erections are still a problem, you may be a candidate for

- Sildenafil (Viagra)

- Vardenafil (Levitra)

- Tadalafil (Cialis)

These medications will not change your sexual appetite but rather have a specific effect on penile blood flow, helping to achieve and maintain erections. An erection will not be achieved with these alone; sexual stimulation must also be employed.

These drugs reflect a new era in medicine, when advertising is directed at the general public rather than physicians. Hence everyone knows about Viagra, Levitra, and Cialis. Testimonials from public figures have helped position these drugs in a positive light; it's okay to use them and this doesn't detract from a macho image.

VIAGRA DOSAGE

The usual dose of sildenafil (Viagra) is a single 50 mg tablet taken approximately an hour before intercourse. It takes an hour or slightly less to start working, with an effect that lasts 3–4 hours. For the best effect, take it on an empty stomach. Those over sixty-five and those with serious liver or kidney problems should start with a 25 mg dose, since their metabolism of the active drug is less, and a lower dose is therefore appropriate. It can subsequently be raised to 50 mg if necessary. The highest recommended dose is 100 mg and this should be tried only if lower doses fail and only on a subsequent day. In other words, if a lower dose does not work, don't take more that day. Only a single dose is advisable per day. This drug comes in three pill sizes: 25 mg, 50 mg, and 100 mg.

LEVITRA DOSAGE

The general principles for using this medication are the same as for sildenafil. A 10 mg dose is taken about an hour before intercourse. If you are over age 65, or have liver or kidney failure, start with half this dose; if that doesn't work, you may then try 10 mg next time. Don't take more than one dose in a day. The maximum dose is 20 mg. Four pill sizes are available: 2.5, 5, 10 and 20 mg.

CIALIS DOSAGE

This drug is similar to the other two except for a longer duration of effect, lasting up to 36 hours. Thus you do not need to time the dose with respect to intercourse, allowing for greater spontaneity. The usual dose is 10 mg, but half this dose if over sixty-five, or if liver or kidney failure. As with the others, only one dose per 24 hours is advised. Three pill sizes are available: 5, 10, and 20 mg. The maximum dose is 20 mg.

CAUTIONS ASSOCIATED WITH STARTING THESE DRUGS

This class of medications lowers blood pressure. This is especially a concern for those with PD since they are prone to low blood pressure (orthostatic hypotension). A drop in blood pressure following a dose of one of these medications may manifest in one of two ways:

- The lowered blood pressure may occur only when you get up, such as when you go to the bathroom. This is typical of the orthostatic hypotension occurring in PD, where the blood pressure drops with standing, but is usually satisfactory when lying or sitting.

- The blood pressure may drop to uncomfortably low levels even in bed (lying down). If you start to feel faint, you may be experiencing this side effect. Furthermore, your sexual performance may suffer (it's difficult to perform if you are on the verge of fainting).

Hence, before taking your first dose, it might be wise to check your lying, sitting, and standing blood pressure. Be sure to do this when your levodopa or dopamine agonist is working (on-state). Remember that levodopa and the dopamine agonists will lower your blood pressure for up to a few hours after each dose. If your pressure readings are around 90/60, this suggests a risk of even lower values and fainting with the additional use of these drugs.

If you have a serious heart problem, especially angina (chest pain due to impaired blood flow to heart muscle), avoid sildenafil, vardenafil, and tadalafil, unless your physician approves. These medications should not be used if your heart condition requires you to take a nitrate drug (i.e., nitroglycerin, isosorbide), although your doctor may allow exceptions.

A number of minor side effects may also develop with use of these drugs and are not worrisome. These include changes in color vision or visual acuity, facial flushing, nasal congestion, nausea, or headache.

BEYOND VIAGRA, LEVITRA, AND CIALIS

There are other options for men with inability to obtain erections. However, they are a little more complicated and consultation with a urologist is necessary. The urologist may first assess the quality of erections by overnight measurement; men tend to get erections during sleep, which can be measured with a special device.

Further options from the urologists include:

- Administration of a medication into the end of the urethra at the tip of the penis (i.e., into the orifice at the end of the penis; the same orifice from which urine passes). This is done with a small applicator prior to sexual activity. When this dissolves into the penis tissue, it causes an erection.

- Injection of a different medication into the base of the penis via a small needle prior to sex. This sounds painful but is actually well tolerated by most men, resulting in an erection lasting several minutes to hours.

- Use of a special vacuum tube that is placed over the penis, resulting in increased blood flow and an erection. A rubber band-like ring is then placed at the base of the penis, which traps the blood and allows the erection to be maintained.

The first two of these options may occasionally result in side effects, so they are initially tried in the urologist's office to make certain everything goes smoothly.

Surgery is also an option for treatment of impotence. Penile implants surgically placed into the shaft of the penis are generally of two types:

- Semirigid rods that produce a permanent erection (they can be easily bent backward to conceal this in one's trousers).

- Inflatable implants that can be pumped to achieve the erection when appropriate. The actual pump is surgically placed in the scrotum and the reservoir with the air for inflation is implanted in the abdomen. These are all well concealed.

Obviously these implants will not precisely duplicate a natural erection.

Female Sexual Function

There is a wealth of medical literature on male sexual dysfunction, including impotence caused by chronic neurological disease. However, much less has been written about the influence of neurological disease on female sexual function. Only recently has the effect of PD on female sexual functioning received any attention in the medical literature. Moreover, women are generally reluctant to discuss sexual functioning with their physicians, especially if the physician is male. Male physicians managing PD are reluctant to ask their female patients about sex and tend to focus on more elementary problems of PD, such as tremor or ability to walk. Hence sexual functioning is usually ignored. I also plead guilty to this shortsightedness.

It is difficult to draw any broad conclusions about the effect of PD on female sexual function because what has been written is either anecdotal or has focused on small numbers of women. Furthermore, some form of sexual dysfunction occurs in the majority of middle-aged women without PD (e.g., reduced libido, lack of orgasm, pain with intercourse, tightness or dryness of the vagina). Hence female sexual dysfunction cannot all be blamed on PD. In limited published studies, women with PD do experience reduced desire for sex, reduced orgasm, and often complain of vaginal tightness, dryness, or pain. To what extent these problems were specifically linked to PD (versus more general factors such as age) is unclear.

Factors related to PD may also play a role in female sexual dysfunction such as depression or medications. Depression dampens desire for many things that we previously found enjoyable, including sex. Medications may also dampen sexual desire or functioning, although this has been poorly studied in women. Sedating medications may reduce female libido. On the other hand, the medications for PD do not appear to have a major influence on female sexual function as best we know; however, this has never been systematically investigated.

What can women with PD do to enhance their sexual desire and function? There are no aphrodisiacs that will magically turn you into a sexual animal. The best we can do is address some general issues that might improve sexual function.

First, female sexual responsiveness is maximal when there are no distractions, stressors, physical pain, or discomfort. Extrapolating from that, it makes sense that female sexuality will be optimized if parkinsonian symptoms are adequately treated. The occasional tendency to defer or limit medications (especially levodopa therapy) may result in a myriad of symptoms that prevent achieving the optimum mental and physical state required for sexual arousal. Undertreatment is often associated with akathisia (inner restlessness; inability to get comfortable), stiffness, and sometimes painful cramps, or other sources of pain; occasionally, frank anxiety results from inadequate treatment. Hence appropriate treatment of PD should also benefit sexuality.

Second, treat psychological depression. Depression is notorious for contributing to sexual dysfunction and loss of libido in the general population. Those with PD are at an increased risk for depression and this is important to recognize and treat (see chapter 22). Parenthetically, the selective serotonin reuptake inhibitor (SSRI) drugs are commonly used to treat depression and may reduce libido and sexual function in some people. If sexual function is a major concern, perhaps another medication from another class of drugs might be tried; an example of a non-SSRI drug that might be appropriate is bupropion (Wellbutrin).

Third, if you are experiencing vaginal discomfort, pain, tightness, or dryness during intercourse, discuss this with your internist or gynecologist. Besides the obvious water-soluble lubricant (e.g., K-Y Jelly), they might also recommend an estrogen cream. Daily use of an estrogen cream applied to the vaginal area increases natural suppleness and lubrication. Also, discuss with your sexual partner the need to increase the time of foreplay to allow the natural lubrication to develop.

Finally, timing is often crucial. Although sexual activity goes best when spontaneous, you can sometimes plan ahead and create the proper time for sex that fits with your biological and parkinsonian cycles. First, libido diminishes when you are tired. Hence, midnight trysts may not be the optimal time for some. Second, if your response to parkinsonian medications fluctuates, make certain that you are in a levodopa on-state at the anointed time. If you lapse into a levodopa off-state, this will disrupt your performance and enjoyment.

Do Viagra (sildenafil) and similar drugs work for women with PD? Only limited studies have addressed this question and none have focused on vardenafil or tadalafil. For women in general, Viagra appears to have a very limited benefit on sexual functioning; in some studies it was largely ineffective. The same cautions provided men are appropriate: avoid it if you have heart disease with chest pain (especially if you are taking nitrates such as nitroglycerin or Isordil for angina) or if you have low blood pressure (orthostatic hypotension).

EFFECTS OF MENSTRUAL PERIODS AND ESTROGEN ON PARKINSONISM

Estrogen and progesterone are the two major female hormones. Before menopause, blood levels vary with the menstrual cycle. Blood estrogen levels especially correlate with a variety of subjective symptoms among all women. A plummeting estrogen level just before and during menstrual periods is associated with the myriad of symptoms that have been termed premenstrual syndrome.

Women with PD may be especially susceptible to the effects of estrogen. Among those who are premenopausal with regular periods, the response to their PD drugs (especially carbidopa/levodopa and dopamine agonists) may decline just before and during their menses. This decline in the response correlates with low estrogen levels. This doesn't happen in every woman, but it occurs frequently. The key is to recognize the pattern. If you do, then a medication strategy can be employed. You may need to plot the pattern for a few menstrual cycles to be certain.

ALTERING YOUR CARBIDOPA/LEVODOPA DOSAGE DURING MENSTRUAL DOWNTIME

If you can identify a monthly pattern when your PD medications are not working well, then the strategy for dealing with this is fairly obvious. The basic principle is to increase medication doses during the time of the month when control of parkinsonism is lost. How much to increase depends on how much you decline during this time. Once this part of the month is over, you can revert to the medication doses you were previously taking.

If carbidopa/levodopa is one of your PD medications, then this is the drug we increase during this downtime of the month. Usually the problem is that carbidopa/levodopa fails to kick in during this monthly downtime (even though it works reliably at other times of the month). To counter this, raise your carbidopa/levodopa doses by a half tablet of the 25/100 formulation during this time of the month. Try this for several doses. If still insufficient, you can raise the dose again by another half tablet. You may continue with these increments of a half tablet if necessary. If you are taking the immediate-release formulation of carbidopa/levodopa, you should not need to exceed a total of three tablets for each dose (i.e., original dose plus the increments). We set this relative limit because it is rare that levodopa doses need to exceed 300 mg to capture their best effect, provided that they are taken on an empty stomach. In most cases, higher doses don't add benefit. If sustained-release carbidopa/levodopa is being used (Sinemet CR), slightly higher doses than this may be necessary (see chapter 12).

MY LEVODOPA EFFECT DOESN'T LAST AS LONG DURING MY MENSES

There is an exception to this strategy for those whose levodopa effect does not last until the next dose. If during menses, your carbidopa/levodopa kicks in adequately but the effect doesn't last long enough, then don't change the dose. Rather, shorten the interval between doses to match the response duration. Obviously if you shorten the interval between doses, you will need to add an extra dose or two each day so that you are not uncovered at the end of the day. This strategy is the same whether you are taking the sustained-release or immediate-release formulation of carbidopa/levodopa.

I'M TAKING A DOPAMINE AGONIST DRUG AND MY PARKINSONISM DETERIORATES DURING MY MENSES

If you are not taking carbidopa/levodopa but rather a dopamine agonist, then we obviously raise the agonist dose to overcome menstrual deterioration. You will need to refer back to the schedules at the end of chapter 13, which provide guidelines for increasing the dose. Unless you are at the end of the dopamine agonist dosing schedule (i.e., using the highest dose), you can raise the dosage by the steps shown in these schedules.

The dopamine agonist drugs take considerably longer to adjust than levodopa therapy and are subtler in their effect. For these reasons, it is difficult to make proper dosage adjustments confined to certain times of the menstrual cycle. Often it works better to simply raise the agonist doses across the board, throughout the entire month. This differs from what was remarked with regard to carbidopa/levodopa therapy, where we only raised the levodopa doses during specific troublesome times of the month. However, if you start to approach the maximum dosage listed in chapter 13 and are still quite disabled during your menstrual time, you may need to start levodopa therapy (see chapter 12).

POSTMENOPAUSAL ESTROGEN REPLACEMENT THERAPY

What can you expect from estrogen therapy (e.g., Premarin, Estrace) if this is started after menopause? How will that affect PD and the response to PD medications? The answer is that it probably will not have a major impact on your parkinsonian symptoms or on the response to carbidopa/levodopa or other PD drugs. If anything, it likely will improve your response to these medications. Any decision to start an estrogen should be made on other grounds.

29

♦ ♦ ♦

Treating Other Problems: Swelling, Skin Rashes, and Visual Symptoms

Several other conditions are common in Parkinson's Disease (PD) that require treatment other than levodopa and related drugs. In this chapter we will address three problems that frequently develop in the context of PD: swollen legs, certain skin rashes, and visual distortions or blurring.

Swollen Legs

Swelling of the legs is common among seniors in general. It is particularly common among seniors with PD but sometimes occurs in younger people with PD as well.

People often worry that swelling is caused by poor circulation *to* their legs. Rather, it is often just the opposite; it results from poor circulation *from* the legs. Let's briefly define terms so that we can consider this in more detail. Arteries carry blood with oxygen and nutrients to the major organs, muscles, skin, and so on. After the oxygen and nutrients have been extracted, the blood flows back to the heart via the veins.

In the case of leg swelling, the problem is not in the arteries; this is not a sign of poor circulation *to* the legs. Rather, the problem is often in the veins, which return blood after it has flowed through the muscles to nourish them.

URGENT: ONE SWOLLEN, TENDER LEG

A blood clot in a leg vein may cause swelling and this is a condition that must be diagnosed quickly, so that the clot does not dislodge and spread to your lungs. This leg vein clot is termed thrombophlebitis. If the clot breaks off and passes to your lungs, it results in shortness of breath and sometimes pain with breathing. This is termed pulmonary embolism. A massive spread of clot to the lungs can be suddenly fatal.

People who are sedentary with pooling of blood in their legs due to prolonged sitting are more susceptible to thrombophlebitis. This is not the only factor in thrombophlebitis; obviously many people have jobs that require sitting at a desk, and few experience this problem. However, people with advanced or undertreated PD not only tend to be sedentary but also may not spontaneously move their legs when seated. This lack of muscle activity contributes to pooling of blood in the feet and legs. Slowly moving blood, pooled in the feet and legs, clots more easily.

Clues that you are experiencing thrombophlebitis, rather than some other cause of leg swelling, include the following:

- Rapid and recent onset: This vein clot typically is noticed as a recent development, as opposed to swelling that has been present for years. Once the clot has obstructed the flow of blood, the telltale swelling develops in a few days at most.

- Pain: The clot and the swelling are often (but not always) painful. Usually the pain is primarily in the calf. This is in contrast to most other causes of leg swelling, which are painless.

- Tenderness: The rapid onset of the clot and swelling makes the calf tender when gently squeezed.

- Affects one leg: Most benign forms of leg swelling involve both legs, whereas thrombophlebitis almost always affects only one leg.

Hence, if you have recently developed a swollen, tender, painful calf, see your doctor today! If he or she cannot see you, then go to the local emergency room to be evaluated. If you have also become short of breath, go directly to your closest emergency room. The doctor may then choose to confirm this with an ultrasound of your leg veins. Treatment is typically with a blood thinner, usually heparin first, then warfarin (Coumadin).

SERIOUS BUT NOT URGENT CAUSES OF LEG SWELLING

Major internal organ failure may be associated with leg swelling. This includes heart, kidney, and liver failure. Typically the swollen legs are associated with other symptoms, such as shortness of breath, extreme lethargy, and often more widespread body swelling. This is often easy for the physician to recognize and then confirm with tests. Most people seen in PD clinics with leg swelling do not experience it for these reasons.

COMMON AND LESS SERIOUS CAUSES OF LEG SWELLING

Leg swelling is common among those with PD, and in the vast majority of cases, it is not a sign of thrombophlebitis or organ failure. The remaining causes are more benign. Remember that we are talking about chronic, painless swelling of both legs. The common causes include one or more of the following.

- Inactivity (with dependency of legs)
- Incompetent veins
- Treatment of orthostatic hypotension (common in PD)
- Certain PD drugs

We will consider each of these, recognizing that most of the time, more than one factor plays a role.

INACTIVITY (DEPENDENCY OF LEGS)

Those with PD are often less active. The more you sit, the more the blood tends to pool in your feet and legs, pulled there by gravity. Over the course of the day, tiny amounts of fluid seep from the veins and, eventually, swelling may become apparent. Leg swelling is common in any neurologic disorder where walking is compromised and people spend most of the day sitting.

INCOMPETENT VEINS

With normal aging, the veins in your legs lose their elasticity and become baggy and often a little leaky. This is the opposite of what happens to arteries with aging; arteries tend to narrow because of arthrosclerosis. Veins become dilated as they age. In some cases, previous clots in the leg veins (thrombophlebitis) exacerbate this. The sequel to these clots is a permanent impediment to the return of blood from the legs. The remaining veins become dilated and the vessel walls stretched and perhaps leaky (e.g., as in the case of superficial varicose veins).

TREATMENT OF ORTHOSTATIC HYPOTENSION

Orthostatic hypotension is a drop in blood pressure occurring when standing. There is a tendency to develop this among many with PD and this tendency is exacerbated by PD medications, as noted in chapter 21. Our first line of treatment is salt and fluids, sometimes in combination with fludrocortisone, which causes salt (sodium) retention. This treatment strategy is often effective, but this extra salt may cause leg swelling. Is this worrisome? No, except in people who have failing hearts and cannot tolerate the extra salt and fluid (their hearts are too weak to pump this extra volume). In that case, the swelling will also be associated with shortness of breath.

PD DRUGS

Carbidopa/levodopa does not predispose to leg swelling, at least not frequently. However, leg swelling occasionally occurs with other drugs used in the treatment of PD, including all the dopamine agonist medications. This is not worrisome and develops in less than one person in five.

Amantadine may cause swelling plus reddish or purple discoloration of the legs. Although this may be unsightly, it is not a serious problem; if it doesn't bother you, it is okay to continue.

TREATMENT OF CHRONIC PAINLESS SWELLING OF BOTH LEGS

If your leg swelling is not due to thrombophlebitis or to heart, kidney, or liver failure, then there are a few simple treatment strategies that may control the problem.

- Salt restriction: If your blood pressure is not low, reducing the salt in your diet may help.

- Elevate your legs: If you sit for prolonged periods, elevate your legs. How high? You need to allow gravity to pull the blood from your feet to the trunk of your body. To promote this, raise your feet to the level of your heart. Note that a low footstool will not be high enough.

- Avoid prolonged sitting: If you have a sedentary job, periodically get up and walk around. The muscle contractions in your legs during walking pumps blood to reverse pooling in your feet. If forced to sit, such as on an airplane, consciously contract the muscles in your legs; for example, repetitively raise your heels off the floor.

- Wear compressive hose: Compressive hose, such as Jobst stockings, will constrict your leg veins and limit the swelling. When purchased, make certain that they are the proper fit; if too loose, they won't do any good. Also, make certain that you don't wear stockings with compressive bands, or held up by rubber bands; these could make the problem worse by impeding the blood flow in veins.

- Diuretics (and a note of caution): Physicians often prescribe a diuretic (water pill) to treat swelling. These cause your kidneys to excrete salt (sodium) and water. However, if you have PD, you must be careful with this strategy. As mentioned, many with PD have a tendency toward orthostatic hypotension and diuretic therapy may push you over the edge. Do not take a water pill if you have already been diagnosed with orthostatic hypotension. Commonly prescribed diuretics include furosemide (Lasix) and hydrochlorothiazide (HCTZ), sometimes in combination with triamterene (Dyazide).

The bottom line is that for most with leg swelling, this is not a worrisome problem. Except in a few of the more extreme cases, it can typically be controlled by simple measures.

Skin Rashes

SEBORRHEIC DERMATITIS

Seborrheic dermatitis is the hallmark rash of Parkinson's disease. Not everyone gets it, but clearly it develops more often among those with PD. Seborrheic dermatitis was even more common before the advent of levodopa; at least it seemed that way. Without levodopa, self-care and personal hygiene were compromised by advancing, untreated parkinsonism. However, seborrheic dermatitis is not just a hygiene problem, and rigorous washing is not the simple answer once it occurs.

Before we discuss this further, let's define a few terms. "Seborrhea" is oiliness of the skin. Usually seborrhea occurs where the skin's oil glands are the most dense, especially the face and scalp. Other areas of relatively higher oil gland density are in regions of skin folds, such as the armpits, under the breasts, groin, and buttocks.

Those with seborrhea may develop seborrheic dermatitis. "Dermatitis" is a general term implying inflammation of the skin. In other words, the oiliness of the skin predisposes to an inflammatory reaction. Seborrheic dermatitis is marked by redness and scaling in addition to oiliness. This occurs especially over the face, where the reddened flaky skin is most apparent on the sides of the nose, eyebrows, eyelids, and over the ears. In the scalp, it tends to generate large dandruff-like flakes. Seborrheic dermatitis may also occur in the skin fold regions where there is a high density of oil glands: arm pits, under the breasts, groin, and buttocks.

Why are those with PD predisposed to seborrheic dermatitis? This is not fully known. Some have speculated that the autonomic nervous system is responsible; among other things, the autonomic nerves regulate certain chemical events in the skin. Others blame it on difficulties with grooming due to the movement limitations of PD. No one knows for certain and it may be a combination of things. There are other neurological and medical disorders where seborrheic dermatitis is also more frequent.

THE CAUSE OF SEBORRHEIC DERMATITIS

Several factors contribute to the development of this skin condition. Obviously the oil (sebum) from skin oil glands is a factor and may act as an irritant if left on the skin. Also, it may interact with microscopic skin organisms to generate irritative products. In fact, the yeast *Pityrosporum ovale* (also termed Malassezia), appears to play a central role in the development of seborrheic dermatitis. This yeast is a normal inhabitant of human skin but, under the right conditions, causes or contributes to this problem. Medications that reduce levels of this yeast, such as ketoconazole, are effective treatments.

TREATING SEBORRHEIC DERMATITIS

If the rash is on your face or scalp and fits the above description, this could well represent seborrheic dermatitis. Have your physician examine your rash. If your physician agrees, you could proceed with a course of treatment. If there is doubt or if treatment proves unsuccessful, a dermatologist should advise.

There are a variety of treatment agents for seborrheic dermatitis and we won't cover each and every one. Rather, we will provide limited suggestions; if your physician prefers other agents, defer to those suggestions.

TREATMENT: SEBORRHEIC DERMATITIS OF THE SCALP, BROWS, AND OTHER HAIRY REGIONS

- Try simple things first: Shampoo two to three times per week with preparations containing either selenium sulfide (e.g., Selsun Blue) or zinc pyrithione (e.g., Head and Shoulders). A product containing a higher concentration of selenium sulfide (2.5 percent versus 1 percent) is also available by prescription. Allow these medicated shampoos to remain in contact with the scalp or face for 5–10 minutes. You could do this by washing, rinsing, and then washing again. In between, use regular shampoo on a daily basis. For milder cases, especially where dandruff is more of the problem than redness, this strategy may be sufficient.

- For more troublesome cases, especially if redness is present, an antiyeast shampoo containing 2 percent ketoconazole (e.g., Nizoral) is appropriate. Leave it on for about five minutes and apply two to three times weekly. You may continue to use the shampoos cited in the previous paragraph two to three times weekly with a regular shampoo the other days. You may also apply the ketoconazole shampoo to your face. This product requires a prescription, although a 1 percent ketoconazole shampoo is available over the counter and might be effective. Improvement will take 2–4 weeks. Once this problem is controlled, you could continue using this once weekly to prevent a recurrence.

- Low potency steroid lotions, gels, or creams may also be applied for up to a few weeks, in addition to the above. These are available over the counter as 0.5 percent or 1 percent hydrocortisone preparations. They suppress the redness (inflammation). They may be applied up to three times daily for brief periods of time if you have intense inflammation. Do not use them continuously because they may cause other skin problems when used beyond a few weeks.

- In addition to the medicated shampoos cited above, a 2 percent ketoconazole cream may also be necessary to eradicate the yeast. Apply this daily after shampooing. It is available alone or combined with hydrocortisone, 0.5 percent or 1 percent. If you use the hydrocortisone combination, do not use this beyond a few weeks unless your physician instructs you otherwise. Continuously applying steroid preparations to the skin over long periods of time may eventually damage it.

- An alternative to the ketoconazole cream is a cream or gel containing 1 percent terbinafine (Lamisil), which is available over the counter. It is applied once or twice daily.

TREATMENT: SEBORRHEIC DERMATITIS OF THE FACE AND OTHER NONHAIRY AREAS

- Washing with a medicated soap is an integral component of treatment. You may choose to wash your face and other affected areas with the same medicated shampoo you use for your hair (see above). For the face, a bar soap containing zinc pyrithione is available (ZNP soap) and may be used with the same general guidelines described above for the hair. You may use this soap or shampoo daily.

- After washing, apply a 2 percent ketoconazole cream (Nizoral) to the affected areas and reapply later in the day. If you have much redness and inflammation, you may use a ketoconazole preparation that also contains 0.5 percent or 1 percent hydrocortisone (but eliminate the hydrocortisone after a few days to weeks). Allow up to four weeks for a response.

- An alternative to the ketoconazole cream is terbinafine (Lamisil), which is sold over the counter as a 1 percent cream or gel. As with ketoconazole, apply this twice daily.

Are there any serious side effects that one could encounter with these skin treatments? Typically not, but if it seems that the agent(s) you are using is causing irritation or in some other way making the problem worse, abandon that treatment and have a dermatologist review. Rare individuals are allergic to sulfites and may experience a reaction to ketoconazole. If you suspect a sulfite allergy, then don't use this unless your physician approves.

RASHES CAUSED BY MEDICATIONS FOR PD

Although the drugs for PD may cause side effects, rarely, if ever, do they cause true allergic reactions. Similarly, these drugs do not cause rashes, with the following exceptions.

- Amantadine frequently causes discoloration of the legs with a mottled (chicken wire pattern) purple or red appearance, often with swelling. It is not dangerous and if it does not bother you, it is acceptable to continue taking amantadine. Rarely the ergot dopamine agonist drugs, bromocriptine and pergolide, cause a similar reaction.

- Carbidopa/levodopa in the 25/100 immediate-release formulation may rarely cause a rash. Importantly, the rash is *not* from either the carbidopa or levodopa, but rather from the yellow food coloring used in the preparation of this particular pill. The other carbidopa/levodopa preparations are formulated with different food coloring and may be used instead: immediate-release 10-100, 25-250 (both blue), sustained-release 25-100 (pink or gray) and 50-200 (tan or gray).

If you are allergic to this yellow dye and wish to start carbidopa/levodopa, use the same schedules shown in chapter 12, but substitute 10-100 tablets for 25-100 tablets. These have the same levodopa content and hence the same potency; they can be used interchangeably. You receive less carbidopa with the 10-100 formulation and consequently are more likely to experience nausea. If nausea develops, take one 25 mg supplementary carbidopa tablet (Lodosyn; orange pill) with each 10-100 pill. See the discussion of supplementary carbidopa in chapter 12.

DISCOLORED LEGS DUE TO INCOMPETENT VEINS

We noted above some of the problems of leg veins that occur with aging. Damaged veins and increased vein pressure often result in slow leakage of fluids and blood products into the leg tissues. When this occurs on a chronic basis, these products may discolor the skin and sometimes this process, along with the swelling, causes a low-grade inflammatory reaction; this has been termed stasis dermatitis. The skin discoloration typically has a brownish appearance and is often distended by the swelling. This bronze or brown discoloration is the clue to this process. Sometimes varicose veins are prominent as well. If this has induced a prominent inflammatory reaction, there may also be redness and scaling of the skin, sometimes with weeping sores.

There is no quick and easy treatment of this problem. The typical strategies include the following.

- Avoid prolonged standing.
- When sitting, elevate the legs to the level of the heart.
- Wear compressive hose fitted to the size of your legs when up and about (e.g., Jobst stockings); take these off at night when in bed.

- If obese, attempt to lose weight.

- If there is a prominent inflammatory component, a corticosteroid cream may be applied 2–3 times daily for a few weeks. With this problem, a higher potency prescription topical corticosteroid is often employed.

If there are open sores, a dermatology consultation is advisable. People with stasis dermatitis are prone to reactions from creams and salves, especially antibiotic ointments. Hence the treatment may become complex.

Water pills (diuretics) are typically a mainstay of treatment to help keep the swelling down. However, those with PD are prone to orthostatic hypotension (low blood pressure when standing). Hence the standing-up blood pressure must be checked before starting a water pill and should be checked periodically after. If you start one of these drugs and begin to feel lightheaded, this is a clue to a low blood pressure (see chapter 21).

DRY SKIN

Dry, flaky skin is a common problem in general, increasing with age. Chronic sun exposure in years past is a major contributor to this. In northern climates, the dry heat from furnaces in the wintertime exacerbates this problem. Those frequently exposed to solvents or soaps (including homemakers doing the dishes) will be prone to this in the exposed areas.

Dry skin can be treated with a variety of measures. Common sense strategies include the following.

- Avoid excessive bathing to involved areas; shower or bathe perhaps every 1–2 days.

- Avoid exposure to solvents, detergents, and soaps as much as possible. Use protective gloves if necessary.

- Apply a moisturizer after washing the body and perhaps again later in the day. A range of moisturizers may be found in your drugstore. The lighter lotions and creams include such names as Keri, Lubriderm, Moisturel, and Nivea. The thicker formulations remain in place longer and hence may be more effective; however, they are messier. These heavier agents include Eucerin, Aquaphor, and various petroleum products (variations on Vaseline).

If you have redness and swelling in addition to dry skin, have your doctor take a look.

Visual Symptoms

PD will not cause you to lose your vision. Impaired visual acuity does occur among people with PD, however, and primarily for three reasons: (1) side effects from medications, (2) problems of the outer eye from reduced tearing and blinking, (3) age-related eye problems that have no direct relation to PD (e.g., glaucoma, macular degeneration, cataracts).

Let's consider each of these problems.

DOUBLE VISION FROM MEDICATIONS

People with PD occasionally experience double vision (diplopia). Neurologists recognize that double vision may be a sign of serious neurological conditions. In the context of PD, however, it rarely has any sinister origins. When double vision occurs, it typically affects those with advancing PD who are taking multiple medications, often in higher doses.

In my experience, the most common PD drugs linked to double vision are the dopamine agonists. Also, any sedating drugs may contribute (e.g., muscle relaxants, prescription pain medications, or the anxiety drugs listed in table 19.2 in chapter 19). If double vision is a problem, you should review your medication list with your physician and eliminate unnecessary drugs. Often, however, the offending drug(s) can't be discontinued.

The cause for double vision is loss of normal eye alignment. Our two eyes normally see things in perfect parallel. Each eye focuses on the same image and these images are superimposed in the brain. Normally the overlap in the brain is precise and we perceive one image. However, if the parallel alignment is lost and the eyes deviate, the images are no longer aligned in parallel. When that occurs, our brain perceives two images (double vision).

If the eye deviation and double vision are constant, it can sometimes be corrected with a prism in your eyeglasses. A prism is an asymmetrically thickened lens that bends the path of light rays. By measuring the degree of your eye deviation, a prism can be fashioned that realigns your visual images in parallel. An alternative for double vision when reading is to buy a pair of cheap reading glasses from the drug or department store and obscure one lens by taping over it; then you will be using only one eye and hence see only one image.

VISUAL BLURRING FROM MEDICATIONS

A wide variety of drugs may cause blurred vision, including those just mentioned. This list can be extended to include all the medications listed in table 23.1 (chapter 23). The anticholinergic drugs are especially noteworthy, including trihexyphenidyl (Artane) and benztropine (Cogentin). They directly affect the function of the lens and pupil.

USUAL CAUSES OF VISION LOSS AMONG SENIORS

As we age, our vision declines in several ways. People with PD are affected, just like everyone else. Let's think about these age-related vision problems.

Visual acuity requires each component of your eyes to be working optimally. These components include:

- The pupil: This is the aperture in the front of your eye that lets in the light. Just like the aperture of an automatic camera, the pupil enlarges or constricts, depending on the amount of ambient light.

- The lens: This is just behind the pupil and focuses the light appropriately on the back of the eye (i.e., on the retina), just like the lens of a camera. The lens changes to refocus as we shift our gaze from near to far.

- The retina: This is analogous to the film in a camera. The lens focuses the light rays on the retina, which registers that image. The image on the retina is then transmitted to the brain.

- The vitreous: This is the water-like fluid inside the eye. The image that the lens focuses on the retina passes through this clear vitreous.

These components and the systems that control them tend to age to variable degrees, affecting visual acuity. The usual conditions that may affect your vision as you grow older include the following.

- Fixation of lens shape: Through early adulthood, the lens shape automatically changes, allowing us to shift focus from far to near objects; by middle age, it loses this flexibility (the reason for reading glasses in middle age).

- Floaters: Debris may collect in the vitreous fluid producing spots that "float" in our visual field. Usually these are benign; however, if massive, this could be a sign of bleeding in the retina and warrants evaluation by an ophthalmologist.

- Macular degeneration: This is a degenerative condition of the retina developing later in life.

- Cataracts: This aging change causes clouding of the lens, which can be surgically treated.

All of these are common among those with PD, but no more common than among the general population of the same age.

GLAUCOMA AND PD MEDICATIONS

Glaucoma is an eye condition in which the pressure inside the eye rises above normal. If the pressure is chronically high, this may result in eye damage. The anticholinergic drugs used in treating PD, such as trihexyphenidyl (Artane) and benztropine (Cogentin), may increase the ocular pressure. Hence they may not be a good idea if you have glaucoma. If used, your ophthalmologist should be aware and monitor the pressure. Theoretically carbidopa/levodopa could worsen glaucoma, but this has not been the general experience. If you have glaucoma and take carbidopa/levodopa, inform your ophthalmologist; simply monitoring your eye pressures should be sufficient.

HALLUCINATIONS

Seeing things that aren't there occurs in PD, usually provoked by medications. This is a problem of brain visual perception centers rather than the eye per se. However, severe vision loss predisposes to hallucinations. We considered hallucinations in chapter 24.

PROBLEMS OF THE OUTER EYE: DRY EYES, EXCESSIVE TEARING

People with PD blink less than normal. Blinking lubricates the surface (cornea) of the eyes, and a slowed blink rate results in reduced lubrication. As a consequence, the eyes may dry out and feel irritated. If this is a minor problem, simply applying artificial tears several times daily may be helpful (e.g., HypoTears, Refresh). Also, if your parkinsonism is poorly controlled, optimizing your PD medications will also help, since this may increase your blink rate back toward normal.

Paradoxically, excessive tearing may occasionally be a consequence of this problem. The reduced blinking from PD results in dry eyes, which triggers a reflexive increase in the flow of tears. Furthermore, because of the reduced blinking, the tears tend to pool on the lower eyelid, overflowing. Tearing may be so pronounced as to run down the face. Ophthalmologists treat this by placing plugs in the tear ducts. With this reduction in normal tears, artificial tears are used as a substitute.

INVOLUNTARY EYE CLOSURE (BLEPHAROSPASM)

People with PD occasionally develop involuntary closure of the eyes, termed blepharospasm (blepharo = eye lid). It is a dystonia—an involuntary spasm or muscle contraction. Hence it is analogous to other forms of dystonia that occur in PD, such as dystonic curling of the toes or foot inversion.

In its mildest form, the blepharospasm of PD is manifest as increased blinking. When more severe, the eyes may tend to involuntarily close. Anything that irritates the eyes, especially drying of the eyes, will exacerbate this problem.

Blepharospasm is not common among those with PD, and when I have encountered it, it most often has been associated with levodopa off-states, or when parkinsonism is insufficiently controlled. It may also be seen in those who have a parkinsonism-plus disorder, most notably progressive supranuclear palsy (see chapter 6).

Treatment of blepharospasm is along two lines. First, an ophthalmologist should determine if an inflammatory eye condition is present or if there has been a subtle injury to the cornea, the outer surface of the eye. Dried or inflamed eyes will tend to involuntarily close for that reason alone. Excessive dryness of the eyes should be treated. Second, control of parkinsonism should be optimized, since this eye dystonia may be a symptom of PD. If blepharospasm occurs only during levodopa off-states, then these fluctuations should be treated as indicated in prior chapters. On the other hand, if your parkinsonism is doing poorly and blepharospasm is one component of that, more aggressive treatment across the board is in order.

Blepharospasm could also be a manifestation of excessive treatment. If it is only present when your levodopa effect is present and goes away when it has worn off, then this is likely. Similarly, if blepharospasm is present only during times of levodopa dyskinesias, it likely is from an excessive medication effect. If you think it is from your medications, you can test this by skipping a carbidopa/levodopa dose and observing whether the blepharospasm goes away when you have been abstinent for 6–8 hours.

Finally, for those who cannot control blepharospasm with simpler measures, botulinum toxin injection is appropriate. It is administered via a tiny needle and weakens muscles at the site of the injection. The effect typically lasts 2–4 months. For treatment of blepharospasm, botulinum toxin is injected into the muscles around the eyes responsible for eye closure. This procedure is typically done by an ophthalmologist or your neurologist.

PART TEN

♦ ♦ ♦

Nutrition, Exercise, Work, and Family

30

♦ ♦ ♦

Diet, Nutrition, and Osteoporosis

Do I Need a Special Diet?

Your diet will not affect PD, but it may affect your levodopa response. As noted in chapters 12 and 17, digested protein products (amino acids) compete with levodopa for transport into the brain. This is easy to avoid in early PD by simply taking the carbidopa/levodopa doses separate from meals (e.g., an hour before each meal if using the immediate-release formulation). Later in PD, short-duration levodopa responses often develop, with fluctuations in control of parkinsonism. At that time, attention to dietary protein may be important and the diet may need to be adjusted; this was addressed in detail in chapter 17. Apart from this, no special diets are necessary. Eat well-balanced meals and try to keep your body weight at the ideal level (avoid obesity). However, there are some general nutritional issues that are important for your overall health and we will address them in this chapter.

Sensible Dietary Supplements

If you have PD and especially if you are a senior, good nutrition is important. However, you don't need all the supplements hyped on TV and in magazines. If you eat a reasonably balanced diet that includes fruits, vegetables, and protein sources, you probably don't need much more. But this is not quite the end of the story.

TAKE A MULTIVITAMIN

If you eat a well-balanced diet, do you need a multivitamin? I recommend this for those with PD. In fact, I typically advise taking one essential multivitamin twice daily. There are two principal reasons for recommending multivitamin therapy, which relate to (1) vitamin D supplementation, which helps prevent osteoporosis—weakening of bones—and (2) homocysteine metabolism. We will examine osteoporosis prevention in detail at the end of this chapter. The vitamin D contained in one or two essential multivitamins is adequate to meet your daily requirement for bone strength. Let us now consider homocysteine, which is a subject foreign to most lay people.

HOMOCYSTEINE AND VITAMINS

Homocysteine is a metabolic by-product of certain biochemical reactions in your body. It is present in measurable levels in your bloodstream. In recent years, homocysteine has gained notoriety for being associated with certain medical disorders. In the general population, those with high homocysteine levels are more prone to strokes, heart attacks, and dementia. This is not to say that those with a high homocysteine level will have a stroke, but simply that their risk is increased. The exact mechanism underlying this process is still under investigation.

Homocysteine levels increase when we become deficient in B vitamins or folate. Conversely, those with high homocysteine levels can effectively reduce them to normal with B vitamin and folate supplementation. This is the standard treatment for people in general with high blood homocysteine levels.

Recent studies have suggested that levodopa therapy tends to raise homocysteine levels in the bloodstream. It doesn't raise levels dramatically, but on the average, they are higher than found in people not taking carbidopa/levodopa. Does this have any adverse consequences? Perhaps not. Studies do not suggest that people with PD are at an increased risk of heart attacks or stroke; in fact, the stroke risk may be reduced. Obviously some with PD will develop dementia after many years, but there is no evidence that levodopa treatment increases this risk. Dementia as a late consequence of PD was common well before the introduction of levodopa, and studies have shown that delaying levodopa treatment does not lower the subsequent risk of dementia.

At present, it is not clear that the somewhat higher levels of homocysteine among those with PD are detrimental, but this continues to be investigated. Since we can lower the level with the B vitamins and folate, why not take a multivitamin to cover this concern?

WHICH MULTIVITAMIN IS BEST?

There are many different brands of multivitamins. Moreover, pharmaceutical companies may include minerals and trace metals in addition to the vitamins.

There are vitamins for seniors, women, men, and so on, with a host of additional substances such as manganese, copper, and zinc. Should the multivitamin you take contain minerals and metals? Should you take a special brand, such as one of those expensive vitamin concoctions sold in nutrition stores or health food catalogs?

If you consume a reasonably well-balanced diet, it is not clear that you need the extra trace metals and minerals that are added to multivitamin formulations. In fact, some investigators believe that at least some supplementary metals may be a bad idea for those with PD. Specifically, higher consumption of iron and manganese has been loosely associated with developing PD, although this is far from proven. Iron and manganese are among the metals added to multivitamins for seniors, women, men, and some of the expensive vitamin preparations. If you are malnourished or dieting, these multivitamins plus minerals may be appropriate for you. Otherwise, a plain essential multivitamin seems appropriate. Besides, these extra minerals and metals add to the expense, side effects (nausea), and pill size (making it harder to swallow).

You do not need to worry that only special brands of vitamins will meet your needs. Some companies advertise their product as being unique or "natural." However, vitamins are vitamins. Why pay more for expensive formulations from health catalogs?

A basic multivitamin should cover any potential vitamin D deficiency and may be sufficient to keep homocysteine levels in the normal range. The ingredients of such a basic "high-potency" multivitamin are shown in table 30.1. For many people, a single multivitamin tablet is adequate, but two tablets may be necessary for others. To hedge our bets, it is reasonable to take one multivitamin tablet twice daily.

If you examine the vitamin shelf at your drug or grocery store, you will find that the ingredients listed in table 30.1 are standard in all multivitamin preparations. The other additives, which are metals and minerals, are not necessary. Multivitamin pills containing only the ingredients listed in table 30.1 are labeled as essential. If the size of the pill is important to you, consider purchasing plain One-A-Day brand multivitamins, which are formulated as small, easy-to-swallow red pills. Your pharmacy may have its own generic substitute for this, which may be a little cheaper. Note, however, that if you purchase the One-A-Day brand for men, for women, and so on, this includes the aforementioned metals and the pill is no longer tiny.

Are there any exceptions to these recommendations for multivitamins? If you have calcium-containing kidney stones, check with your physician (vitamin D enhances calcium absorption). Also, those who take the heart drug digoxin (Lanoxin) should have their calcium levels checked after starting vitamin D or calcium medications, since digoxin side effects may occur if the blood calcium is out of line.

Will two essential multivitamins be sufficient to keep your homocysteine within the normal range? This is easy to check by a simple blood test. If the

Table 30.1.   Basic Ingredients Contained in a High-Potency Essential Multivitamin

Vitamin	Vitamin Content*	Daily Doses Recognized As Potentially Toxic**
Vitamin A	5000 units	100,000 units
Vitamin D	400 units	Variable***
Vitamin B-1 (thiamine)	1.5 mg	–
Riboflavin	1.7 mg	–
Vitamin B-6 (pyridoxine)	2 mg	50 mg****
Vitamin B-12	6 mcg	–
Vitamin C (ascorbic acid)	60 mg	–
Niacin	20 mg	Variable
Vitamin E	15 units	–
Folic acid	0.4 mg	–

*None of these amounts are close to any toxic ranges.

**Where blank, these vitamins have no recognized toxicity when taken in reasonable doses. Typically, your body excretes excesses.

***Vitamin D is necessary for normal calcium absorption. If you are prone to calcium-containing kidney stones, then you should check with your doctor before taking vitamin D supplements. If you are taking the heart medication digoxin (Lanoxin), you should have your calcium checked after starting any vitamin D or calcium supplements since high calcium might result in digoxin toxicity.

**** High vitamin B-6 doses may cause a disease of nerves with numbness, tingling in the limbs, plus unsteadiness. When this has occurred, it was with doses of 500 mg daily or more, although rarely with doses as low as 50–75 mg daily.

homocysteine is higher than normal, despite the multivitamin supplementation, a slightly more aggressive vitamin program is then appropriate. In that case substitute one of your two multivitamin tablets with a single tablet of a supplement such as Foltx, which contains 2.5 mg of folic acid, 2 mg (2000 mcg) of vitamin B-12, and 25 mg of vitamin B-6. Folgard Rx 2.2 is a similar drug.

One note of caution: do not take daily doses of vitamin B-6 much beyond 30 mg daily. Chronic high-dose B-6 ingestion has been associated with neurological disorders of nerves with numbness, clumsiness, and walking problems. This has been primarily with doses exceeding 500 mg daily but rarely with lower doses, perhaps even as low as 50 to 100 mg daily. High doses of folic acid and vitamin B-12 have not been associated with any toxicity.

VITAMIN B-6 AND MULTIVITAMINS

When levodopa therapy was introduced about three decades ago, it was recognized that levodopa metabolism could be accelerated by administration of vitamin B-6 (pyridoxine). This reduced its effectiveness. However, this was no longer a problem after the subsequent addition of carbidopa to make carbidopa/levodopa. Since carbidopa/levodopa is the form of treatment we all currently use, we don't need to worry about the vitamin B-6 in our diet or the small amount in standard multivitamins. Hence those with PD do not require special multivitamins. In fact, levodopa treatment tends to lower vitamin B-6 levels, which might increase homocysteine. Hence a little extra vitamin B-6, as found in a couple of multivitamins, is probably a good idea.

VITAMIN E

Vitamin E is an antioxidant vitamin and tends to protect against excessive chemical reactions in the body that involve oxygen. These are ongoing in every cell, and we have a variety of inherent mechanisms that protect us against excessive oxidation reactions. However, some believe that excessive oxidation is a factor in the development of PD. This view is speculative but predicts that antioxidant vitamins might be beneficial.

Very high doses of vitamin E (2000 units daily) were administered to hundreds of people with PD in a large clinical trial a number of years ago. This supplementation turned out to be no more effective than a placebo (sugar pill). Hence there is no objective evidence to recommend this to those with PD. Moreover, a composite analysis of all controlled vitamin E trials revealed a slight but significantly increased mortality risk with doses of 400 units daily or higher.

COENZYME Q$_{10}$

Health food advocates push a wide variety of products for every illness, including PD, most without any proof. The exception is coenzyme Q$_{10}$, discussed in chapter 9. Although we don't know if it slows PD progression, it did prove beneficial in one study compared to placebo. More investigations are forthcoming to address its role in PD treatment.

The dose of coenzyme Q$_{10}$ found effective in this single study was 300 milligrams (mg) four times daily (1200 mg per day). Lower doses (300 or 600 mg daily) were not beneficial. Hence, if used, it would make sense to take the dose that provided benefit, 1200 mg daily. In this study, the side effects with this dose were essentially the same as with the placebo, at least over the sixteen months of this investigation.

Coenzyme Q$_{10}$ is not a prescription drug and can be purchased in health food stores and drug stores. The 1200 mg dose is quite expensive, costing at least $100 monthly. Unfortunately your pharmacy plan will not cover this supplement, since it is not a prescription drug.

Preventing Osteoporotic Fractures

Bone density decreases as we age. When bone mass is severely lost through this process, it is termed osteoporosis and bones become susceptible to fracture.

This is typically the underlying process when seniors fall and fracture a hip. Prevention of osteoporosis is a relevant topic to most people with Parkinson's disease, since balance may be impaired with risk for falls.

CALCIUM METABOLISM AND OSTEOPOROSIS PREVENTION

Calcium is the primary element that is crucial for bone strength. It is a ubiquitous substance in our bodies and is required for a variety of important metabolic processes. Blood levels of calcium are tightly controlled by various internal regulatory mechanisms. A constant blood level of calcium is crucial for normal physiology. The vast majority of our body stores of calcium are maintained in our bones. The body's regulatory mechanisms pull calcium out of bones if blood levels decline. If insufficient quantities of calcium are supplied through diet, it is reabsorbed from the bones to keep the blood levels constant. This can lead to osteoporosis.

ADULT DIETS DEFICIENT IN CALCIUM

Children are typically encouraged to drink their milk. However, as we become adults, we often do not consume much milk or dairy products. Studies indicate that most Americans over fifty receive inadequate amounts of dietary calcium. This can come back to haunt us as seniors when the cumulative effects of insufficient calcium ultimately result in osteoporosis and risk for bone fractures.

LACK OF EXERCISE AND OSTEOPOROSIS

Inactivity also promotes calcium reabsorption from bone. This renders bone less dense and therefore more prone to fracture. Hence those with PD who have curtailed their physical activities may be especially susceptible to osteoporosis.

VITAMIN D

The absorption of calcium from our diet takes place in the gut, and vitamin D is required for this to be done in an efficient manner. Ingested vitamin D is biochemically changed by the body's internal biochemical mechanisms to make it more effective. One important step in this processing of vitamin D requires skin sunlight exposure. This helps convert it into a metabolically active form. Not a lot of sun exposure is required, but for those who are sedentary in northern climates, this could be a problem.

Where does one get vitamin D? It comes from our diet. Certain beverages, especially milk, are fortified with this vitamin and this is listed on the label.

Some evidence suggests that those with PD may not have optimal vitamin D absorption and metabolism. Hence people with PD may need slightly more vitamin D than average.

MILK

Milk is a good source of calcium and vitamin D. However, it is also a source of protein, and the protein content could be a problem for some with PD. Specifically, levodopa taken with milk may result in less levodopa reaching the brain. As explained in chapters 12 and 17, when dietary protein is digested, it is broken down into smaller units, amino acids. Levodopa is also an amino acid and competes with diet-derived amino acids for transport into the brain.

Is milk ingestion a problem for all who take levodopa? Not necessarily; if the dose of levodopa is not taken with milk, this should be okay. (Actually, you shouldn't take your carbidopa/levodopa dose within one hour of milk ingestion or two hours after.) This only becomes a problem if levodopa doses are required at short intervals to maintain a good effect (e.g., every two hours). For those with frequent levodopa needs, milk intake should be restricted to mealtimes. For those whose levodopa response is very sensitive to meal effects, milk intake may need to be limited. These individuals require other sources of calcium and vitamin D.

OSTEOPOROSIS RISK AND PD

As noted, the typical person with PD is particularly prone to the development of osteoporosis for one or more reasons.

- Osteoporosis is a condition of aging and PD is more common among seniors.

- A sedentary lifestyle, as may occur in PD, facilitates the development of osteoporosis. Physical activity is necessary to maintain bone strength. Also, those who tend to stay inside with no sun exposure may have inadequate levels of metabolically active vitamin D.

- Milk intake is often low in middle age and beyond. For those with PD whose levodopa response is severely compromised by dietary protein, milk may be eliminated from the diet.

- Absorption and metabolism of vitamin D to the fully active form may be mildly insufficient among those with PD, based on recent studies.

Finally, if you have orthostatic hypotension and have increased your salt intake, this can lead to increased calcium excretion in your urine. This could also contribute to osteoporosis in the long run.

SYMPTOMS OF OSTEOPOROSIS

Osteoporosis occurs over years. There are no symptoms until the bones become so weak that they fracture. It is the bone fractures that result in the pain that is sometimes attributed to osteoporosis. However, during the years and decades when the bones are weakening, there are no symptoms.

Osteoporosis may sometimes be suspected when bones seem to fracture in the context of mild or even no trauma. It may also be suspected from routine X rays. However, the standard form of assessment is with a particular type of bone scan called a bone density study. Bone density scans are relatively painless; a substance is injected by vein that binds to bones and provides an index of bone mass and strength. Internal medicine physicians order bone density scans for individuals who are at risk for osteoporosis. This is appropriate for many with PD.

HOW TO PREVENT OSTEOPOROSIS

Because developing osteoporosis has no symptoms, it is wise to take preemptive measures as early as possible. Routine measures to prevent osteoporosis include adequate daily intake of both vitamin D and calcium.

We already commented that your vitamin D requirements can be supplied by one of many over-the-counter multivitamins, which typically contain 400 units per tablet. For those middle-aged and beyond, 400 to 800 units daily is generally recommended. Because of the multiple risk factors for osteoporosis associated with PD, the larger amount, 800 units of vitamin D daily, is an appropriate intake. If a multivitamin is your sole vitamin D source, then take two multivitamin tablets daily. Vitamin D is also contained in some calcium supplements. If the small print on the labels is confusing, ask your pharmacist to advise regarding the recommended amounts above. General guidelines for calcium and vitamin D are summarized in supplement 30.1 at the end of the chapter (you may photocopy it).

How much calcium intake is adequate? This varies slightly depending on several factors. For men and premenopausal women, approximately 1200 milligrams (mg) of elemental calcium daily is optimal. For postmenopausal women or anyone with known osteoporosis, 1500 mg of elemental calcium daily is appropriate.

Why is *elemental* calcium specified in the above recommendations? Because the amount of calcium may be measured in one of two ways and this specifies which method we are using. Calcium in pill form is attached to another substance, such as gluconate, phosphate, lactate, or carbonate. Unless elemental calcium is specified, the measurement may include both calcium and the substance to which it is combined; in other words, it may relate to the total compound of calcium carbonate, calcium gluconate, and so on. The term "elemental" indicates that only the element calcium is being specified. The above recommendations of 1200 to 1500 mg of daily calcium are appropriate for only elemental calcium requirements (i.e., calcium alone).

In what form should calcium be taken? If milk and calcium-fortified juice intake are substantial, much of the daily requirement may be met. The content is listed on the container label. For those who do not drink much milk or fortified juice, calcium supplements are the primary option. These are available at grocery and drug stores. Antacids such as Tums tablets or the generic equivalent supply calcium. Other formulations may include vitamin D with the calcium, such as Os-Cal + D, Citracal + D, and a wide variety of equivalent over-the-counter products.

Occasional individuals are prone to kidney stones, and calcium is a major component of kidney stones, although not in every case. Those susceptible to calcium-containing kidney stones may have to avoid excessive calcium. If you have developed kidney stones, discuss this with your doctor.

MENOPAUSE AND OSTEOPOROSIS

Women after menopause are more likely to develop osteoporosis. This relates to the loss of estrogen. Multiple studies have demonstrated that estrogen supplementation in postmenopausal women increases bone strength. Hence this is often one of the treatments considered for osteoporosis.

TREATMENT OF DOCUMENTED OSTEOPOROSIS

When bone density scans reveal osteoporosis, the treatment goes beyond simple calcium and vitamin D supplementation. Medications that increase bone density are prescribed. This may include biphosphonate drugs such as alendronate (Fosamax) or risedronate (Actonel), as well as calcitonin nasal spray (Miacalcin), or the parathyroid hormone analog, teriparatide (Forteo). It may also include the addition of an estrogen in post-menopausal women. Internists or those who specialize in bone metabolism typically prescribe these drugs.

Supplement 30.1.

Recommendations to Prevent Osteoporosis Among Those with Parkinson's Disease

(These guidelines may not be appropriate if you have a history of calcium-containing kidney stones.)

For Premenopausal Women and All Men

1. 1200 mg of elemental calcium daily

2. Vitamin D, 400–800 units daily (1–2 multivitamins daily or another source)

3. Consider a bone density scan as appropriate (discuss with your physician)

For Postmenopausal Women

1. 1500 mg of elemental calcium daily

2. Vitamin D, 800 units daily (two multivitamins that contain 400 units each or another vitamin D source)

3. Consider a bone density scan

For Men And Women with Osteoporosis Confirmed on Bone Density Scan

1. 1500 mg of elemental calcium daily

2. Vitamin D, 800 units daily (two multivitamins that contain 400 units each, or another vitamin D source)

3. Consult your internist or specialist for supplemental medication.

31

◆ ◆ ◆

The Role of Exercise, Physical Medicine, and Physical Therapy

In our society much of what we do is passive. Many of our jobs are performed behind desks and counters with little expenditure of physical energy. Our recreation has become increasingly passive with television, computers, and electronic games. But our Western culture is paying a price for this couch potato lifestyle with rising obesity. We are now recognizing that this passivity translates into increased rates of diabetes mellitus, heart attacks, and strokes. Moreover, the complications of normal aging are exacerbated by this easy lifestyle. Osteoporosis is accelerated by lack of physical activity, with consequent hip fractures. As we age, our muscles tend to lose their tone and strength, and this is exacerbated by lack of physical activity. Our tendons and ligaments lose their elasticity with age, and a sedentary lifestyle increases the symptoms of stiffness and aching. The old adage, "If you don't use it, you lose it," is an irrefutable fact of aging. Graceful aging requires that we stay physically (and mentally) active to preserve our bodies as best we can.

Parkinson's disease (PD) is inextricably tied to aging. It usually starts in middle age or beyond and parallels the aging process; the longer you have PD, the older you get. Thus people with PD need to fight both their disease and normal aging. It turns out that exercise is a key element in both of these battles.

The Goals of Your Exercise Program

PD is a heterogeneous disorder. Some are quite impaired from PD with substantial immobility. Others function physically at the same level as their peers. Most are somewhere in between. Furthermore, the ages of those with PD obviously vary, as does their general medical condition. Hence, when we are addressing exercise, there is no one-size-fits-all program.

There are several goals for exercise:

- Maximize and maintain flexibility

- Maintain muscle strength

- Maintain capacity for good balance (also a function of the degree of PD and effect of medications)

- Optimize exercise capacity (which will increase your energy)

- Engage in aerobic exercise to the extent possible to improve heart function, avoid obesity, and counter atherosclerosis

How to do all of this? Many of us can meet these goals without major deviations from our lives, but with a simple commitment to staying physically active. How much of a formal exercise program is required depends on the severity of your of parkinsonism, age, and general medical state.

Exercise puts demands on the body that result in long-term gains but in the short term may unmask problems lurking beneath the surface. Hence there are a few caveats to consider regarding exercise.

- If you have a heart condition, you will need clearance from your internist, family physician, or cardiologist to start a new exercise program.

- Some people have heart problems without knowing it. If you experience chest pain while exercising, this could be a sign that your heart is receiving inadequate blood to meet the demands of exercise. That is a worrisome sign and requires immediate attention. If that occurs, stop exercising; if the chest pain continues, have someone take you to the nearest emergency room. However, if it abates, you still need to see your physician on a semiurgent basis for further evaluation.

- Faintness (feeling like you might pass out) may occur while exercising. That is typically a sign that your blood pressure is low. Stop the exercise. If you feel very faint, lie down. Check your pulse and, if possible, have someone check your blood pressure. Your physician then needs to address this. More is said about this below. Vertigo, which is a spinning sensation in your head, is not a sign that your blood pressure is low and usually reflects an inner ear condition (see chapter 21).

- If you have problems with balance, avoid exercise routines that increase your risk of falling.

However, don't let these notes of caution dissuade you from exercise. It is important to your long-term well-being.

Exercise for Those with Well-Controlled Parkinsonism

If your parkinsonism is fairly well controlled and you have no other medical limitations to exercise (i.e., no heart or lung problems that prevent it), you may meet your exercise goals as others do of your age. For some, work (e.g., farming, construction) or hobbies (gardening, yard work, sports) may go a long way toward meeting these goals. These shouldn't be discounted. For most with the capability of being active, our society provides exercise options, such as health and fitness clubs (including YMCAs), exercise classes, and activities such as bicycling, hiking, and so on. You don't need a formal Parkinson's exercise program if you can engage in the usual exercise outlets that are available to all of us. However, you will need to choose activities and exercises that involve your entire body. Hips, knees, shoulders, back, and neck tend to get stiff and tight with both aging and PD; all these major joints need activities that put them through the entire range of motion.

Exercise gurus advise stretching before and after exercising, and this is especially important for those with PD; remember to stretch all four limbs, back, and neck. Health clubs, YMCAs, and the like typically have staff that can advise you about this.

If you have limitations, such as bad knees or a painful shoulder, obtain medical advice so that your exercise regimen incorporates activities that appropriately rehabilitate those troubled limbs or joints. This may include consulting a physical therapist or sports medicine specialist regarding an appropriate stretching and exercise program.

One key element of these exercise programs is to choose activities that you will maintain. It doesn't help you in the long run to exercise fanatically for six weeks, get bored, and then give it all up. Switching from one type of activity to another is a good way to maintain your interest. For example, if you belong to a health club, you may elect to ride an exercise bicycle for several weeks, then switch to a rowing machine and perhaps some weight training. If that starts to get old, you might swim laps or join an appropriate aerobics class. Remember that life is a marathon, not a sprint. Exercises that are onerous are hard to continue indefinitely; it is easy to talk yourself out of exercising. Hence, anything you can do to make it interesting will help in this lifelong endeavor. If you have been leading a sedentary lifestyle, start your exercise program slowly with limited immediate goals. However, as you acclimate to your new program after a few weeks, push yourself a little and increase those exercise goals. Part of the fun of exercise is seeing yourself reach new heights. However, this is never immediate and you need to be patient.

How important is exercise if you have PD? In my PD clinic, I have had the distinct impression that those with a strong commitment to exercise have fared substantially better in the long run.

Exercise for Those with Incompletely Controlled Parkinsonism

Some people with PD have movement problems that preclude the usual fitness programs. Something more tailored to their capabilities is necessary. If your limitations are not too severe, you might still avail yourself of fitness options in the community, simply avoiding what is outside your abilities. For example, if imbalance is your primary problem, treadmills may not be a good idea, whereas an exercise bicycle may work just fine. However, for some, it is not that simple. If your parkinsonism is limiting in a major way, then you will need advice tailored to your problem. A physical therapist can advise you about this. Let your therapist know that you would like instruction in both stretching and exercise. The goal is to provide you with a program that you continue on your own (it's less expensive that way). Also, ask your therapist if there are any resources in your community that would be appropriate. For example, Tai Chi classes, which enhance flexibility and balance, or water aerobics classes may be available through community centers, YMCAs, and so on.

Levodopa Responses and Exercise

People with PD get the most out of exercise when their medications are optimally adjusted. If you are underdosed, exercise is difficult or impossible.

After a number of years of PD, people taking carbidopa/levodopa begin to experience levodopa responses time-locked to each dose (short-duration responses). Hence there is a tendency for the effect to wear off a few hours or less after every dose. If you experience such a fluctuating response to carbidopa/levodopa, there are a few principles that you need to know to make your exercise regimen go as smoothly as possible.

- Exercise goes best when you are in your levodopa on-state. When the effect has worn off, it is hard to exercise and stretch.

- If you are taking carbidopa/levodopa and fluctuating between being underdosed or overdosed with dyskinesias, try to adjust your doses so that you are not underdosed during exercise; do this even if dyskinesias result. Exercise typically goes much better in an overdosed, dyskinetic state. The only exception is perhaps among people who experience severe dyskinesias.

- When exercising, you use up your levodopa effect faster. Countless people have told me that their levodopa response does not last as long when physically active. If you normally experience a three-hour response to each dose, it may only last two hours when exercising. This is important to recognize. The treatment strategy is to take your carbidopa/levodopa doses at shorter intervals during exercise. If you know the levodopa effect is due to run out at two, instead of three hours, take a dose early to prevent that.

Remember that energy levels are highest and fatigue lowest during levodopa on-states.

Orthostatic Hypotension, Dizziness, and Exercise

Some people with PD are prone to a drop in their blood pressure when they stand. This is termed orthostatic hypotension, discussed in chapter 21. Most people with PD do not experience this but it is problematic in a distinct minority. People with orthostatic hypotension will feel lightheaded when on their feet due to this low blood pressure. If it drops too low, they might pass out.

The primary reasons for orthostatic hypotension are medications (all the PD drugs) and PD-related autonomic nervous system dysfunction, as already noted. It is often a problem only when your PD medications are working (levodopa on-states). A large meal will also tend to exacerbate this tendency.

Symptoms of orthostatic hypotension may occur during vigorous exercise. If you become hot during this exercise, this is even more likely. If you feel faint when exercising, have someone check your blood pressure and pulse at that time. If your blood pressure is less than 90/60, then the faintness is due to too low a blood pressure. Don't try to continue with the exercise (we don't want you to faint). Treatment is discussed in chapter 21. Remember that this tends to be a problem in the erect position (standing, walking, running). If this is a persistent problem, despite treatment, you might be able to engage in sitting exercises, such as a rowing machine, and so on.

It is also important to check your pulse if you feel faint because a problem of heart rate could also be the cause. If your rate is very slow, for example less than forty beats per minute, this should be semiurgently discussed with your physician. Exercise will raise your heart rate, but among those middle-age and beyond, it should not be much above 150; if you feel faint and your heart rate is much greater than that, this also needs to be addressed by your physician.

Freezing

The word "freezing" makes most people think of a cold day. Those with PD use the term to address a momentary paralysis of movement due to parkinsonism. In the vernacular of PD, "frozen gait" relates to an inability to move your feet; they are stuck in place as if magnetized to the floor. Such freezing may also affect hand movements and sometimes speech. However, it is the frozen gait that is the most troublesome and deserves special comment.

People with gait freezing are unable to take a step, as if their feet were nailed to the floor. This typically occurs when they are about to take their first step. Once they get started, they often are able to walk as long as they continue at a reasonable pace. However, once they stop or even slow down, freezing recurs. Turning around or turning corners also provokes freezing. Interestingly, walking through doorways, even if the pace is maintained, typically causes freezing. Stressful situations or walking in crowds seem to exacerbate this tendency. For most, having frozen feet is a momentary problem and, after a few seconds or less, they get going. However, with severe gait freezing, you may get stuck in place and require help to start walking again.

Why in the world should your feet get stuck to the floor, and then seconds later be able to walk almost normally? This presumably relates to the fact that the brain has separate motor control circuits for initiating walking and maintenance of walking. This act of gait *initiation* seems to be especially susceptible to the effects of PD.

As you might guess, the first thing to do if you are troubled by frozen feet is to adjust and optimize your PD medications. If the freezing occurs during levodopa off-states, then you need to focus on drug adjustments to eliminate off-states. If freezing is independent of your levodopa doses, then you may benefit from more aggressive carbidopa/levodopa dosing. If you are not taking carbidopa/levodopa, then you probably need to start. These are issues discussed in earlier chapters and the details about medication adjustments won't be repeated here.

Rarely, freezing occurs with excessive doses of medications. I have only encountered this among people taking dopamine agonists, and even then very rarely. Nonetheless, if you are on higher doses of a dopamine agonist drug with prominent freezing, try cutting your dose in half for two days. In my experience, that has been a sufficient trial to provide clues whether this is responsible. Typically, you can tolerate a 50 percent dose reduction for a couple of days or so; if freezing fails to improve on this lower dose, revert back to the prior dose.

Unfortunately in some people, gait freezing persists, despite aggressive dosing of PD medications. For them, however, certain physical therapy tricks may be helpful. The theoretical intent is to use a different area of your brain to substitute for the malfunctioning motor control circuit.

Initiating walking is an unconscious act, just like swinging your arms when you walk. Let's focus on arm swing to gain some insight into these types of problems. People with PD tend not to swing their arms but they can, if they think about it. If the brain's unconscious arm-swinging circuit doesn't work properly, you can use a conscious brain motor circuit to override this. In other words, think about swinging your arms and they will swing.

Similar to consciously swinging your arms during walking, you can make a conscious effort to initiate walking when your feet are frozen. It requires thinking the right thought to do this. Simply thinking about walking is ineffective. You need to think about a different movement that will unleash that first step. Once you get started, then the walking typically can continue (the brain area that *maintains* walking then takes over). Here are a few tricks that physical therapists might suggest to successfully take that first step.

- Swing one leg forward. Think about swinging the leg rather than walking. Start with a long leg swing that will place that leg far in front of you (but not so far that you fall).

- Try goose-stepping. This was the marching gait of German soldiers. They would stiffly lock their knees and march by taking long stiff steps. Envision what they looked like and keep this thought as you take your first step.

- Think about a drum major's marching step, raising one leg straight up off the ground before placing it forward. Envision that same movement when you get stuck.

- Think about a drill sergeant's marching cadence: "one-two, one-two, one-two . . ." You might even count out loud. This might get you started and help you mentally envision a marching step.

- Thinking of a certain musical tune may be helpful. For example, a gliding first step may come more easily if you hum "Blue Danube" in your mind and imagine a ballroom dancer gliding in that same way. A boogie or rock and roll tune that brings a dance step to mind may also work.

- Find a target on the floor and step on it. Sometimes people imagine they are stepping on a fly in front of them. Look for an imaginary fly on the ground and try to crush it; this may get your gait started.

- A variation on this involves using a laser pointer to create a target to step on. If you point the laser light 1–2 feet in front of you and then think about stepping on that tiny lighted spot, that may get you going. Laser pointers are used by professors and lecturers and may be purchased at bookstores.

This is not an exhaustive list but is meant to illustrate the concept of mental imagery to get you going. You are left to your own creative ideas about what strategies might work best for you. The idea is to have a mental image that you can call on repeatedly throughout the day. When you freeze, momentarily relax and think that thought, then go.

Falls

Early in PD, imbalance is minimal or nonexistent. With PD progression imbalance may slowly develop and if prominent, result in falls. Normal aging also contributes to this problem; about one-third of aged (non-PD) adults fall yearly according to one study. Imbalance sufficient to cause falls does not develop in all with PD; however, if you live long enough, it probably will be an issue sooner or later.

Falling is one PD symptom that may not consistently respond to aggressive medical treatment. However, PD medication adjustments should be tried if imbalance and falls are occurring.

A physiatrist or physical therapist is important when imbalance becomes a problem. He or she can address several factors that lend themselves to treatment:

- Avoiding situations that put you at risk for falling. Falls often occur when distracted or when trying to do two things at once. When on your feet, it may be necessary to avoid thinking about other things or engaging in other tasks. Also, since many falls occur when changing positions or postures, the therapist may work with you to maintain proper body mechanics in those situations. If gait freezing seems to provoke falls, then the strategies outlined above are appropriate, as well.

- Muscle weakness and deconditioning. If you have been leading a sedentary lifestyle and your muscles have weakened as a consequence, they will be less able to compensate for minor missteps during walking. Maintaining muscle strength is important to compensate for imbalance. Depending on your general medical condition and other factors, your physiatrist may even recommend a weight training program.

- Exercise as a component of a weight loss program. Obesity exacerbates problems of imbalance. If you are carrying around an extra 50–100 pounds of fat, overcoming minor imbalance that leads to falls is more difficult. Weight loss requires both dieting and calorie-burning exercise.

- Balance training. Balance exercises help. However, a balance exercise program must be designed that meets both your needs and your capabilities. As you make gains, the goals can be increased as you work with your therapist.

- Gait aids. As mentioned above, there are a variety of aids that compensate for imbalance, but they are not appropriate or necessary for everyone. Depending on your specific problem, a physiatrist or physical therapist will choose what meets your needs, from a cane to a wheeled walker.

- Optimizing the home to avoid trips, falls, and injuries. Physiatrists look at the big picture and will consider with you the things in your home that might exacerbate the tendency to fall, such as throw rugs or slippery floors. They also can advise about minor home modifications, such as grab bars in areas where you might be stepping over impediments (bathrooms, or the step from the garage to your house). Certain aspects of your home may also need to be considered, such as hard floors or sharp furniture corners, which put you at an increased risk for injury if you do fall; these are modifiable.

- Safety aids. If you have imbalance and especially if you have osteoporosis, hip pads may prevent a hip fracture. These can be purchased at medical supply stores and your therapist can advise. Other sorts of pads and protections can be used, depending upon the area of your body at risk.

If imbalance and falls are present, you should pay attention to the previous chapter, where we consider osteoporosis prevention. Obviously strong bones are especially crucial if your balance is impaired.

Stooped Posture

PD often results in a stooped posture. Sometimes this is written off to normal aging or incorrectly attributed to osteoporosis. However, just as tremor, rigidity, and bradykinesia are due to changes in brain motor control mechanisms, so is stooped posture. PD medications may partially improve your stance, and physical therapy strategies may also be helpful.

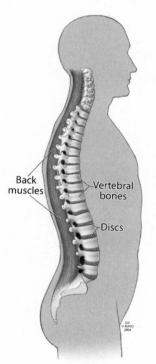

Back muscles

Vertebral bones

Discs

The spinal column is made up of a series of vertebral bones, stacked one on top of another, similar to a tower of children's building blocks (figure 31.1). Each vertebral bone is shaped like a flat oil drum and is separated from the adjoining vertebrae by cushioning discs. This tall column of vertebral bones and discs is surrounded by muscles that stabilize it, as illustrated in figure 31.1.

The configuration of the spinal column is primarily regulated by the contraction of the surrounding muscles. The brain normally adjusts the tone in the muscles so that we stand erect and tall but also with a little curvature at our neck and lumbar regions (lordosis). A blueprint for this posture is imprinted in the motor control area of your brain, which generates the signals that produce it. Voluntary bending and twisting of the

31.1 The bones of the spinal column are called vertebral bodies and are separated by discs. These, and the joints behind, allow mobility. Muscles control, align, and stabilize the spinal column. The muscles in front of the spinal column are not shown.

trunk and neck is accomplished by appropriate contraction of these spinal muscles. These volitional trunk and neck movements are accomplished through other brain motor control regions that program our routine movements.

Among those with PD, malfunction of the unconscious programming of the spinal muscles causes stooping. Instead of producing an erect posture, these muscles revert to a default motor program, resulting in a flexed posture. Despite this, the capacity for voluntary movements of the trunk remains fairly intact (i.e., you can bend and flex your trunk and neck).

This is analogous to other involuntary and unconscious movements that suffer in PD, such as arm swing and facial animation. Those with PD can stand up straight, swing their arms, and frown their faces. However, unless they think about it, the posture tends to become stooped, arm swing diminishes, and facial animation dampens.

The physical therapy strategy for countering this is to consciously think about pulling your shoulders back and standing straight. Your spouse may have already told you to do this (perhaps too often). For this strategy to be effective, you need to constantly think about it. When distracted, there is a tendency to revert to the stooped pattern. Nonetheless, you can train yourself to stand straighter if you focus on it.

Stooped Posture and Low Back Pain

A stooped posture is probably not the primary cause of low back pain in most people. However, if you have a tendency toward lumbar pain, stooping may contribute. Why? Think about the work that your back muscles must do to maintain your trunk in the forward, stooped position. Compare that to the work required if you are standing straight up. When standing erect, your vertebrae are resting one on top of another (see figure 31.1); in that position, the supporting muscles of the back don't need to do much work, other than stabilize. Compare that to the spine that is programmed by the brain to stoop forward. This position requires the back muscles to pull against gravity to keep you from doubling over on yourself. Such overworked muscles begin to ache after a while. If you have an inherent tendency toward low back pain, this will add to it.

32

◆ ◆ ◆

Family, Friends, the Workplace, and Caregivers

Should I Keep My Diagnosis a Secret?

Should your PD diagnosis be disclosed to friends and family? Clearly your spouse needs to know, and rarely are there exceptions to this axiom. Disclosure beyond that, however, is a personal choice and depends on circumstances. Let's think about some of the factors that weigh in this decision.

If your PD is well controlled and you are experiencing no compromise of activities, it is not necessary to reveal the diagnosis. The PD medications are often effective in abolishing the signs of PD; others may not notice that anything is wrong. You may feel more comfortable not talking about your diagnosis of PD and that is perfectly fine. Sometimes it is easier to downplay the illness and focus on the positives in life.

For some, it is important to talk about PD. Perhaps your sense of immortality has been shattered by the prospect of a chronic disease; if the mental burden weighs on your mind, then by all means, share this with appropriate friends and family. Talking about things that bother us helps make peace with ourselves and confront our shortcomings.

For those whose PD is compromising function or causing conspicuous signs, it's wise to let friends, coworkers, and the boss know. You may need them to cut you a little slack, but they can't do this unless they know what is going on.

Reduced Energy May Necessitate Reduced Demands

Even when PD is otherwise well controlled, there is often a drop in energy and stamina. Medicines may not fix this. If you have been a high-energy, multitasked go-getter all your life, you may not be able to keep up as you once did. You may need to tell this to your friends, family, and employer. Their expectations of you may need to be reduced; you can no longer do three things at once. Disclosing that you have PD is a good excuse for turning down yet another committee or volunteer job.

Workplace Decisions

Parkinson's disease does need not to force you into retirement. Many with PD have worked for years after diagnosis. Obviously the demands and requirements of your work are a factor. A cardiac surgeon or a jet fighter pilot has little margin for error and may be sidelined by minimal problems. On the other hand, most jobs in the workplace are compatible with PD, at least in the milder stages. My view is to continue working as long as you are able to comfortably meet the demands of your occupation. In general, we are all happier and most fulfilled when busy and challenged with responsibilities.

Optimize your medication regimen for best performance at work. It's okay to limit your PD drugs if functioning well. However, if your job is suffering, it is a mistake to arbitrarily restrict medications in hopes of saving the best responses for later. Your medication responses are not bankable. Failing to take advantage results in lost opportunities. Restricting your medications so that they will work better later is like trying to save your youth for later.

Physical Challenges in the Workplace

If your job is more physical than mental, PD symptoms will provide a greater challenge. Climbing ladders, walking on roofs, and heavy labor are not possible indefinitely if you have PD. Problems with walking, balance, or slowness may force you into more sedentary work, or disability and retirement. Usually it is obvious when you can no longer keep up. It is important to recognize this in a timely fashion if there are safety concerns.

Subtle aspects of PD also challenge the worker, especially the reduced energy and increasing fatigue that often accompany PD. Although these may be partially treatable with medications directed at PD (or poor sleep, depression), they rarely can be completely reversed. PD also tends to interact with normal aging to exacerbate aches and pains in muscles and joints that may make it tough to do physical tasks.

There is a sixty-year-old farmer who comes to see me every fall after the crops are in. Despite ten years of PD, he runs a large farm mostly on his own. He builds his own fences, repairs the farm machinery, plows the fields, and so on. When he asked me, "I love what I'm doing; can I go another five years?" I responded optimistically. His parkinsonism is stable and well controlled. I do not expect any dramatic decline in the next several years. I see many farmers, carpenters, and skilled laborers in my practice who similarly keep up with the demands of their work. Hence PD can indeed be compatible with physically demanding jobs, although not in every case.

White-Collar Work

Sedentary jobs without physical demands are more compatible with PD. However, there are a variety of problems that can make sedentary occupations difficult:

- Fatigue

- Reduced dexterity, compromising writing or computer keyboarding

- Inability to do two things at once, so-called multitasking

- Reduced ability to handle stress (stress is inherent in every job)

- Softer voice, making it more difficult to communicate

- Slowed thinking (bradyphrenia), paralleling slowed movements

- Cosmetic issues, such as a prominent tremor or dyskinesias that distract you or your customers

- Walking problems, making it difficult to travel on business

- Unpredictable off-states that immobilize

- Disrupted nighttime sleep, resulting in daytime drowsiness

Thus no job is safe from PD, although with optimum medical treatment, it may be possible to limit these problems. Again, if your job is being compromised, take full advantage of PD drugs and ignore suggestions to withhold or limit treatment.

Disability and Retirement

If the demands of work are beginning to exceed your capabilities, then it may be time to consider disability or retirement. Before proceeding, you will need to discuss this with at least three people:

- Your doctor, to make certain that you have not missed some therapeutic opportunities that might make you better able to cope

- Your employer, who may be able to modify your job to better accommodate your needs

- Your spouse, and perhaps others in your family, since this will result in a shared lifestyle change

Disability status is not automatic with the diagnosis of PD. You will need a physician's statement on the appropriate paperwork to qualify. However, if your doctor is able to document disability from PD, it is unusual for the disability to be disallowed.

Your Rights

What if you believe that your job performance has not suffered from PD, but your employer disagrees and is threatening to fire you? What recourse do you have? You obviously need to consult an attorney to obtain the correct advice. However, I can summarize the basic legal doctrines that bear on this matter. The federal statute that covers this is the Americans with Disabilities Act, and most states also have similar laws on the books. If your parkinsonism is sufficiently advanced to compromise your activities of daily living and is confirmed by a medical opinion, you should be covered by these statutes. Those who meet these disability criteria cannot be fired just because they have a disability. It is incumbent on your employer to make reasonable accommodations to allow you to do your job. However, you, the employee, must be able to perform the essential functions of your job, with or without these accommodations. If you can't perform despite these accommodations, and if your employer cannot reassign you to another job, then you can be fired. Hence you are protected to a certain degree, but you also need to be able to meet reasonable work standards.

If you are fired, where can you plead your case? You may file a complaint with the Equal Employment Opportunity Commission. You do not need an attorney to do this, but the chances of success increase with the help of a knowledgeable employment attorney. Another avenue is via the Department of Human Rights in your state, which may be consulted for advice.

Late in PD: Providing and Accepting Care

Many with PD do well for years and the stress on the family is never substantial. However, there may come a time when family and especially your spouse become a crucial and necessary part of your care. The good news is that PD is treatable and we can keep people active and ambulatory for many,

many years. The bad news is that eventually we all get old and PD adds to the burden of aging.

Some people cringe at the thought of depending on someone else for anything. "I don't ever want to be a burden on my wife (or husband, children, etc.)!" We typically go through our lives with a self-image of strength and independence; we can do anything necessary for our families and ourselves. We have been the pillars and the caregivers. Now the tables turn. What an embarrassment! What a humiliation!

This perspective seems very shortsighted to me. We are looking at the natural cycle of life. Most people who live long enough will develop some condition later in life that requires help. Even if you are in the peak of health, you can still fall, break a hip, and be stuck in a wheelchair. These are things we cannot change; they have been written in our genetic codes. We live our lives as best we can, but when the time comes for us to get old or develop illnesses, we need to accept this.

Depending on others is not all bad for either the afflicted or the caregiver. Some great love stories have come through my clinic. These will never be recorded in literature, but a partner's devotion to an affected spouse tops the stuff of best-selling novels. I have been witness to husbands who bring their frail parkinsonian wives to the clinic, attending to their every need and treating them like the sixteen-year-old beauty queens they once were, sixty years ago. I have been humbled by wives who fawn over their ailing parkinsonian husbands, even though they no longer are the handsome athletes who won their hearts in their youth.

The cycle of life ties children to their aging parents. There is a beauty to this cycle. Think about the mother who stays up countless nights nursing her baby, then worrying and sacrificing, as she lovingly raises her child to adulthood. For children to return that love as a caregiver later in life can be very fulfilling and enriching.

Becoming a caregiver is no small task and my point is not to trivialize the work and sacrifice. However, it can be rewarding and enriching and we shouldn't lose sight of that.

Caregiving

PD is a progressive condition and after ten or twenty years, many lose at least some of their independence. Furthermore, since this is a disease that typically starts later in life, the problems of aging are superimposed. As time passes, it is often crucial to have someone who can help with the activities of daily living. Many need only limited assistance, but a few need extensive help. The family, especially the spouse, typically becomes the major caregiver. If the necessary assistance is not substantial, this may be an easy transition. Unfortunately that is not always the case.

The Challenges and Stresses of Caregiving

Entire books have been written about caregiving. These issues are not restricted to PD, since there are a multitude of disorders that chronically compromise lives, especially later in life. PD is so heterogeneous that you cannot
predict what caregiving requirements, if any, will ultimately be necessary.
However, let's consider a few basic principles that apply primarily to spouses
(occasionally children) who are challenged with an intensive caregiving relationship. If you are in the role of the caregiver and this necessitates a major
commitment of your time and energy, you should give some thought to the
following.

- What you are doing is heroic. Recognize this and don't take your efforts
  for granted, even if everyone else does (including your spouse with PD).
  In your quiet moments, tally up the things you have done for your
  loved one that day and congratulate yourself. No one is required to
  become a caregiver. We are free to abandon that person if we choose.
  Those who stay and fight the battle are special human beings. Keep that
  in mind.

- Don't expect thanks or outward signs of reward. What you are doing
  may require a huge sacrifice of your time and effort. However, in chronic
  ongoing relationships of this type, a spoken thank-you is rare.

- Roles are invariably reversed in caregiver relationships and sometimes
  this is a source of stress. Men who are used to managing the finances or
  driving the family automobile may resent relinquishing these tasks to
  their wives. Women who took pride in their homemaking may complain about the bland food now cooked by their husbands or the lower
  standard of housekeeping. In caregiving situations, new roles are borne,
  and this needs to be recognized.

- Don't expect perfection in the caregiving role. The person with PD will
  come up short on some tasks and that needs to be accepted. Roll with
  the punches and accept what you've got.

- Don't forget to look around and see the beauty in the world. Enjoy the
  morning sunlight and the birds singing. Appreciate the leaves in the fall
  and the sunsets in the summer. It is too easy to get carried away with all
  the responsibilities of caregiving and forget those things that can bring
  us a moment of joy.

- Maintain your own interests and make time for them. Don't make
  caregiving a 24/7 task. Set aside time for the things that you need as
  necessary perks in your life. Caregiving is a long road and you should
  not ignore yourself.

- If your caregiving requirements are intense, program regular respites into the schedule. Get away for a few hours every day if possible, or at least two or three times weekly. Don't feel guilty about this. It may seem inappropriate to go out and play golf for a few hours when your spouse is stuck at home. However, this is okay. You need time for yourself! This is necessary to cope with the demands of caregiving. If your loved one has problems staying alone, there are community resources to help with this, such as senior centers or perhaps a hired assistant. Don't be reluctant to arrange for caregiving help.

- Maintain relationships with friends and community. There is a tendency to abandon these relationships as we get bogged down with the responsibilities of the day. If your life becomes too restricted to the loved one you are caring for, you lose perspective and it's easy to get discouraged. We need friends and other relationships to keep going.

- Have someone you can talk to when your life becomes stressed. This may be a close friend or other family; it could be clergy. Sometimes it is hard to be objective when we are stuck in our own little world. Most of us occasionally need others to talk or ventilate to; this is necessary for our own sanity and to maintain a broad perspective.

- It's okay to get angry at your loved one. Caregiving relationships are challenging because of the limitations that PD imposes. Frustration is an integral part of these relationships. Accept your anger when it occurs and don't feel guilty about it. However, avoid carrying that anger, since that would be detrimental to both of you in the long run. If you can't shake the anger, find someone to talk to about it.

- Get enough sleep. PD often results in poor sleep for not only the patient but also the sleep partner. All sorts of things may occur during the night, ranging from acting out dreams (REM sleep behavior disorder) to the repeated need to urinate. It is common for the person with PD to keep a spouse or family up at night. A sleep-deprived caregiver will find coping even more difficult. If your loved one with PD is keeping you awake, there are strategies for improving his or her sleep and these have been discussed in previous chapters. Be certain that your physician addresses these as best as possible.

- Address your own physical and mental needs. Caregivers are not immune from illness. They also need annual medical examinations. When you go for this annual exam, this will also provide one opportunity to bring up your own mental health. Caregivers get depressed and for good reason; their life has taken an unanticipated and unfortunate turn. Depression may need to be treated and this is not a sign of weakness.

- Live one day at a time. There is a tendency to worry about the future and ruminate about things over which we have no control.

Caregivers may also benefit from local PD support groups. Most communities have groups where caregivers may share their experiences.

PART ELEVEN

◆ ◆ ◆

Surgery and Procedures for Parkinson's Disease: Present and Future

33

◆ ◆ ◆

Brain Surgery for PD Symptoms: Thalamotomy, Pallidotomy, and Deep Brain Stimulation

In this chapter, we consider surgeries that can be performed to treat the symptoms of Parkinson's disease (PD). These are not experimental and currently are being done at many hospitals in the United States and around the world. The surgeries described in this chapter are generally covered by standard health insurance policies, provided that you meet the criteria.

The surgeries we will address are employed for specific problems encountered in PD. They fall into two general categories: brain lesioning and deep brain stimulation. There are three different targets inside the brain for these procedures:

- Thalamus
- Globus pallidus (pallidum)
- Subthalamic nucleus

These brain nuclei are shown in figure 33.1.

Lesioning Procedures

The term "lesioning" implies destruction. Surgical lesioning of the brain involves destroying a small, well-defined area of brain tissue. The specific procedures are named on the basis of the targeted brain area. Thalamotomy implies destroying (lesioning) a small area of the thalamus; pallidotomy similarly

473

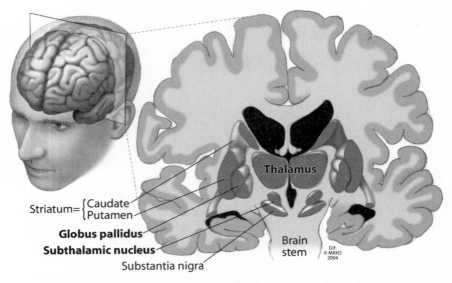

Striatum = { Caudate
              Putamen

Globus pallidus

Subthalamic nucleus

Substantia nigra

Thalamus

Brain
stem

D.F.
© MAYO
2004

33.1 Three different sites have been targeted in lesioning or stimulation surgery to treat Parkinson's disease: thalamus, globus pallidus (pallidum), and subthalamic nucleus. These structures are highly interconnected with the dopaminergic nigrostriatal system (substantia nigra, putamen and caudate).

implies lesioning a region inside the pallidum. Neither the entire thalamus nor the whole pallidum is destroyed with these lesioning procedures; rather, only a limited portion of brain circuitry is destroyed.

Destroying brain tissue to treat movement disorders is not a new idea. The original surgeries of this type date back to the late 1930s. In the 1950s and 1960s, brain lesioning was frequently performed as treatment of PD. With the advent of levodopa therapy about 1969, lesioning procedures were abandoned, only to be rediscovered more recently.

Why should destroying brain tissue improve PD? After all, the symptoms of PD are due to loss of brain cells. Shouldn't a surgical lesion to the brain add insult to injury? The explanation lies in the complex interplay of brain circuits. The brain has many circuits that work in concert and provide checks and balances on one another. Some components of circuits facilitate certain movements, and this is counterbalanced by other components that inhibit these movements. If one component is lost, as is the case with PD (i.e., loss of the nigrostriatal system), there may be a shift toward too much activity in another component of the system. Hence a small destructive lesion in the right place may help reset balance in the circuitry. Our understanding of these circuits and their precise interactions is crude, and the effects of these lesions can be explained only in very general terms.

Lesioning is done by implanting an insulated wire with an exposed tip. The tip is heated for a brief time (typically about a minute) to a certain specified temperature. This cauterizes (destroys) a small amount of tissue in a concentric circle around that site, and a small hole in the brain is created. There are other ways in which lesioning has been done, but cauterization is the method currently employed by most neurosurgeons.

Deep Brain Stimulation

Deep brain stimulation is really an extension of lesioning procedures and has supplanted them in many cases. It was borne of the recognition that electrically stimulating the brain through the exposed tip of an insulated wire ("electrode") could turn on or off brain cell activity. High-frequency stimulation turns off neurons, as shown in figure 33.2. This has the same effect as lesioning, except that it is reversible; when the stimulation stops, the brain cells resume their baseline activity. The advantages of deep brain stimulation over lesioning include the following:

- Less damage to normal brain tissue (although some damage occurs from insertion of the electrode).

- Potential to make adjustments in the electrical current and other parameters to optimize the effects.

There are some advantages to lesioning, however:

- The effect is permanent, which is desirable if the surgery was successful.

- There are no wires, batteries, or computer circuitry to malfunction or replace.

Currently most physicians believe that the relative advantages of deep brain stimulation favor this approach over lesioning. Hence, this is now done much more frequently than the lesioning procedures.

Although deep brain stimulation is done at the same brain sites as thalamotomy and pallidotomy, it is also performed at a different brain location, the subthalamic nucleus (see figure 33.1), which is now the brain target most often used for surgical treatment of PD. The thalamus and pallidum are primarily targeted for treatment of tremor or levodopa-induced dyskinesias. More is said about these indications below.

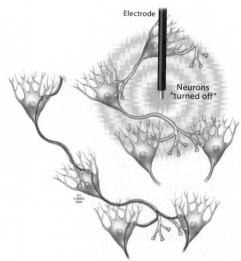

33.2 Deep brain stimulating electrode inside the brain. The high frequency stimulation turns off the activity of neurons in the vicinity.

What to Expect

Both lesioning and deep brain stimulation are complex, daylong events involving numerous physicians and technicians. Space age technology has provided us with the complex gadgetry needed to perform these procedures with the necessary precision. Let's consider the typical surgery from the standpoint of the patient.

The procedure starts with placement of the head frame. This is done under mild sedation and with local anesthetics, as depicted in figure 33.3. The head frame is firmly attached to your skull with small bolts or pins (it cannot be allowed to move). It has a three-dimensional coordinate system with markers that are detected during subsequent brain scanning (either MRI or CT). It allows the surgeon to convert the anatomy of the brain into a three-dimensional grid system. With this head frame in place, any given brain site can be specified in numerical coordinates (e.g., X millimeters from the midline, Y millimeters from a reference point in the front-to-back plane and, similarly, Z millimeters in a top-to-bottom plane). This is termed stereotactic brain surgery.

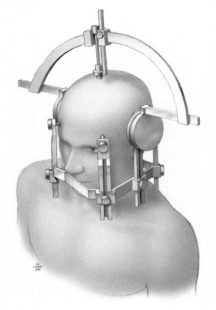

Next the brain is scanned, using either conventional MRI (magnetic resonance imaging) or CT (computed tomography). The computer integrates the scanned brain images with the markers on the special head frame. With this, the computer is able to provide exact three-dimensional coordinates for any given brain locus. The coordinates are with respect to specific points on the head frame.

33.3 The stereotactic surgical head frame is fastened to the skull with small bolts.

In the operating room at the time of the actual surgery, a small hole is made in your skull, exposing the brain. For the remainder of the surgery, only mild sedation and pain-relieving medications are employed. Deep anesthesia would prevent the surgical team from monitoring brain cell electrical activity or assessing the preliminary effect of the electrode placement on your parkinsonism. The anesthesiologists, however, can keep you fairly comfortable with medications through the intravenous line.

Many surgeons employ electrical brain recording to confirm the proper site for either lesioning or implantation of the stimulating electrode. This brain recording is done by inserting a small recording-wire into the brain, insulated except for the tip. This picks up the normal electrical activity of brain cells in the region of the tip. The pattern of brain cell activity provides clues to the surgical team about the location inside the brain. Sometimes several passes of this recording electrode are made to confirm the target. The recording electrode is ultimately withdrawn. With knowledge of the proper coordinates, the final stage is to either make the lesion or implant the deep brain-stimulating electrode into the designated site.

To perform lesioning, the surgeon inserts the electrode and properly positions it at the targeted site. The electrode tip is heated for the predesignated time and then the outcome is evaluated. A member of the surgical team assesses certain aspects of your parkinsonism (e.g., tremor, rigidity, etc.) to determine the effect of the lesion. The lesion may be enlarged, depending on what is learned from this assessment. Once satisfied, the surgeon withdraws the lesioning electrode and closes the operative hole in the scalp. This concludes the lesioning surgery and you are now ready to leave the operating room.

To perform deep brain stimulation, the surgeon implants a permanent stimulating electrode with the tip at the targeted brain site. It is attached to a wire that will ultimately be connected to the stimulating unit. As with lesioning, you must be awake, which allows the surgical team to assess the effects of the stimulation on your parkinsonism. The wire leading from the electrode will be tunneled under your skin to the site of the neurostimulating unit. This stimulating unit is also implanted under the skin, usually just below your collar bone (clavicle); this is illustrated in figure 33.4. General anesthesia is employed for this subsequent implantation of the wire and stimulating unit. This is often done a day to a few days after the brain surgery.

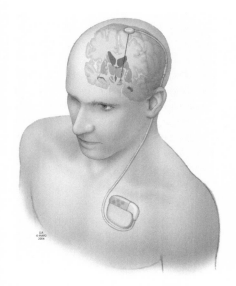

Deep Brain Stimulation Devices

The neurostimulating unit is similar to a heart pacemaker in both appearance and function (figure 33.4). It delivers electrical impulses that are transmitted to the brain electrode. The parameters of the electrical stimulation are programmed from this unit; the stimulation characteristics are adjusted to maximize the response while minimizing side effects.

33.4 Deep brain stimulation. The programmable neurostimulating unit is implanted in the upper chest, under the skin (like a heart pacemaker). Current from the unit passes via the insulated wire (under the skin) to the stimulating electrode within the brain.

This programming is done with a small external computer that your doctor or stimulation-nurse uses to optimize the response. Although the programming can be done immediately after the surgery, often it is delayed for a week to a few weeks. This allows healing and stabilization of the site inside the brain where the electrode is situated. You will not be provided with a device that allows you to change the settings of your stimulating unit; however, you will be given a magnetic switch that allows you to turn the stimulator off and on, if you desire.

Programming the stimulation is complex, with a variety of parameters that can be modified. The electrode within the brain has four separate stimulation sites and the device can be programmed to stimulate from any of those four. Also, the properties of the electrical current can be adjusted in numerous ways to produce the best response. This includes changing the frequency of the pulse, which is typically set to fire at a very rapid firing rate (about 130–150 stimulation bursts per second). The magnitude and the duration of the burst are also adjusted to produce the best response.

Like a heart pacemaker, this neurostimulating unit contains a battery. The battery needs to be replaced every few years. This is done via minor surgery, opening the skin at the site of the neurostimulating unit in your upper chest wall.

Later Problems with Deep Brain Stimulation

The neurostimulating units have proven to be reliable. However, the wires connected to the units have been known to break, albeit infrequently. This requires minor surgery to replace. But, if the brain electrode malfunctions, replacement is not minor. Also, as with any implanted foreign material in the body, infections can occur. This is infrequent and usually involves the wire under the skin.

Reprogramming the stimulator may subsequently be necessary. Usually this is not a frequent requirement once the initial programming has captured a favorable response. If there is a decline in parkinsonian control, adjusting the stimulation parameters may well recapture the lost benefit.

The potential for malfunction and the occasional need for reprogramming make it desirable to have ready access to the medical team. Hence, if it is impossible to travel on short notice from your home to the center performing the surgery, you may not be an ideal candidate for this procedure. Typically, the medical center performing the surgery takes subsequent responsibility for reprogramming and any stimulator repair. Many medical centers are reluctant to take on patients who have had a stimulator implanted elsewhere. Hence, proximity to your surgical center needs to be considered when considering deep brain stimulation.

Caveat

Physicists and electrical engineers are well aware that electromagnetic fields induce electrical currents in wires. This phenomenon occurred with disastrous consequences in one patient with a deep brain electrode. This individual received electrical diathermy treatment from his oral surgeon after extensive tooth extractions. Diathermy uses high frequency electromagnetic fields to induce deep heat and promote healing. Unfortunately the diathermy electrical field induced an electrical current in this person's brain electrode, resulting in severe and permanent brain damage. This is an exceptional case. However, it should serve as a reminder that anyone with a brain electrode should not receive diathermy or be treated with any other concentrated sources of electromagnetic energy.

Am I a Candidate for Brain Surgery?

Only a small minority of people with PD need to consider brain surgery. Why not offer surgery to all with PD? There are several reasons.

- Brain surgery is *not* low risk.

- Some people with parkinsonism are at a high risk for surgical complications or failure.

- Not all problems linked to PD respond to surgery.

- Medical treatment is quite good in most cases.

Let's think about this in more detail.

General Factors Predicting Failure or Complications

Certain characteristics put you into a category of a high likelihood of failure or surgical complications:

- Dementia. This is likely to worsen with any of these surgeries for PD. Most surgeons will not offer any of these brain surgeries to those experiencing substantial problems of thinking and memory.

- Advanced age. The older you are, the greater likelihood of problems. First, problems of a general medical nature can occur, such as heart attacks, blood clots in your lungs, and so on. Second, the brain slowly shrinks over a lifetime, constantly losing brain cells to the aging process. Hence there is less brain reserve—destruction of brain cells from the surgery cannot be as easily compensated by remaining brain circuits. Advanced age is a relative concept and you might negotiate this with your surgeon. For most people, age 80 places them into an especially high-risk category, but the risks start to rise years before this.

- Other serious medical problems. A variety of medical conditions outside the brain may make these surgeries too risky. This includes failure of major organs, such as heart, liver, kidneys, or lungs. Any bleeding problems or requirement for blood thinners obviously increases the risk of a brain hemorrhage during surgery (unless the blood thinner can be safely stopped for a period).

Symptoms Not Helped by These Surgeries

What problems fail to benefit from any of these surgeries? There are, unfortunately, a variety of conditions that surgery will not help:

- Dementia (may make it worse)
- Psychological problems (depression, anxiety)
- Hallucinations, delusions (may worsen)
- Sleep disorders
- Urinary or bowel symptoms
- Fatigue
- Sexual dysfunction
- Pain (unless dystonic pain)

Moreover, if you have one of the parkinsonism-plus syndromes, such as progressive supranuclear palsy, multiple system atrophy, or corticobasal degeneration, these surgeries will not help (see chapter 6).

Indications for Brain Surgery

So who are the good candidates? One of these surgeries may be appropriate for you if you fit into one of these categories:

- Severe tremor is your most troublesome problem and it cannot be controlled with medications
- Levodopa-induced dyskinesias (involuntary movements) are severe, disabling, and cannot be reduced by lowering your medications without resulting in unacceptable parkinsonism

- Fluctuations in your levodopa response result in much parkinsonian off-time, which cannot be controlled by medication adjustments

However, just because you qualify on these grounds does not mean that you should undergo surgery. For some, medical treatment is still the best option and this needs to be individualized.

Which Surgery, and Which Brain Target?

Currently the surgery most commonly employed for the general treatment of PD is deep brain stimulation of the subthalamic nucleus. However, there are specific circumstances where the thalamus or the pallidum might be targeted. Also, there are occasional people who would prefer lesioning rather than implanted electrical gadgetry; hence, they might opt for thalamotomy, pallidotomy, or even a lesion of their subthalamic nucleus.

For each of these surgeries, I have attempted to provide some crude estimates of benefits and risks. This will obviously vary depending on your particular case and the experience and expertise of the surgical team. Your surgeon can provide more specific risk-benefit statistics based on his or her own track record. We will address the thalamus and pallidum first before focusing on what is now the most popular surgery: subthalamic nucleus deep brain stimulation.

Choosing the Thalamus: Thalamotomy or Thalamic Deep Brain Stimulation

The primary reason for targeting the thalamus is for control of tremor. Tremor of any type, whether due to PD, essential tremor, multiple sclerosis, or traumatic brain injury, can be subdued with thalamotomy or thalamic deep brain stimulation. If tremor is indeed the major and overriding problem and the thalamus is targeted, usually a deep brain stimulation procedure is performed. Although thalamotomies have been done for tremor for the past fifty years, they are now done much less frequently with the advent of deep brain stimulation.

The brain has a right half and a left half. The right brain controls the left body and vice versa. Thalamotomy or thalamic stimulation on one side will reduce or abolish tremor on the opposite side of the body. Procedures done on only one side are termed unilateral, as opposed to bilateral, meaning both sides. Unilateral thalamotomy or thalamic stimulation markedly reduces or abolishes PD tremor on the opposite side in about 80 percent of cases.

Unilateral thalamotomies can be performed without high risk of complications. The risk of a permanent neurologic deficit (e.g., weakness or clumsiness of a limb, speech problems, etc.) is less than 15 percent, with most not severe or disabling. However, if thalamotomy is done on both sides of the brain (bilateral), then the risks increase substantially, especially speech problems. Hence thalamotomy is usually done on only one side of the brain.

If tremor is severe on both sides of the body and bilateral surgery is thought necessary, thalamic deep brain stimulation is appropriate. This can be performed without the greater risks of bilateral thalamotomy.

The thalamus is an appropriate target only if chronic tremor is the predominant problem. The slowness, walking problems, or reduced dexterity do not improve with surgeries targeting the thalamus. Since tremor is the primary problem in only a small minority of people with PD, other brain sites are usually chosen for surgery. Thalamotomy or thalamic deep brain stimulation may also reduce levodopa-induced dyskinesias and rigidity, but if these are substantial problems, the pallidum or subthalamic nucleus is the preferable surgical site.

Pallidotomy

Lesioning the pallidum to treat PD was first done extensively about a half century ago. The early experience was inconsistent, which is not surprising, given the surgical equipment of the 1950s and 1960s, plus the lack of brain imaging (i.e., MRI, CT brain scanning). About ten to fifteen years ago, pallidotomy was rediscovered as a treatment for PD. With modern surgical equipment and techniques, more precise and properly localized lesions can be made, allowing for more consistent results. In the early to mid-1990s, pallidotomy gained momentum and was the most popular surgery for PD at that time. With the advent of deep brain stimulation, pallidotomy is now performed only infrequently for symptoms of PD.

Pallidotomy done on one side of the brain (unilateral) primarily benefits parkinsonian symptoms on the opposite side of the body. Clearly the most dramatic and consistent benefit from pallidotomy is the reduction of levodopa-induced dyskinesias; typically these are completely abolished on the opposite side of the body. Tremor is also markedly reduced, although perhaps not as consistently or completely as with thalamotomy. The other aspects of parkinsonism also improve, but only partially and less consistently. With a unilateral pallidotomy procedure, parkinsonism improves by about 25–30 percent, as assessed with the usual PD scoring scales.

Risks tied to a unilateral pallidotomy are similar to those of thalamotomy. Ballpark figures from published reports of complications include stroke-like problems in less than 5 percent, speech problems in up to 10 percent, and death in less than 1 percent. Visual field blind spots were common when pallidotomies were first done since the brain's visual pathways traverse close to the pallidum. However, with increasing attention to this problem, the risks to the visual system are now usually less than 10 percent. In published series, the overall risk for permanent neurological deficits after unilateral pallidotomy is about 10–15 percent, with many or most of these deficits being mild. However, bear in mind that what is published typically represents the better outcomes; surgical teams tend not to report results when things don't go well.

Pallidotomies done on both sides of the brain (bilateral) carry a different set of potential benefits and risks. One might expect that bilateral pallidotomy would double the benefits of unilateral (single-sided) pallidotomy; however, that is not the case. With surgery on the second side, the additional improvement in parkinsonian scores is only about 10–15 percent, although dyskinesias will likely be markedly reduced or abolished on both sides of the body. Offsetting this, however, are the potential side effects of bilateral surgery. As with thalamotomy, lesioning on both sides of the brain substantially increases the risks of permanent deficits. With bilateral pallidotomy, impaired speech is a substantial risk; permanent deterioration in speaking may occur in 25–50 percent of those operated on. Furthermore, a decline in certain aspects of thinking and memory may also occur. With the advent of deep brain stimulation, bilateral pallidotomy is rarely performed because of this side effect spectrum.

Do the benefits of pallidotomy persist? There are few published reports of long-term follow-up and, even then, observations have been limited to a few years. Measurable improvement seems to diminish at least slightly over time (compared to the presurgical state). This probably relates at least partially to the normal progression of PD, which is not halted by the surgery.

Pallidotomy improves parkinsonism scores in those with levodopa-responsive PD. If you have one of the parkinsonism-plus disorders (see chapter 6) or if you are unresponsive to carbidopa/levodopa, then neither pallidotomy nor pallidal deep brain stimulation is likely to be of benefit.

Deep Brain Stimulation of the Pallidum

Pallidal deep brain stimulation should capture the benefits of pallidotomy, but without as much risk. The experience seems to bear this out. With pallidal deep brain stimulation, the surgery can be done on both sides of the brain, but with a lower frequency of permanent neurological deficits. Published reports of bilateral pallidal deep brain stimulation indicate that PD scores improve about 40 percent, on the average. Moreover, levodopa-related dyskinesias are markedly improved or abolished.

Although complications appear to be less with deep brain stimulation, they do occur. For example in one recent larger series of bilateral pallidal deep brain stimulation, 10 percent of patients experienced a brain hemorrhage, sufficient to result in a stroke-like deficit in most of them (weakness on one side of the body). Less frequent problems include seizures and speech difficulties.

The stimulation may also cause side effects such as tingling in the limbs, impaired movement, or difficulty in speaking. However, these can be reversed by adjusting the stimulation parameters.

Programming the stimulator to capture the best responses is sometimes a time-consuming task. This may require days to complete, in which the stimulator is adjusted and then reprogrammed later after a period of observation.

Parkinson's disease medications, including carbidopa/levodopa, are still necessary in full doses for those with pallidal deep brain stimulation. Since dyskinesias are markedly reduced or eliminated, however, one can be more aggressive with levodopa treatment, which may add to the benefit.

Longer-term follow-up of pallidal deep brain stimulation has been published, ranging up to five years. Although dyskinesia control persists, there is a decline in control of PD symptoms after the first year; by three to five years, parkinsonism returned nearly to baseline, despite attempts to reprogram the stimulators.

Deep Brain Stimulation of the Subthalamic Nucleus: The Preferred Surgery

Among the available surgeries for PD, deep brain stimulation of the subthalamic nucleus appears to be the most effective. Medical centers specializing in PD surgery now offer primarily this over the other surgical options. There are three advantages of deep brain stimulation of the subthalamic nucleus versus the pallidum.

1. Subthalamic nucleus stimulation appears to be more efficacious in reducing parkinsonism, at least to a mild degree (see below).

2. The benefits appear more likely to be sustained, based on five-year follow-up studies.

3. Medication doses, including carbidopa/levodopa, can be markedly reduced and occasionally eliminated with the subthalamic nucleus surgery.

Subthalamic nucleus deep brain stimulation does not directly reduce dyskinesias, as occurs with pallidal stimulation. However, dyskinesias are substantially reduced consequent to the markedly lower levodopa doses necessary after the subthalamic nucleus surgery.

To capture the best benefits, subthalamic nucleus deep brain stimulation is done on both sides (bilaterally). The improvement with unilateral stimulation is rather modest compared to bilateral surgery. Hence, subthalamic nucleus surgery is usually planned for both sides, although the surgeries may be staggered (i.e., one side is done first, and the second done a few months later). The general estimates provided below for risks and benefits relate to bilateral subthalamic nucleus deep brain stimulation.

The Benefits of Subthalamic Nucleus Deep Brain Stimulation

The effect of subthalamic nucleus stimulation is comparable to your best levodopa response. In other words, if your levodopa dose is optimally adjusted, subthalamic nucleus deep brain stimulation will capture the peak effect of that response. However, it will not make you any better than that. The obvious benefit is that it can sustain your response without wearing-off or off-states. If you are a severe fluctuator with a brief levodopa response, this surgery will keep you in your best levodopa on-state. This avoids the ups and downs of the medication effect. Added to this are reduced dyskinesias as a consequence of lower levodopa doses. Carbidopa/levodopa doses can be reduced by about 40–60 percent, on the average.

Thus the primary candidates for subthalamic nucleus deep brain stimulation are those who have an excellent levodopa response but a response that markedly fluctuates or is compromised by dyskinesias. This is illustrated by Mr. Samuel:

> Mr. Samuel had a two-hour response to each dose of carbidopa/levodopa. About a third of his doses failed to kick in, resulting in immobility. When his levodopa did work, he could walk but had moderate imbalance; moreover, his gait was degraded by dyskinesias. Dopamine agonist therapy helped only a little and entacapone worsened his dyskinesias. He subsequently underwent bilateral subthalamic nucleus deep brain stimulation. He now is in an on-state all the time; he no longer lives in fear of a carbidopa/levodopa dose failing to kick in. He has reduced his carbidopa/levodopa doses by half, which has almost abolished his dyskinesias. However, he still has moderate imbalance.

To summarize, this surgery won't make you any better than your best levodopa response, except for the reduction of dyskinesias. If you don't respond to levodopa, then this surgery won't help you.

What if you haven't responded to carbidopa/levodopa because you have trouble tolerating it? Will this rule out a response to surgery? Sometimes intolerance to carbidopa/levodopa is a red flag for one of the parkinsonism-plus disorders discussed in chapter 6. These do not respond to subthalamic deep brain stimulation. However, some people experience only a partial response to carbidopa/levodopa because they can only tolerate low doses due to severe nausea, low blood pressure (orthostatic hypotension), or some other persistent side effect. In this case, they may still be candidates.

A comment about orthostatic hypotension is in order. When low blood pressure is a treatment problem for someone with PD, medications are typically the primary culprits, especially carbidopa/levodopa and the dopamine agonists. Subthalamic nucleus stimulation allows a dramatic reduction in the carbidopa/levodopa doses, which should allow the blood pressure to return to more normal levels.

Will the benefits of subthalamic nucleus stimulation persist? One recent study reported sustained benefits to five years of follow-up. However, it was apparent from the data that this did not halt the progression of PD.

There is risk to undergoing subthalamic nucleus deep brain stimulation. In one large series, brain hemorrhage with stroke-like symptoms occurred in 3 percent of patients and seizures in another 3 percent. Also, a confused, disoriented, and sometimes agitated state may occur for the first week or two after the surgery, primarily among seniors. As with pallidal stimulation, there may be side effects from the subthalamic nucleus stimulation per se. This includes tingling in the limbs, double vision, or speech problems. However, in most cases, the stimulation parameters can be adjusted to minimize such side effects.

Programming subthalamic nucleus deep brain stimulation is complex and is further complicated by the need to reduce PD medications. The initial programming may take up to several weeks before the best stimulation and medication parameters are established.

Lesioning the Subthalamic Nucleus: Subthalamotomy

If subthalamic nucleus deep brain stimulation can improve parkinsonism, what about simply lesioning the subthalamic nucleus? This would eliminate the wires and electronic gadgets and the need for programming. This has been done in limited numbers of patients, primarily outside the United States. There is some risk for involuntary movements similar to the most marked dyskinesias provoked by levodopa therapy. However, with optimally placed lesions, these seem to occur in only a minority of people. Overall, there has been insufficient experience with this surgery to form any conclusions. It should be regarded as experimental.

34

◆ ◆ ◆

Experimental Treatments: Fetal and Stem Cell Implantation, Neurotrophic Hormones, and Gene Therapy

Cell Transplantation Using Fetal or Stem Cells

If neurons in the substantia nigra are degenerating, why not replace them with new cells? Makes good sense. With modern technology, we should be able to implant healthy brain cells into the areas of degenerating neurons and reverse Parkinson's disease (PD). Sounds simple, and in fact it does work to some extent. However, there are some impediments to this strategy. We can better understand the obstacles if we consider how the complex circuitry of the brain initially develops.

Development of the Brain

The brain is far more complicated than the most sophisticated computer conceived by scientists. It contains about 10 billion neurons and many of these neurons have thousands of connections with one another. These connections are the wiring circuits, conceptually like a computer circuit. As we learned in chapter 2, connections to distant areas in the brain are made via axons, which are the wire-like extensions from neurons (see figures 2.1 and 2.2 in chapter 2). Axons transmit signals to other neurons and may extend to far reaches of the brain. For example, a primary neuron located in the cortex (outer layers of the brain) may send a long axon all the way down to the bottom of the brain (the brain stem) or to the spinal cord. Moreover, there may be connections all along this path. Not all brain neurons, however, have distant connections. Some interact only with neurons in their own region, but perhaps with thousands of connections.

The receiving end of the neuron is equally complex. Recall that signals from neuron to neuron are transmitted through synapses, where a neurochemical such as dopamine is released (see figure 2.2, chapter 2). The receptors for this neurochemical signal are often located on dendrites, which are the wire-like extensions from the cell body. These dendrites do not travel long distances like axons; however, they may form extremely complex networks. For example, a single neuron in the cerebellum may receive 150,000 synaptic connections through its dendrites.

The brain's wiring is very, very complex. Not only are there 10 billion neurons, but they interact with one another through perhaps thousands of synaptic connections.

This complicated brain did not happen all at once. It was built slowly in the mother's womb (although brain development continues through the early years of life). It is in the womb that the fundamental brain wiring is formed. This occurs through a cascade of events. In this cascade, each step depends on the previous. Immature cells divide in the center of the brain to form neurons and these new neurons then migrate outward. The areas in the middle of the developing brain where these cells replicate are called germinal zones. In these germinal zones, neurons destined to be located in distant areas of the brain are being formed. These newly formed cells then physically move outward (migrate) to their ultimate destination. Certain neurons go first, another type next, and so on. There is a vast array of ever-changing chemical-hormonal signals that guide each step and direct this process of migration. The DNA blueprints of these cells organize all of this development; certain chemical signals are activated at precisely the right time in development to stimulate each developing cell to do the proper thing. Later that chemical signal is turned off and supplanted by another appropriate chemical signal for the next step. As the neurons are moving outward to their destination, they do not have any physical impediments to this migration, as will be the case once the brain is fully developed and packed with cells. This entire process proceeds in countless steps, with wave after wave of new neurons moving to their correct location in the developing brain and then forming the appropriate synaptic connections. The sequence and timing of this process is crucial. This developing network of brain cells can only proceed if each component of the overall process occurs at precisely the right place and time in the sequence.

What does this have to do with cell implantation for PD? If you understand the complexity of brain development, you can appreciate the challenges to researchers. The obstacles are those of time and space.

1. Time. The wiring of brain circuits is programmed early in our lives by a precise sequence of events, with each event triggering the next. These

complex brain connections only occur when the process proceeds in the proper order and at the right time in brain development. To date, we have no sense of how to replicate this precisely programmed cascade of cellular events.

2. Space. Once the brain wiring is in place in the mature brain, there is no extra space. Neurons and glia are tightly packed together along with the connections (axons and dendrites). Of the entire volume of the brain, perhaps only 15–20 percent is not occupied by some cellular element. Thus there are physical impediments to forming connections (synapses) with other brain cells, except in the immediate vicinity. In the mature brain, if an axon were to grow, it would be blocked from extending very far by the surrounding cells and cellular elements.

What are the implications for cell implantation? If new neurons were implanted into the adult brain, we would currently have no means of inducing these cells to form the appropriate complex connections that occur in normal brain development. This would require a cascade of chemical signals, one after the other and in exactly the right location to make this happen. Moreover, there is no space in the adult brain for transplanted neurons to physically grow axons to distant targets. Implanted cells do indeed survive, form synaptic connections with the native neurons, and release neurotransmitters. However, these may not be the right connections or provide the right neurotransmitter for that particular location.

Current Implantation Techniques

With present technology, there are two basic strategies that could be employed for therapeutic implantation of cells into the brain.

1. Cells can be implanted that release a specific neurotransmitter, for example, dopamine-secreting neurons.

2. Cells that release "neurotrophic hormones" that nourish brain cells can be implanted. Neurons can be made more robust and healthy with certain neurotrophic substances found in the normal brain. These neurotrophic hormones may even induce mature brain cells to form new synaptic connections. These neurotrophic substances are like the fertilizer you put on your lawn; grass can grow without it, but it grows better and is healthier with the proper concentrations of fertilizer. Cells can be genetically programmed to manufacture and release specific types of neurotrophic substances. Neurotrophic hormones will be discussed later in this chapter.

To date, implantation for PD has primarily been directed at replenishing dopamine within the striatum. Although complex synaptic connections cannot be programmed with current implantation technology, we can implant cells that release dopamine. With certain types of implanted cells, synaptic connections do develop with the native neurons in the immediate vicinity of the transplant.

Treatment Limitations in Advanced PD

With progression of PD, the dopaminergic nigrostriatal system continues to degenerate, which ultimately may result in instability of the levodopa response, with motor fluctuations and dyskinesias. However, as long as the degeneration is confined to this dopamine system, we can still treat the symptoms of PD with medications; there may be ups and downs, but people still respond.

Unfortunately for some with PD, the degeneration may not be confined to the dopamine systems. Other brain cells and circuits may also succumb. When these other circuits degenerate, the additional symptoms do not respond to dopamine medications. But, neither will they respond simply to implantation of brain dopaminergic neurons. It is this degeneration in other brain systems that is responsible for dementia, which is found in about a third of people with PD. It is also responsible for the parkinsonian symptoms that don't respond to medications in any dose (e.g., imbalance and other refractory gait problems in advanced PD).

Implanting dopaminergic neurons won't help if the symptoms are the consequence of degeneration in nondopaminergic systems. At the present time, it is not yet known how to restore these other brain circuits with implantation technology. This places distinct limits on what we can expect to achieve with brain cell implantation.

Avoiding Rejection of Implanted Brain Cells

The body's immune system recognizes the presence of foreign cells. It identifies, attacks, destroys, and disposes of them. This is what allows us to defend ourselves from viruses and bacteria. However, this process is an impediment to cell implantation. Fortunately the general surgical experience that has accumulated over the past couple of decades has generated strategies for attenuating this problem. Obviously, lungs, hearts, kidneys, and livers are now routinely transplanted and survive. This survival is with the use of antirejection drugs that dampen the activity of the immune system. This does come at a price, however. An immune system that has been attenuated will not fight infections as effectively. Thus people with transplanted organs walk a fine line with these antirejection drugs, whereby the immune system is turned down just enough to allow the transplant to survive, but not so much that overwhelming infections threaten their lives.

There has been ongoing debate about the need for rejection drugs in human cell implantation for PD. We do know that the immune system is not as aggressive inside the brain (due to the blood–brain barrier). Hence cells implanted into the striatum of someone with PD may be able to survive and grow, even without the use of antirejection drugs. However, it is less clear whether that survival is sustained indefinitely.

There has been considerable experience with cell implantation for PD over the past fifteen years. Cell lines that have been implanted into people with PD have included adrenal cells, fetal brain cells, pig brain cells, and now we are moving into the era of stem cell implantation. Let's review what we have learned.

ADRENAL-BRAIN TRANSPLANTATION

Adrenal-brain transplantation was the first attempt to treat PD by implanting cells into the brain. The first surgeries were done in the mid-1980s, and by the late 1980s this procedure was being performed at many major medical centers in North America and Europe.

Adrenal-brain transplantation involves removing one of your adrenal glands and implanting part of this into your brain. The inner portion of our adrenals produces dopamine and related substances. Scientists recognized that this inner adrenal tissue could be used to replenish dopamine in the striatum among those with PD. Potential rejection by the immune system should not be a problem since your own adrenal is the source of transplanted tissue. We all have two adrenal glands, one perched on top of each kidney. Since you don't require two adrenal glands, one could be taken for transplantation.

Clever idea! Unfortunately, despite initial optimism, it turned out to be a failure. Some patients may have benefited, but it remains unclear whether this was a placebo effect. Most patients did not improve substantially. The primary reason for the poor success became clear within a few years when several of the transplanted patients died due to natural causes, accidents, and so on. Brain examination revealed no surviving adrenal cells. Thus the surgery seemingly failed because the adrenal cells died. This surgery is no longer performed.

FETAL TRANSPLANTATION

Young cells tend to be more robust than old cells. This was the rationale for choosing fetal brain tissue for implantation. Fetal brain cells should have a much better chance for survival. Presumably the old adrenal cells used in adrenal-brain transplantation were near the end of their normal life span. They simply could not withstand the rigors of transplantation surgery.

Fetal substantia nigra neurons would seem to be the ideal source of tissue to implant for PD. Not only do they secrete dopamine, but they are precisely the cells that have been lost due to the PD degenerative process. In other words, we are replacing the degenerated neurons with brand-new cells of the same vintage.

The procedure obviously requires a fetus and specifically a fetus aborted early in pregnancy (older fetal brain cells do not survive as well). The specific tissue chosen for implantation is dissected from the fetal brain under a microscope. The desired dopamine-containing cells are found in the midbrain, and it is the midbrain that is extracted and implanted. Because the fetal midbrain is small and provides only limited numbers of cells, tissue from several fetuses is used for each patient.

The initial attempts to implant fetal brain cells came on the heels of the adrenal-brain transplantation experience. By the mid-1990s a number of medical teams had implanted fetal brain tissue and reported at least some success in improving parkinsonism. Encouraging reports of fetal brain implantation for PD were tempered by concerns that the results were not being objectively analyzed. Furthermore, placebo effects could have been playing a role, as was undoubtedly the case with adrenal-brain transplantation.

How effective is fetal transplantation? Answering this question would require a prospective clinical trial with independent, dispassionate evaluators and measures to control for the placebo effects. In fact, two such trials, funded by the federal government, have been performed, and we now have objective data.

Both of these fetal cell implantation clinical trials were remarkable in their design. PD patients who volunteered were randomly assigned to one of two groups, receiving either the fetal cell implant or sham surgery. Patients were informed that they might not receive the actual fetal implant (the sham surgery). Neither patients nor clinicians evaluating the outcomes knew whether fetal tissue had been implanted in any given patient. This controlled for possible placebo effects. Those who had the sham surgery had a hole drilled in their skull but no implant. Those undergoing the actual surgery had midbrain tissue from multiple fetuses implanted into their putamen. This implant contained dopaminergic substantia nigra neurons. Immunosuppressive treatment was used in all of the patients in one of these two studies.

Unfortunately, the outcomes of these fetal transplantation trials were a bit discouraging. After 1–2 years, the groups of patients who had received the fetal implants had parkinsonism scores that were only slightly better than the sham surgery groups. Statistically the differences were so small that they could have been due to chance. In one study, it seemed that benefits were confined to people less than age 60. In the other study, benefits seemed to be among those who had milder parkinsonism at the start of the study. Even more discouraging was the development of dyskinesias in half of the patients in one study and 15 percent in the other; these persisted despite no medications. In several patients, further brain surgery was necessary to control these dyskinesias.

This lack of striking success was not due to poor implant survival. To the contrary, the implanted fetal midbrain tissue not only survived but grew into mature-looking dopaminergic cells. This was apparent from special imaging studies (positron emission tomography, PET) as well as brain examination of patients who subsequently died. If fetal cell implantation were an appropriate treatment for PD, it should have been apparent in these well-designed, carefully conducted studies.

PORCINE (PIG) TRANSPLANTATION

One of the concerns of fetal cell implantation has been the availability of human fetal tissue. In the trials described above, brain tissue from several fetuses was used for implantation into each person with PD. To provide a more available source of brain tissue, fetal pig brain has been suggested. In fact, there are currently ongoing trials of pig brain tissue implanted into people with PD. Given the rather limited benefit experienced by those who were implanted with human fetal tissue, it is hard to believe that pig brain tissue will be the answer. However, this might change with new developments in the laboratory, especially new insights into genetic programming of cells.

STEM CELL IMPLANTATION FOR PD

What are stem cells? These are the most immature cells. They have not yet taken on the defining characteristics of neurons, muscle cells, kidney cells, and so on. The excitement about stem cells for implantation is that they can reproduce themselves and hence proliferate in test tubes. They could thus provide an unlimited supply of cells for transplantation.

Where do you get stem cells? Those most favored for human implantation come from newly fertilized human eggs (ova). We now routinely fertilize human eggs in the laboratory to assist women who cannot get pregnant; this is called in vitro fertilization. In this procedure, eggs (ova) are taken from a woman's ovary through a minor surgical procedure and placed in a test tube. Then they are combined with sperm, which fertilize the eggs. A fertilized egg is then implanted into a woman's womb (uterus) and develops into a baby. When gynecologists perform this procedure, they often have fertilized eggs left over (they always prepare more than one). This can be the source of embryonic stem cells.

These embryonic stem cells have not yet taken on any definite characteristics; thus they are not differentiated into neurons, muscle cells, and so on. It is these cells that have an almost unlimited capacity for self-renewal in the laboratory. With certain techniques, it is possible to induce them to become neurons (or other types of cells). This procedure has been the subject of ethical debate, since these same fertilized eggs could also become human beings if placed in the proper environment of the uterus.

Can stem cells also be found in older embryos (fetuses) that have been aborted? Indeed they are present, but with these slightly older cells, the differentiation process has already started. Consequently the cells are more limited in their capacity to proliferate and develop into desired cell lines, although they can be induced to do this with certain laboratory strategies.

Adults also have stem cells present in bone marrow. But they are even more restricted in their capacity to reproduce, and it has been difficult to induce them to develop into neurons for implantation. However, research laboratories are working on this.

Whatever the source of stem cells, the goal is to grow them in the laboratory and implant whatever numbers of them are necessary to treat PD. But is it that simple? Clearly not, regardless of the ethical debate. Why should we expect stem cell implantation to be more successful than fetal cell implantation? In the fetal implantation investigations described above, the transplanted fetal embryonic tissue should have been a perfect replacement for what was lost; fetal substantia nigra dopaminergic neurons were used to replace the same cells that had degenerated due to PD. Despite the fact that these cells survived and became integrated into the native brain, the benefits were modest at best. If replacing substantia nigra neurons with new substantia nigra neurons doesn't effectively treat advancing PD, why should stem cells fare any better?

This is not a hopeless endeavor and there is hope for the future with stem cell technology. However, scientists must better understand how to control and program these cells to better replace degenerated brain circuitry. Simply placing dopamine-secreting cells in the brain appears to be an insufficient treatment strategy. Thus stem cell implantation is likely years away from providing us with a practical and useful treatment for PD.

NEUROTROPHIC HORMONES AND GENE THERAPY

There are many potential avenues where medical science may take us in our endeavor to treat and even cure PD. Some of these are in the conceptual stages. Further clarity awaits the discovery of the cause(s) of PD, which could occur in this decade. It is difficult to know where medical science will take us. However, let's consider several treatment avenues that may come to fruition in the future.

NEUROTROPHIC HORMONE INJECTION

We already considered neurotrophic hormones. Briefly, these are substances present in the brain that cause brain cells to thrive and grow, acting much like fertilizer in your flower garden. Several of these have been discovered and studied.

One neurotrophic factor that has undergone therapeutic scrutiny is GDNF (glial cell line-derived neurotrophic factor). This is one of the most potent growth factors for dopaminergic neurons. There was sufficient evidence from animal studies to justify administration of this into the brain ventricles of people with PD in a small clinical trial. The ventricles are the slits that we all have in the center of our brains where we make most of our spinal fluid (depicted in figure 3.5 in chapter 3). In this clinical trial, a tube was maintained in the brain ventricles through which the GDNF could be injected. This treatment turned out to be a failure; there was no benefit and only side effects. Two subsequent studies of GDNF brain infusion have generated mixed results. In these trials, the GDNF was injected directly into the striatum of several PD patients, with the infusion tube connected to an implanted pump. The first trial demonstrated significant improvement, but this could not be replicated in a controlled study.

OTHER MEANS OF ADMINISTERING GDNF OR OTHER NEUROTROPHIC HORMONES

These neurotrophic hormones are large molecules that cannot cross into the brain. They are excluded by the blood–brain barrier. Moreover, these hormones do not remain in place indefinitely but are degraded and eliminated by normal brain clearance mechanisms. How then can we provide such hormones to critical brain areas on a continuous basis? A constant infusion through a pump was the strategy employed in the studies just described. However, to do this over many years is potentially fraught with methodological problems. One alternative has been to genetically program a virus to make and secrete the neurotrophic hormone and then implant the virus into the brain. Several "safe" viruses are available for this purpose and this has been done in animals. However, there are a number of practical issues to be addressed before this can be done in humans.

GENETIC PROGRAMMING

Theoretically, genetic programming as treatment for PD is not limited to neurotrophic hormones. In fact, this general strategy might be used in a wide variety of ways to treat PD. For example, genes have been introduced into animal brains inducing the cells to manufacture dopamine. However, loss of dopaminergic neurons is only one component of PD. If we were able to manipulate the genetic code more effectively, we conceivably could induce native brain cells to reproduce and form new synaptic connections. Thus, we could restore the brain's computer circuitry that had been damaged by PD.

Genetic programming of cells for the treatment of PD could be accomplished in several ways.

- Genes could be introduced directly into the brain to modify the function of the native brain cells. Thus, neurons already in place could be genetically reprogrammed and transformed to restore lost brain circuitry. This could be done with viruses carrying an appropriate genetic code. As we discussed, there are several viral candidates for this strategy; these candidate viruses are known to be benign and not infectious.

- Stem cell lines grown in culture could be genetically modified. These stem cells could be induced to make dopamine, form certain synaptic connections, etc. Once optimally genetically programmed, they could be implanted into the brain.

- Living cells from the person with PD could be biopsied and then genetically programmed; once genetically modified, they could then be implanted into the brain. For example, bone marrow cells are easy to obtain with a syringe. They could then be genetically transformed in a test tube. These genetically modified cells could then be injected into that same person's brain. Using one's own cells would reduce the likelihood of the immune system rejecting the implanted cells.

The technology is in place for genetically programming cells. In fact, scientists have been rewriting the genetic codes of cells for many years through several standard techniques. The challenge, however, is to decipher the codes of the complex mechanisms that create not only unique brain cells but also the unique interconnections between the cells.

ATTACKING THE CAUSE OF PD

I have saved for last what I regard as the most exciting prospect. It probably should be last since we don't have proof of the cause of PD. However, as summarized in chapter 8, alpha-synuclein, the protein abundant in Lewy bodies, is looking like the bad actor. Circumstantial evidence is pointing to an accumulation of alpha-synuclein as perhaps the primary inciting factor in PD. Excessive or abnormal alpha-synuclein is the cause in certain rare families with inherited PD. In other families where alpha-synuclein is genetically normal, the cause has been impaired breakdown of proteins, including alpha-synuclein.

The alpha-synuclein story parallels the beta-amyloid story in Alzheimer's disease. It now seems very likely that the primary cause of Alzheimer's disease is brain accumulation of the abnormal protein beta-amyloid. Parallel to PD, the cause in rare families with Alzheimer's disease has been a genetic defect resulting in brain beta-amyloid accumulation. The brain cannot dispose of this protein because of its insoluble nature. This accumulation appears to stimulate a cascade of events that ultimately leads to death and destruction of brain cells, in this case, Alzheimer's disease.

Alzheimer's research is one step ahead of PD. Strategies are now being tested to stop or reverse the brain production of beta-amyloid. Vaccination against brain amyloid was the first clever strategy. In fact, this was dramatically effective in reducing brain amyloid levels in experimental mice. The vaccine stimulated the body's immune system to attack and destroy beta-amyloid. The initial trial in humans may have reduced brain amyloid levels, but unfortunately resulted in brain inflammation in a minority of test subjects.

Although this vaccination strategy is now on hold, it opens the door to other approaches to reduce brain amyloid. Currently, pharmaceutical companies are developing drugs that block the brain enzymes that produce the toxic form of beta-amyloid. Other drugs are being investigated that induce the brain to manufacture enzymes to break down the beta-amyloid. Finally, antibodies are being developed that specifically target beta-amyloid; it is hoped that these would not cause the brain inflammation that was provoked by stimulation of the immune system with the amyloid vaccine. These antibodies would be generated in test tubes and then injected. The challenge is to get these across the blood-brain barrier where they can attack the brain's amyloid.

If we can do this with amyloid, why not with alpha-synuclein? If indeed alpha-synuclein accumulation is the inciting factor in PD, we could use similar strategies for reducing the burden of brain alpha-synuclein.

Currently my research colleagues at Mayo are developing an RNA molecule that targets the DNA blueprint for alpha-synuclein. RNA (ribonucleic acid) is chemically similar to the genetic material, DNA. RNA is present in normal cells and functions in conjunction with DNA to carry out the synthesis of necessary cell constituents. RNA has a chemical configuration that complements DNA. In fact, specific RNA sequences will bind to DNA that has the same genetic code. The strategy is to develop a short strand of RNA that has the same genetic programming sequence as the alpha-synuclein DNA code. The RNA then binds specifically to only the alpha-synuclein DNA, and by doing this, inhibits it. This has been termed small interfering RNA. Again, the challenge will be getting this across the blood–brain barrier. This is but one means of shutting off production or inducing breakdown of brain alpha-synuclein.

THE FUTURE

Transplanting cells into the brain to reverse symptoms of PD holds promise, but the onus is on medical science to develop this into a practical and effective treatment strategy. Scientists are now learning how to rewrite the genetic code of cells. Thus cells can be genetically reprogrammed to do things beyond their original capability. Such genetically modified cells could be implanted into the brain to form crucial synaptic connections in their normal pattern, rather than haphazardly. This, however, is for the future. With present techniques, the benefits of neuroimplantation are limited and this strategy should currently be considered experimental.

How close are we to finding the cure for PD? If we can land a man on the moon . . .

PART TWELVE

◆ ◆ ◆

Parkinson's Disease Information Sources

35

♦ ♦ ♦

Support and Advocacy Groups, and the Internet

Local Support Groups

Many communities have well-organized Parkinson's disease (PD) support groups that meet regularly. These meetings allow people with PD and their families to exchange information and share ideas for dealing with common problems. Frequently guest speakers (doctors, nurses, therapists, etc.) are invited to discuss topics of interest. These groups additionally provide a social outlet and a chance to meet people in similar circumstances. If you are unaware of a PD support group in your community, check with your doctor's office, clinic, or hospital for information.

Not every local support group is appropriate for each person with PD. The mix of people differs from group to group. People generally feel most comfortable where they are similar in age and PD severity to the other members of the group. Some regions have special support groups tailored to specific segments of the PD community, such as young-onset PD. If your local group does not fit with your needs, you always have the option of organizing your own support group.

National PD Advocacy Groups

Several national PD groups provide a variety of services, including disseminating information, lobbying the government for research funding, and providing seed money for researchers starting new projects. The major groups are listed at the end of this chapter. They have excellent websites; you may also call, write, or e-mail to receive information and educational material.

The Internet

The Internet is a great source of information as well as misinformation. You must be discriminating. The websites for the national PD groups listed at the end of this chapter provide reliable, up-to-date information. Medical societies can also be excellent sources. I highly recommend the websites of the Movement Disorder Society and the American Academy of Neurology.

The Movement Disorder Society is a large international professional group open to all physicians and scientists with an interest in Parkinson's disease and other disorders of movement. It also maintains a special website targeted to the lay audience—www.wemove.org—which provides useful information about not only PD but also the Parkinson's-plus syndromes mentioned earlier in this book.

The American Academy of Neurology also has a website for the lay public: www.thebrainmatters.com. You may select from a variety of topics, including PD. The academy has additionally recognized the interest of the public in learning about new medical findings as they are published. To address this interest, it has created a patient page linked to the journal *Neurology* (the official journal of the academy). This includes summaries written for the lay public of just published articles in *Neurology*. Parkinson's disease is one of many topics covered in this journal. You can access it by going to the journal's home page: www.neurology.org. Click on the patient pages icon to find abstracts summarizing the most recent papers in this twice-monthly journal. It also contains links to other relevant sources of information.

National PD Advocacy Groups

American Parkinson's Disease Association, Inc.
1250 Hylan Boulevard
Staten Island, NY 10305
Phone: (800) 223-2732 or (718) 981-8001
Fax: (718) 981-4399
E-mail: apda@apdaparkinson.org
Website: www.apdaparkinson.org

Michael J. Fox Foundation for Parkinson's Research
381 Park Avenue South, Suite 820
New York, NY 10016

Phone: (212) 213-3525
Fax: (212) 213-3523
Website: www.michaeljfox.org

National Parkinson Foundation, Inc.
1501 N.W. 9th Avenue
Miami, FL 33136
Phone: (305) 547-6666
Fax: (305) 243-4403
E-mail: mailbox@npf.med.miami.edu
Website: www.parkinson.org

Northwest Parkinson's Foundation
P.O. Box 56
Mercer Island, WA 98040
Phone: (877) 980-7500
E-mail: nwpf@nwpf.org

Parkinson's Action Network (PAN)
1025 Vermont Avenue NW, Suite 1120
Washington, DC 20005
Phone: (202) 638-4101
Fax: (202) 638-4105
E-mail: info@parkinsonsaction.org
Website: www.parkinsonsaction.org

Parkinson's Disease Foundation
833 W. Washington Boulevard
Chicago, IL 60607
Phone: (800) 457-6676 or (312) 733-1893
Fax: (312) 733-1896
E-mail: UPF_ITF@msn.com
Website: www.pdf.org

Parkinson's Disease Foundation
1359 Broadway, Suite 1509
New York, NY 10018
Phone: (800) 457-6676 or (646) 388-7600
E-mail: pdfpmc@aol.com
Website: www.pdf.org

Parkinson's Disease Foundation
710 West 168th Street 3rd floor
New York, NY 10032

Phone: (800) 457-6676 or (212) 923-4700
Fax: (212) 923-4778
E-mail: pdfcpmc@aol.co
Website: www.pdf.org

Glossary

Acetylcholine: A widespread neurotransmitter, relevant to PD, memory, bowel and bladder function.

Agonist: A drug that activates a specific receptor (e.g., dopamine agonists activate dopamine receptors).

Akathisia: Inner restlessness; unable to comfortably sit still.

Alpha-synuclein: A protein normally found in neurons, and present in high concentrations in Lewy bodies. A genetic mutation is the basis for an inherited form of parkinsonism.

Amantadine: A drug used in the treatment of PD. Its primary role is in the treatment of levodopa-induced dyskinesias. It is a mild and partial blocker of glutamate.

Amino acids: The building blocks of protein, and also the class of biologic chemicals that includes levodopa.

Amitriptyline: An antidepressant medication from the tricyclic class that is also used for other purposes, such as a sleep aid.

Antagonist: A drug that blocks a specific receptor (e.g., a dopamine antagonist blocks dopamine receptors).

Anticholinergic: Drugs that block acetylcholine receptors.

Apomorphine: A dopamine agonist available for injection under the skin (subcutaneous); used for a quick response when in a levodopa off-state.

Aspiration: Inappropriate passage of food or liquid into the lungs.

Ataxia: Incoordination, as occurs in problems involving the cerebellum.

ATP (Adenosine triphosphate): A high-energy substance manufactured by the mitochondria inside cells, which is necessary for multiple metabolic processes.

Autonomic nervous system: The internal nervous system that controls bladder, bowels, sweating, sexual function, and blood pressure.

Axon: A wire-like extension from the neuron that transmits an electrical signal from the cell body to the terminal, where the neurotransmitter is released.

Basal ganglia: A term for the combination of striatum, globus pallidus, and interconnected nuclei (including substantia nigra and subthalamic nucleus).

Benserazide: A drug that is identical in its function to carbidopa. This drug is available in certain countries outside the United States, including Europe.

Benztropine (Cogentin): An anticholinergic drug.

Beta-blockers: Drugs that block one type of adrenalin-like responses. These are used in the treatment of tremor, high blood pressure, certain heart conditions, and migraines.

Biphasic dyskinesias: Levodopa-induced dyskinesias that occur twice during the levodopa on-cycle, transiently at the beginning and again at the end. Also called the DID response.

Blepharospasm: Dystonia of the eyes, manifest as involuntary eye closure.

Blood–brain barrier: The lining around the blood vessels of the brain that prevents undesirable substances within the bloodstream from entering the brain.

Bradykinesia: The slowness of movement that is typical of PD.

Bradyphrenia: Slowness of thought.

Brain stem: The lowest end of the brain that interfaces with the spinal cord. Tracts passing from higher brain centers to the spinal cord pass through the brain stem, and vice versa. The brain stem contains nuclei that control elementary functions, such as breathing and eye movements.

Bromocriptine (Parlodel): A dopamine agonist drug from the ergot class.

Carbidopa: A drug that blocks the conversion of levodopa to dopamine in the circulation but not in the brain (it does not cross the blood–brain barrier).

Catechol-O-methyltransferase (COMT): One of the enzymes that break down levodopa and dopamine. Blocking this enzyme is a PD treatment strategy.

Caudate: This brain nucleus forms the front half of the striatum.

Cerebellum: A brain structure located just above the brain stem. Damage to this area causes ataxia (incoordination).

Chemoreceptive trigger zone: A small region in the brain stem that senses certain substances circulating in the bloodstream. When stimulated by one of these substances, nausea results. Since there is no blood–brain barrier at this site, circulating dopamine can stimulate this region and cause nausea.

Cholinergic: Neurons that release acetylcholine as the neurotransmitter.

Chorea: Involuntary movements characterized by their rapidly flowing, chaotic pattern. These are the primary movements caused by an excessive levodopa effect.

Choreiform: A descriptive term implying that the appearance is that of chorea.

Clonazepam (Klonopin): A sedating medication from the benzodiazepine class that is used to treat REM sleep behavior disorder.

Clozapine (Clozaril): A medication used to treat hallucinations and delusions. It is very effective but has significant side effects.

Coenzyme Q (Coenzyme Q_{10}): A substance that participates in the chemical reactions of mitochondria. It may be deficient in people with PD, and preliminary research suggests that it may have a role in PD treatment.

Colon: The large intestine where feces form.

COMT inhibitor: Drugs that block the enzyme catechol-O-methyltransferase, thereby prolonging the action of levodopa.

Cortex: Outermost layers of the brain, which are most highly developed in humans. Complex human thought, language, and behavior are conceived and programmed here.

Corticobasal degeneration: A neurodegenerative condition that has some resemblance to PD.

Corticospinal: One of the primary brain and spinal cord systems involved with controlling movement. This is spared in PD.

CR (controlled-release): The sustained-release form of carbidopa/levodopa (Sinemet CR).

CT scan: Computed tomography scan, which is used to image the brain.

Deep brain stimulation (DBS): Therapy employing high frequency stimulation of a specific brain region through a device similar to a heart pacemaker.

Delusions: Beliefs that are inappropriate, patently false, and sometimes bizarre.

Dementia: Loss of intellectual abilities, usually due to a neurodegenerative disorder.

Dendrites: Short, wire-like processes on neurons that receive neurotransmitter signals from axon terminals.

Diaphoresis: Sweating.

Diastolic: A blood pressure parameter corresponding to the second number in blood pressure readings (such as 80 in the reading 120/80).

Diffuse Lewy body disease (Lewy body dementia, dementia with Lewy bodies): A condition in which the neurodegenerative changes, including Lewy bodies, are widespread, affecting both the substantia nigra (resulting in parkinsonism) and in the cortex (resulting in dementia).

Diplopia: Double vision.

Diuretic: A water pill (increases urine output).

DNA: Deoxyribonucleic acid, which is the molecule used to write the genetic codes of living cells.

Dominant inheritance: The inheritance pattern in which a trait is passed from one generation to the next. Half of the offspring in any generation tend to display the trait (if it is fully expressed).

Donepezil (Aricept): A medication that increases brain levels of acetylcholine, which is used to treat memory disorders.

Dopa decarboxylase: The enzyme that converts levodopa into dopamine.

Dopamine: The neurotransmitter that is deficient in PD.

Dopamine agonist: Synthetic drugs that behave like dopamine.

Dopaminergic: Neurons that release dopamine as their neurotransmitter.

Dysarthria: Impaired precision of speech.

Dyskinesias: In the context of PD, these are involuntary movements provoked by medications, primarily levodopa. These are especially characterized by flowing, dancing movements (chorea) of the limbs, trunk, neck, or face.

Dysphagia: Impaired swallowing.

Dyspnea: Shortness of breath.

Dystonia: A muscle contraction state resulting in an abnormal posture of foot, hand, toes, and so on. This is caused by abnormal motor programming in the central nervous system. Among those with PD, this is usually a parkinsonian symptom rather than a medication side effect.

Dysuria: Painful urination.

Entacapone (Comtan): A COMT inhibitor that prolongs the levodopa effect and is used to enhance the carbidopa/levodopa response.

Enzymes: Cellular molecules used to transform or modify biochemical substances. An example is dopa decarboxylase, which transforms levodopa into dopamine.

Ergot: A class of drugs that includes bromocriptine, pergolide, and cabergoline. These have unique side effects not shared by other dopamine agonists.

Esophagus: The passageway from the mouth to the stomach.

Essential tremor: The most common cause of tremor, sometimes confused with PD. People with this condition experience no other neurological symptoms other than tremor.

Extrapyramidal: A term for the basal ganglia and its connections. The term originated to distinguish this from another movement control circuit, the pyramidal motor system.

Fluctuations: Variations in the levodopa response, with transitions between on- and off-states.

Fludrocortisone (Florinef): A medication used to elevate the blood pressure, which works by causing the kidneys to excrete less sodium (salt).

Freezing: Transient paralysis of movement. In PD, this most often relates to walking, where the feet become stuck to the floor.

Gene: A DNA code for a specific protein.

Glia: The supporting cells of the nervous system. They perform a variety of metabolic and housekeeping tasks that are critical to neurons.

Globus pallidus: This nucleus is located between the striatum and thalamus. Most of the striatal output is to this nucleus, which, in turn, has important projections to the thalamus.

Glutamate: A brain neurotransmitter.

Glutamate antagonist: Drugs that block the brain neurotransmitter, glutamate.

Hallucinations: Seeing things that are not there.

Hesitancy: Slowed, hard-to-start urination.

Homocysteine: A metabolite normally present in the bloodstream. Elevated concentrations are a risk factor for atherosclerosis.

Hypokinetic: The type of speech problem (dysarthria) found in PD.

Hypophonia: The soft voice of PD.

Hypotension: Low blood pressure.

Immediate release: The regular formulation of a medication, distinguished from sustained-release products. Carbidopa/levodopa comes in two forms, immediate-release and sustained-release.

Lesioning: Surgically destroying a small area of brain tissue.

Levodopa: The amino acid that is the precursor to dopamine.

Levodopa treatment: This implies carbidopa/levodopa treatment. Plain levodopa without carbidopa is no longer used.

Lewy body: Round collections of amorphous material inside certain brain neurons in PD. They are especially frequent in the substantia nigra.

Lewy body dementia: *See* diffuse Lewy body disease

Long-duration levodopa response: A sustained effect from levodopa, which develops over about one week. If levodopa is discontinued, this effect conversely dissipates over a week.

Madopar: The brand name for benserazide/levodopa, which is used in some European countries.

MAO-B inhibitor: A drug that blocks one of the two major forms of monoamine oxidase (the B-form). This results in slightly higher brain dopamine levels. The primary drug in this class is selegiline (Eldepryl; formerly known as Deprenyl).

Midodrine (ProAmatine): An adrenalin-like drug that elevates blood pressure but spares the heart.

Mirtazepine (Remeron): An antidepressant medication.

Mitochondria: Components of all cells that carry on crucial oxidative chemical reactions that generate ATP.

Monoamine oxidase (MAO): An enzyme that breaks down dopamine. Blocking it will enhance PD treatment.

Motor: Term for movement and action, for example, brain circuits that program motor function.

MRI: Magnetic resonance imaging, which generates high-resolution views of the brain.

Multiple system atrophy (MSA): A neurodegenerative disorder that may resemble PD.

Nadolol (Corgard): A beta-blocking drug that does not cross the blood–brain barrier, which is used to treat tremor.

Neurodegenerative: A class of disorders in which certain brain systems slowly die (degenerate); this includes conditions such as Parkinson's disease, Alzheimer's disease and Lou Gehrig's disease (ALS).

Neurogenic bladder: A malfunctioning bladder due to impaired nervous system control.

Neuron: The primary brain cell, of which there are approximately 10 billion in the normal brain. Neurons contain a cell body with a nucleus and an axon extending from that cell body.

Neurotransmitter: The chemical released by nerve terminals used to signal the next neuron in the brain circuit.

Neurotrophic hormone: A class of chemicals found in the nervous system that enhances the growth and viability of neurons.

Nigrostriatal: The projection from the substantia nigra neuron to the striatum. Each nigrostriatal neuron has a cell body located in the substantia nigra, with an axon extending to the striatum.

Nocturia: Urination during the night.

Norepinephrine: A neurotransmitter, also called noradrenalin.

Normal pressure hydrocephalus (NPH): A disorder of senior citizens in which the brain ventricles expand; this impairs the function of nearby brain circuits. The symptoms include a parkinsonian gait, urinary incontinence, and cognitive dysfunction.

Nortriptyline (Pamelor, Aventyl): An antidepressant medication that is sometimes used for other purposes, such as a sleep aid.

NSAIDs: Nonsteroidal anti-inflammatory drugs, such as ibuprofen, naproxen, plus a variety of prescription pain relievers.

Nuclei: Collections of neurons grouped together in a somewhat homogeneous brain structure.

Off: The state when levodopa is not working.

Olanzapine (Zyprexa): A medication used to treat hallucinations and delusions. It may induce parkinsonism.

On: The state when levodopa is working and parkinsonian symptoms are relieved.

Opioid: A drug with narcotic properties.

Orthostatic: Standing, as in orthostatic hypotension, where the blood pressure is low when erect.

Osteoporosis: Weakening of bones.

Oxybutynin (Ditropan): An anticholinergic medication used to treat urinary urgency.

Pallidotomy: Surgically lesioning the pallidum to treat PD.

Pallidum: Another name for the globus pallidus, a target of one form of PD surgery.

Parcopa: A new formulation of carbidopa/levodopa that dissolves in the mouth and is then swallowed. Water or other liquid is not necessary to take this pill.

Parkin: A component of the ubiquitin-proteasome system. Mutations of the gene coding for parkin are responsible for many cases of parkinsonism starting before age 40.

Parkinsonism: Implies that the clinical appearance resembles Parkinson's disease; however, it may or may not be PD.

Pergolide (Permax): An ergot dopamine agonist drug.

Peristalsis: Contractions of the gut that move food products through gastrointestinal system during digestion.

PET scan: Positron emission tomography, a nuclear medicine scanning technique. With certain injected substances, dopaminergic neurons are imaged.

Placebo: A sugar pill used in clinical trials.

Polymorphisms: Normal variations of genes.

Pramipexole (Mirapex): A dopamine agonist drug.

Praxis: Programming of smaller motor movements to make a more complex movement.

Progressive supranuclear palsy (PSP): A neurodegenerative condition often mistaken for PD.

Propranolol (Inderal): A beta-blocking drug sometimes used to treat tremor. It is also used to treat high blood pressure, certain heart disorders, and migraine.

Protein: A class of biologic chemicals composed of strings of amino acids.

Putamen: The back half of the striatum. This region sustains greater loss of dopamine than the caudate in PD.

Quetiapine (Seroquel): A medication used to treat hallucinations and delusions.

Receptor: The region of the synapse that binds a specific neurotransmitter.

Recessive inheritance: Traits that occur within a generation but are not passed from one generation to the next (except in rare situations). The trait is expressed only when both genes of a pair are affected; that is, both the mother and father contribute an abnormal gene.

REM sleep behavior disorder: Acting out dreams during rapid eye movement (REM) sleep. Normally the body should be limp during this stage of sleep, except for eye movements.

Rest tremor: The typical tremor of PD. When affecting the hands, it is present when they are not being used, such as in the lap, or at one's sides when walking.

Restless legs syndrome: A creepy-crawly feeling in the legs when trying to sleep, associated with the urge to get up and walk to gain relief.

Reuptake: The mechanism whereby neuron terminals control the duration and intensity of a neurotransmitter effect. The presynaptic terminal sucks up the neurotransmitter after release to prevent the effect from being excessive.

Rigidity: The increased tone of limbs seen in PD.

Ropinirole (Requip): A dopamine agonist drug.

Selegiline (Deprenyl, Eldepryl): An MAO-B inhibitor drug, which tends to enhance the levodopa effect.

Serotonin: A brain neurotransmitter, which may be deficient in some cases of depression.

Short-duration levodopa response: A one- to six-hour response that is time-locked to each levodopa dose.

Sinemet: The brand name for carbidopa/levodopa.

Sleep apnea: Impaired breathing during sleep.

SPECT scan: Single photon emission computed tomography, which can be used to image brain dopamine systems when certain chemicals are injected.

Spinal cord: This, along with the brain, makes up the central nervous system. It is an elongated extension of the brain, extending downward from the brain stem. Tracts from the cortex and subcortex pass through the brain stem to the spinal cord, which is the final common pathway controlling movement. Conversely, sensory information (e.g., touch, pain) passes in the opposite direction via other tracts, up to the brain.

SSRI (selective serotonin reuptake inhibitor): A class of antidepressant medications; the effects are mediated by blocking the reuptake of serotonin.

Stalevo: A combination drug containing entacapone, carbidopa, and levodopa.

Stem cell: A very immature cell with potential to differentiate into a wide variety of cells, including neurons.

Striatum: The brain region that receives the dopaminergic projections from the substantia nigra. The striatum is comprised of two components: putamen and caudate.

Subcortex: Brain centers located underneath the cortex, which tend to have more elementary functions than cortical circuits. The basal ganglia is subcortical.

Substantia nigra: Neurons containing a black pigment and located at the upper end of the brain stem, in the midbrain. This degenerates in PD.

Subthalamic nucleus: A nucleus located just beneath the thalamus, which is intimately connected with the striatum and globus pallidus. Strokes here cause involuntary movements. It is a target for neurosurgical treatment of PD.

Sustained-release (SR): Formulating a medication to make it dissolve very slowly; hence, the effect is delayed and prolonged. Sinemet CR is a sustained-release formulation of carbidopa/levodopa.

Synapse: The interface between a nerve terminal and a receptor. The terminal releases a specific neurotransmitter into the synaptic cleft, which then binds to the receptor.

Systolic: A blood pressure parameter corresponding to the upper number in blood pressure readings (such as 120 in the reading 120/80).

Terminal: The end of the axon, which releases a neurotransmitter.

Thalamotomy: Lesioning the thalamus, primarily done to treat tremor.

Thalamus: A centrally located brain nucleus with widespread connections to the cortex. It receives extensive input from the globus pallidus, as well as from a variety of other brain regions.

Tolcapone (Tasmar): A COMT inhibitor drug that enhances the levodopa response.

Tolterodine (Detrol): An anticholinergic medication used to treat urinary urgency.

Tracts: Collections of axons running together like a telephone cable.

Transporter: A component of cells that moves (transports) a chemical across a cell membrane. For example, the dopamine transporter is responsible for the reuptake of dopamine from the region of the synapse.

Trazodone (Desyrel): An antidepressant medication often used as a sleep aid.

Tremor: A rhythmic (back-and-forth) movement.

Tricyclic: A class of antidepressant medications.

Trihexyphenidyl (Artane): An anticholinergic drug.

Trimethobenzamide (Tigan): A medication used to treat nausea. This does not worsen parkinsonism, as do the other prescription nausea drugs.

Ubiquitin: A cellular molecule that is used to tag proteins destined for degradation.

Ubiquitin carboxy-terminal hydrolase: An enzyme that recycles previously used ubiquitin. A mutation of this enzyme was identified in one inherited form of parkinsonism.

Ubiquitin-proteasome system: A complex system within cells for disposing of unwanted or abnormal proteins.

Ureter: The conduit from the kidneys to the bladder.

Urethra: The conduit out from the bladder, through which urine externally passes.

Urgency: An enhanced sense that one must urinate.

Vertigo: One form of dizziness, characterized by a subjective sense of spinning or movement within the head.

Wearing-off: When the levodopa beneficial effect is declining, typically before the next dose.

Wilson's disease: A rare disorder of copper metabolism, with liver and neurologic problems. Tremor and parkinsonism may occur in this condition.